The Horse Doctor Is In

A Kentucky Veterinarian's Advice and Wisdom on Horse Health Care

Brent Kelley, DVM

Illustrations by Jane Thissen

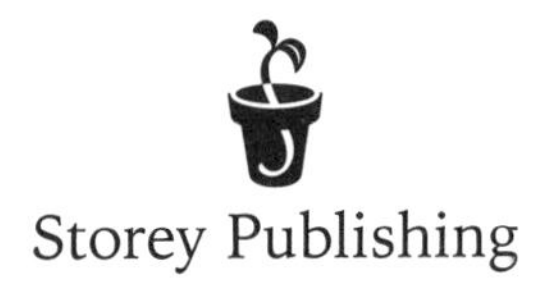

Storey Publishing

The mission of Storey Publishing is to serve our customers by publishing practical information that encourages personal independence in harmony with the environment.

Edited by Marie A. Salter and Deborah Burns
Copyedited by Sue Ducharme
Art direction and cover design by Meredith Maker
Text design by David Lane
Text production by Kelley Nesbit
Indexed by Susan Olason/Indexes & Knowledge Maps

Storey books are available for special premium and promotional uses and for customized editions. For further information, please call 1-800-793-9396.

Printed in the United States by Edwards Brothers, Inc.
10 9 8 7 6 5 4 3

Library of Congress Cataloging-in-Publication Data

Kelley, Brent P.
The horse doctor is in : a Kentucky veterinarian's advice and wisdom on horse health care / Brent P. Kelley.
p. ; cm.
Includes index.
ISBN 1-58017-460-4 (alk. paper)
1. Horses—Diseases—Anecdotes. 2. Horses—Health—Anecdotes. 3. Veterinary medicine—Anecdotes. 4. Kelley, Brent P. 5. Veterinarians—Kentucky—Anecdotes. I. Title.
[DNLM: 1. Horse Diseases—therapy. 2. Animal Husbandry.
SF 951 K29h 2002]
SF951.K325 2002
636.1'089—dc21

2002005558

For Jennifer

*Maybe this will help you
in your practice*

Contents

III. Breeding and Foaling

IV. Care and Management

Preface

I DON'T KNOW WHY BECOMING A VETERINARIAN didn't occur to me sooner than it did. I was always around animals. In fact, I preferred the animals to most people. (I still do.) My family had horses, dogs, cats, and goats ever since I can remember.

My brother showed American Saddlebreds, and I liked them, but I liked Thoroughbreds more. I liked the idea of racing, so I decided to become a jockey.

But genetics did me in. By the time I was twelve, only the stoutest horse could have run very fast with me in the saddle.

So then I changed my plans. I would become a major league baseball player. It took several years to realize that genetics was against me again. I didn't have the talent.

So I was forced to go to college. Unfortunately, I found college to be horrendously boring, so I didn't study. I flunked out of two schools.

This brought about the worst possible thing that can happen to a person: I had to work for a living. I drove a truck. I was a night watchman. I was a disc jockey. I became an electronics draftsman.

But none of those jobs satisfied me. They were work, and they were boring. I still liked horse racing, so I took all my money and became a gambler. I spent a year going from track to track betting on the horses. Expenses were high, but I did okay. I stayed ahead, until one day I bet a bundle on a horse that couldn't lose. Of course, you know what he did: by a whisker.

I took that as an omen. I needed to find an honest but interesting and enjoyable way to make a living. My brother, eight years my senior, had zoomed through school, had his bachelor's degree at twenty, earned his master's at twenty-two. He was established and successful in business. I was twenty-six and getting nowhere.

One day he asked me, "Are you ever going to amount to anything?"

I told him I hoped so. We were in his barn at the time, grooming his horses.

"You've always liked horses. Have you ever thought of working with them?" he asked.

"That would be great, but doing what?"

"Be a trainer. Or a vet."

A vet! Of course!

I went back to college. I had to get excellent grades to bring up the clunkers I had gotten in my two previous tries. (I'd had a 0.9 GPA.) Veterinary schools place more emphasis on grades than on anything else, and in those days the competition was stiff. There were at least ten or twelve applicants for every student accepted.

I got in and I stayed in. When I graduated, I couldn't find a position in an equine practice, so I went to work for a general large-animal practice in another state. After a year and a half, I was able to make the move to Kentucky and start my own practice. I was warned that beginning one's own practice was a lot of work, but it wasn't. Being a veterinarian definitely beats working.

My own practice began on the racetrack, where the horses were wonderful but the work wasn't fulfilling. In many cases, a trainer was just trying to hold a horse together for "one more race." And if he got that one more, he wanted to hold him together for "just one more." This meant we were giving pain relievers and steroids instead of resting and repairing the horses.

But some of the trainers also had breeding farms, and in time I was asked to work on them. This was great, and in a short while I had developed a breeding farm practice.

The horses were still dollar signs to most owners, but on breeding farms a veterinarian can do more than just hold a horse together. High-priced mares and their higher-priced foals require good veterinary care to get the mares in foal and to maintain healthy foals.

Working with Thoroughbreds as I do, it's easy to equate the horses with money, and I admit that I tend to be guilty of that at times. But I also work on pleasure horses — horses that are worth perhaps a few hundred dollars but are priceless as well-loved pets. I try to treat both the million-dollar broodmare and the backyard pony the same.

I have always worried that I don't know enough and that other veterinarians know more than I do. My wife assures me that that isn't the case, but the practice of veterinary medicine is a constant learning experience. Toward this end, I have acquired lots of veterinary books over the years. Some are textbooks; others are geared toward the horse owner. The textbooks use big words and are boring. The horse owners' veterinary "guides" are all "cookbooks" and are equally boring.

I began writing twice-a-month columns for *Thoroughbred Times,* a weekly horse racing and breeding publication. One column is called Veterinary Topics. I try to write in a non-boring manner, because the readers can find boring things to read in lots of other places.

Many times as I write, I find it necessary to refer to textbooks and other references. It isn't so much to find out what I'm writing about (although such cases have arisen from time to time); it's more to make sure that I don't omit something or state it incorrectly. And those books use lots of technical terms (i.e., big words). I have to translate them so I can figure out what it is that I'm reading.

I remember once in veterinary school a teacher was telling us about the particular problems of brachycephalic dog breeds.* When he said "brachycephalic," everyone in the class immediately exchanged questioning glances, but no one said a thing. When it became apparent that no one was going to speak up, I figured that I had to. "What's that?" I asked.

*Brachycephalic dogs, by the way, are those with pushed-in faces, such as boxers, bulldogs, pugs, and similar breeds. I have seen a brachycephalic horse, and the tale is related later in this book (see page 267), but it's unlikely that I'll ever see another one, and I have therefore learned a big word for naught.

"What's what?" the professor replied.

"Brachycephalic."

He gave me a look somewhere between pity and disgust. "Look, Kelley," he said sternly, "you have to be able to speak in technical terms. It makes communicating with other veterinarians so much easier."

I should have told him that no one else in the class knew what it meant, either, but instead I said, "Ninety percent or more of our communicating will be with the owners of the animals. If I say 'brachycephalic' to some housewife with two screaming kids hanging on her, she won't have any idea what I'm talking about, and the next time she may well go to a vet who speaks English." Then I added, "Are there brachycephalic horses?"

Knowing what it's like not to understand what you're reading, I try to use non-technical terminology when possible, but occasionally as I write I find myself slipping into a mild scientific mode. For this reason, an extensive glossary is included at the back of the book. But the value of easily accessible language cannot be overstated; there are readers who are comfortable with the most demanding terminology, but there are more readers who aren't, hence the need to make things understandable for the majority. This isn't a slap at horse folks; if a person has no need to use words such as *reticuloendothelial* and *goniometer,* it is unlikely that he or she will learn what they mean.

"What the world needs," I said to myself one day, "is a horse vet book that is pleasant, entertaining reading. And not boring."

I hope this is it. It's based on my columns for *Thoroughbred Times.* This book is not comprehensive, nor is it intended to include every veterinary topic. But it covers the important issues, and it covers a few things that aren't seen every day. I think it will be both interesting and educational — at least I hope it will be.

In reading these pages, some may conclude that I have limited competence. That may be true, but I don't think it's any more limited than that of most of the other equine veterinarians. I just feel that relating tales of things that went as planned has little or no educational or entertainment value and, after all, that is the purpose of these missives. Another purpose is to make me wealthy. If the education and entertainment being put forth is as successful as this latter goal will probably be, I am missing on those scores, too.

For twenty years, we owned a farm where we boarded mares for clients as well as two or three of our own. Keeping decent employees became increasingly difficult, so we sold the farm and now have a place with a few acres where we keep a couple of pleasure horses along with two llamas, a donkey, a Scottish Highland steer, and two emus. I'm semiretired now, and writing keeps me out of trouble.

Part I
Diseases

Prevention and management

I

Preventable Diseases

Vaccinations

Every owner knows that horses need to be vaccinated, but very few know for what and when. Unfortunately, in many cases a proper schedule is not adhered to. People forget, and when reminders are sent by their veterinarian, they set them aside and just don't get around to them.

Vaccinations are important. It's a whole lot easier and cheaper to prevent a disease than it is to treat it.

But what to vaccinate for and when? The schedule on page 376 will benefit you and your horses. Other veterinarians' schedules may differ slightly from this, but they won't deviate much.

A vaccination program has no real starting point. It's a continuous effort, but ideally a horse's first immunizations begin while it's still in its dam's uterus (see page 222 for more information). When vaccinations are started before birth, protection is passed to the foal through *colostrum,* or first milk. Then boosters are given at appropriate times, and immunity remains. A proper vaccination program, therefore, is ongoing and is a regular part of the horse's life. Keep good records to ensure that boosters are given at proper times.

Viral Encephalitis

BACK IN THE EARLY 1970S, when an outbreak of Venezuelan equine encephalitis occurred in the southern United States, all horses where I was were required to be vaccinated. I'm not sure if it was a national requirement, but it sure was a state requirement.

But, boy, did the horse owners fight it! We told all of our clients of the requirement. To be fair, many understood and complied with no complaints. But many just didn't want to do it. Eventually, though, everyone let us give the initial dose of the vaccine.

Then we had to come back three weeks later and do it again. Even some who agreed willingly to the initial vaccination balked at the follow-up. The common argument put to us was, "If the government requires it, why doesn't the government pay for it?"

My employer countered with, "You're required to have a license plate and you have to pay for that." But it didn't stop the grumbling.

Over the years I've found that encephalitis vaccinations are the most difficult to sell. For some reason, people just don't fear encephalitis. It's one of the diseases that should be feared the most, however, because it can infect people.

What Is Viral Encephalitis?

There are three of these viral diseases: eastern equine encephalitis (EEE), western equine encephalitis (WEE), and the aforementioned Venezuelan equine encephalitis (VEE). All three encephalitides are spread by mosquitoes. The viruses are always present in wildlife, including birds, reptiles, and small mammals. These hosts don't show signs of the disease, however, and the mechanism by which the viruses exist in these hosts without causing disease isn't known.

VEE occurs in the southern states, especially Florida, and throughout central South America. EEE occurs primarily east of the Mississippi River and into southern Canada and also appears in central South America. WEE occurs west of the Mississippi into southern Canada and throughout most of South America.

The diseases are spread after mosquitoes feed on the blood of the wild hosts and then bite horses or people. The occurrence, naturally, is highest during mosquito season: June to November, in most of the United States.

In many cases the virus is shed after it enters a horse, but any residual viruses infect highly vascular organs, such as the liver and spleen. Infection of the central nervous system follows within five days.

Clinical Signs

Acute signs are nonspecific and include fever, anorexia, depression, and muscle stiffness. In less than a week, these signs pass, and in the case of WEE there is sometimes no further progression of the disease.

If the disease does progress, within a few days there is intermittent fever followed by signs of cerebral involvement. These signs include depression, compulsive walking, and somnolence (sleeping) in most cases, but some are just the opposite: the horse may exhibit aggression and excitability.

As the disease becomes chronic, symptoms include head pressing (placing the head against an object and pushing forward), circling, compulsive walking, blindness, head tilt, and muscle twitching. The tongue, pharynx, and larynx may become paralyzed. The horse will lie down and die within a week, usually less.

Treatment

Treatment typically consists of supportive therapy (nutrition), nonsteroidal anti-inflammatory drugs, tender loving care, and crossed fingers. The prognosis is poor. Recovery is rare but it does happen, though few animals return to normal after having this disease.

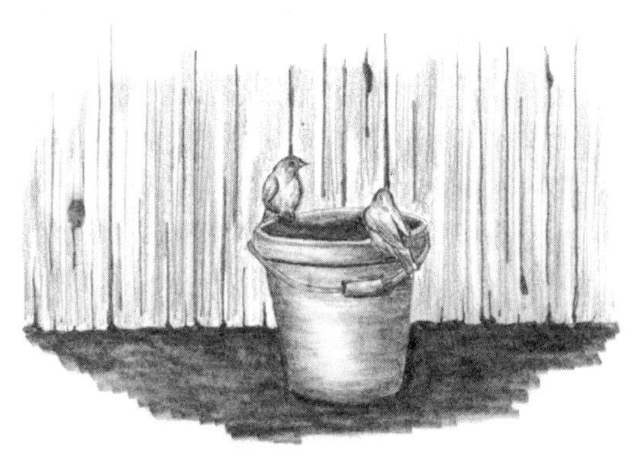

Birds are hosts to viral encephalitis. Mosquitoes that have bitten the infected birds spread the virus to horses.

Prevention

There is no excuse for not vaccinating against viral encephalitis. Excuses may be made for not vaccinating for other diseases (an only horse with absolutely no outside contact, for instance), but the risk caused by mosquitoes can never be ruled out. The encephalitis vaccine is an initial series of two shots administered three weeks apart, followed by annual boosters.

Eliminating areas of standing water where mosquitoes breed is one way to reduce the mosquito population and hence the risk.

Equine Influenza

A CLIENT, HAVING ALL FIFTEEN OF HIS HORSES IN TRAINING laid up with coughs and runny noses, asked me to tell him all there is to know about equine influenza. That made me think, an uncomfortable experience.

Too many times we veterinarians tell clients, "Vaccinate! You must vaccinate!" but we don't tell them why. Each disease has its own story, and if that story is known, perhaps a better understanding of the problem will be attained. And then — ta-da! — we veterinarians will be able to vaccinate more horses to safeguard them against the onset of preventable disease.

What Is Equine Influenza?

Equine influenza is a real zapper. Of all the equine viral respiratory diseases, it probably has the most debilitating effects. Once introduced into a susceptible population, spread is extremely rapid and morbidity (the percent infected) approaches 100 percent. To the best of my knowledge, however, no horse has ever died of uncomplicated equine influenza, hereafter to be referred to simply as *flu.*

Flu outbreaks occur most commonly where large numbers of horses from different backgrounds are gathered in a single location, such as at racetracks, sales, and shows. One infected horse can enter a congregation of five hundred healthy, susceptible ones, and within a week they will all be sick.

Spread is by inhalation, and the virus can be carried on the wind a great distance to affect horses beyond the airspace of the infected animal(s). The incubation period is short, a day to a week, and the spread is tremendously rapid. Young horses (up to three years) are most commonly affected.

Clinical Signs

The first sign is a high fever — often 104° to 105°F — followed shortly (hours to a day) by a harsh, dry, hacking cough and nasal discharge. Other signs typically include decreased or no appetite, decline in performance, lethargy, depression, muscular soreness, leg edema, and/or swollen lymph nodes under the jaw, though not all of these symptoms may appear. Pneumonia can result from secondary bacterial invasion, which is common. Stress, including exercise, bad weather, and shipping, is likely to worsen matters.

If a horse has been vaccinated within the previous year, the clinical signs are usually not as severe, and there may actually be none if the vaccination was recent. The more recent the vaccination, the less severe the infection. Spread is considerably slower in a vaccinated population, and secondary bacterial infections are less likely to occur.

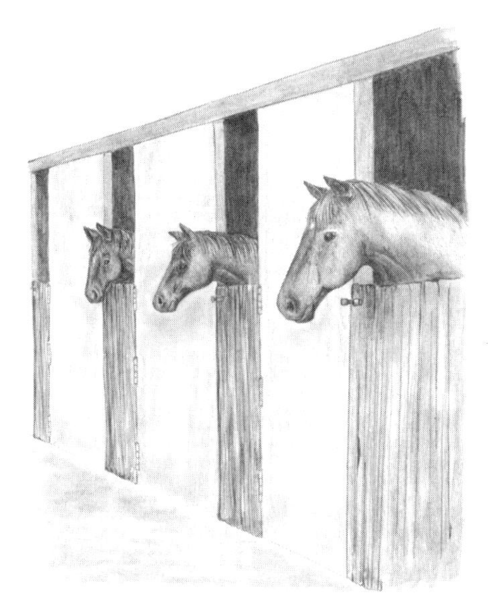

Flu outbreaks occur most commonly where large numbers of horses gather.

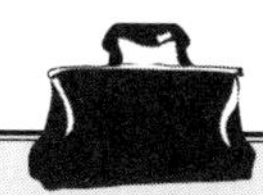

The Flu and You

Several years ago there was a widespread outbreak of flu at a training center here in central Kentucky. At the same time, some sort of flu bug had hit the human population of this area as well. Everyone, both equine and human, at this particular training center was sick, including me. Go back to the first paragraph under Clinical Signs — that described me to a T.

I am not a virologist by any stretch of the imagination, and the only research I ever do concerns rather obscure baseball history, so what I am about to say is based not on any hard scientific evidence, just personal observation. I believe that horses and people can share and spread the flu virus to one another.

On other occasions than the aforementioned flu outbreak, I have seen a high correlation between sick horses and sick people. I don't know which species became sick first, but I'm pretty sure the disease in both went together.

So I guess the bottom line is this: if you have horses, you need a flu shot as much as they do.

Diagnosis

The physical signs previously described, accompanied by rapid spread and high morbidity, are enough for a presumptive diagnosis, but milder cases may be confused with other viral infections such as herpesvirus and rhinovirus, as well as bacterial respiratory infections. A definitive diagnosis, however, can be made by viral isolation from a nasal swab or by paired serum samples drawn ten days to two weeks apart. In the latter, the *antibody titer* (the body's response to the virus as measured in a blood sample) will be increased four to ten times in the second serum sample if the animal has the flu.

Treatment

Tender loving care is really all that can be done for a horse with flu. It is probably a good idea to place unvaccinated horses on antibiotics. Nonsteroidal anti-inflammatory drugs, preferably phenylbutazone ("bute"), may be administered to control fever.

Management is extremely important. Training and shipping should be stopped. A generally advocated rule of thumb is a week of rest for every day of fever. The return to work must be gradual.

Prevention

A good vaccination program will either prevent or reduce the severity of flu. A proper program should begin before a foal is born. The mare should be vaccinated in the last trimester of her pregnancy. This will give the foal protection through the colostrum. There is some debate as to when the new foal should receive its first vaccination. Some recommend beginning the vaccination program at six months of age, while others advocate ninety days. Regardless, boosters need to be given every three to four months from the first vaccination throughout the young horse's racing or performance career. Once the horse is retired, twice-yearly vaccinations are usually sufficient.

It is especially important to maintain the biannual program on breeding and boarding farms, and on farms where there are many horses coming and going. The transient population of a seasonal boarding operation and the comings and goings of mares to be bred on a breeding farm are marvelous sources for the introduction of flu, as well as just about every other disease known to veterinary science.

Rabies

I HAD BEEN OUT OF SCHOOL ONLY A FEW DAYS, maybe a week, and I was still riding around with my employer, learning the area and the clients. We were called to see a backyard pony that was acting "weird." *Weird* is a description I've heard a lot over the years, and usually it's correct.

When we got there we were shown a Shetland-sized pony that was trotting around his small paddock in an uncoordinated manner, occasionally bumping into the fence or into a tree.

"What do you think it could be?" my employer asked me.

"I don't know. Some sort of encephalitis, I guess," I replied. "Or maybe some sort of poison."

"How about rabies?" he asked.

"I don't know. Could it be?"

"It has to be considered."

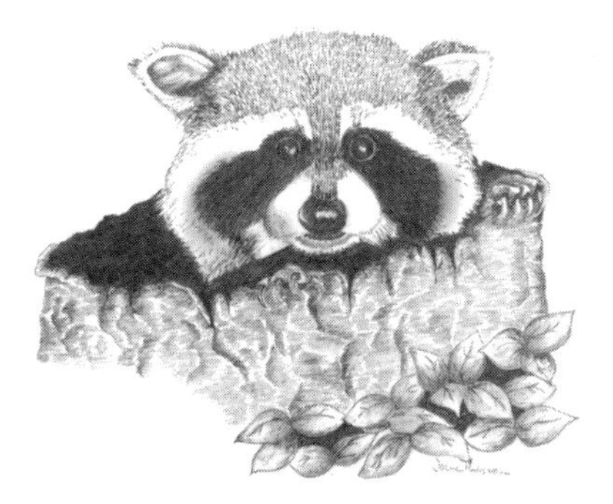

Rabies most commonly infects skunks, foxes, bats, and raccoons.

He had us put on rubber gloves, then he roped the pony (she couldn't be caught otherwise), and we tranquilized her and took blood samples. Nothing was found. Two days later she went down and couldn't get up, although she would try, and we couldn't get her up. There was no choice but to put her to sleep. The postmortem examination of the brain showed that it was, indeed, rabies. The family of four that owned her had to undergo treatment for rabies, which they truly hated, and my employer asked me if I had been vaccinated against the disease.

I had. We had been advised in school that those of us intending to work on large animals and wildlife must be vaccinated and that all veterinarians should be vaccinated. I guess the vaccine is better than the disease (I'm still alive), but, boy, is it something! My arm swelled up to twice its normal size and turned as red as a stoplight and was so painful that I could hardly lift it for days. Since then, I've had boosters, and I react the same way each time, but, as I said, I'm still alive.

Number one on the list of diseases that you don't want your horse to get is rabies. It's a one-way street, and human infection is a serious risk. It's downright scary. I've seen five rabies cases since that first one.

What Is Rabies?

Rabies differs from most other diseases in that it isn't species specific. Any warm-blooded animal can contract it, although among wild animals the most commonly infected are skunks, foxes, raccoons, and bats. Among domestic animals, cattle once had the highest incidence, but that is no longer the case. The latest statistics indicate that cats are now first among domestic species, and this has significant implications for a horse operation. (For more on barn cats, see page 305.)

The cause of rabies is a virus, and entry into an animal is via salivary contamination of an open wound. A bite from an infected animal is the usual source, but salivary contamination of a small cut will do it, too. Other reported routes of infection are inhalation and oral and transplacental transmission to a fetus from an affected pregnant mare.

The rabies virus proliferates at the site of entry, then travels on the axons of peripheral nerves (it isn't blood-borne) until it reaches the brain stem or spinal cord. How quickly this occurs depends on the site of entry; if the virus enters on the face or muzzle, signs may develop within two or three weeks, but if entry occurs on a hind ankle, it may be many weeks or even months before clinical signs begin.

Once the virus reaches the brain, it's disseminated throughout the central nervous system (CNS). The cranial nerves carry it to the salivary glands before clinical signs occur, and herein lies the risk for handlers. Simply placing a bit in an infected horse's mouth or washing off a hand in the water bucket of an infected horse could result in the virus entering your body through any break in the skin, even a hangnail.

Clinical Signs

Signs that may be associated with early rabies but that are *not* specific for the disease include depression, lameness or ataxia, colic, vocal alteration, paralysis, and mania characterized by hyperexcitability. It progresses rapidly from this point, and within four or five days the horse will die. In the terminal stages, there may be urine and fecal retention, knuckling or inability to stand, inability to swallow, and the classic "rabid" form of the disease, in which the horse cannot be restrained and charges people or other animals, biting itself and others. Violent thrashing occurs shortly before death.

Diagnosis

The disease is impossible to diagnose in the live animal but should be considered in any horse that shows peripheral or CNS problems. A differential diagnosis would include any of the several encephalomyelitides, any of several poisonings, brain trauma, and tetanus.

Treatment

There is no treatment for rabies, although if a bite from a rabid animal occurs, don rubber gloves, then debride and thoroughly cleanse the site; disinfect the bite using iodine or 7 percent alcohol. Keep the lesion clean and open; do *not* suture it.

If the horse has been previously vaccinated, it's probably a good idea to revaccinate immediately, but if there is no history of previous vaccination, a vaccination at this point isn't indicated, as it's likely to slow the progression of the disease, which would be cruel to the horse. If the biting animal can be captured, it should be submitted for observation or examination. If it is determined that the biter must be killed, do *not* shoot it in the head; the brain is needed for diagnosis. Likewise, if a horse dies that is suspected of having rabies, the brain must be examined to verify the diagnosis.

Also, if a horse is suspected of having rabies, all people who have handled it should be treated. If rabies has occurred in the area, it isn't a bad idea for those who work with the animals to be vaccinated. This is unpleasant, as I have pointed out already, and expensive, but it's preferable to death and less costly than a funeral, the two outcomes of a rabies infection.

Fortunately, a bite, even from a rabid animal, may not result in rabies. If a horse is bitten and the biter is identified as rabid, the bitten horse must be quarantined for six months. It's a good idea to quarantine a horse that is known to have been bitten by a wild animal, even if the animal was not captured. Public health officials will outline how the quarantine is to be accomplished and will review precautions necessary for the horse's handlers. If at any time during the six-month evaluation period the horse shows presumptive signs of rabies (see Clinical Signs), both the quarantine and the animal should be terminated.

Prevention

Vaccination of horses is recommended. It's a cheap precaution and may well avert a potential disaster. Foals may be vaccinated initially after ninety days of age and should receive booster shots annually. Older horses can be started at any time and should receive booster shots annually as well. The vaccine should be given by a veterinarian, because not all rabies vaccines are intended for use in horses, and the precise site of vaccination is important.

All horses should be vaccinated. Horses at pasture are at greatest risk because they're more apt to have contact with wild species.

Unfortunately, some believe that horses in a "closed" situation — racetracks or show barns, for example — aren't in danger of contracting rabies, but this isn't true. Cats are a common adjunct to any horse operation, and the feral cat population around the United States is uncountable. These facts, coupled with the documented increase in feline rabies, mean that it's equally important to vaccinate "inside" horses and "outside" horses. Vaccination of barn cats is also essential.

Remember: as with any infectious disease, prevention is the key to controlling and combating rabies.

Tetanus

A LOT OF WHAT WE (VETERINARIANS) DO — *most* of what we do — is routine and repetitious, so much so, in fact, that we (I, anyhow) forget that these things are not necessarily routine *or* repetitious for others. Clients, for example.

One time a new client asked me, "Why do I need to vaccinate for tetanus? What *is* tetanus?"

Wow, I thought, where has this guy been?

Within a week, another client, this being one of several years' standing, asked, "What if a horse gets tetanus? What is it?"

Well, I knew where this guy had been, so maybe, I thought, there is a communication problem of some sort. I had assumed that everyone knew what tetanus is and why we vaccinate against it, but obviously this isn't the case.

So, on the odd chance that there are others out there not familiar with tetanus and the reason we vaccinate, here's the story.

What Is Tetanus?

Tetanus is caused by the bacterium *Clostridium tetani.* (*Clostridium* is a fun genus; diseases caused by other clostridial species include botulism, anthrax, and gas gangrene.) The disease can occur in all animals, but the horse is the most susceptible, which is problematic because *C. tetani* is a normal inhabitant of the equine intestinal tract. Every time a horse defecates, it unwittingly introduces the organism into its environment.

Although tetanus is classified as an infectious disease, it cannot be spread from animal to animal. *C. tetani* is an *anaerobe,* meaning it grows in the absence of oxygen, so outside the body where oxygen is plentiful it is not a problem. The organism, which resides virtually everywhere in the horse's environment, enters a wound that satisfies all of its requirements for reproduction and proliferation: that is, no air and devitalized tissue. Puncture wounds are the major point of entry for the disease, especially punctures of the sole of the foot, but any integumentary alteration (lesion in the skin or feet) provides a potential access route. (A puncture by a rusty object, such as a nail, contaminates a wound more readily than does a puncture by a clean object.)

The organism itself doesn't actually cause the disease; as it grows, a toxin *(tetanospasmin)* is produced and released into the tissue, where it is spread by both the blood and retrograde axonal migration (it travels up the nerve axons) to the central nervous system (CNS). It eventually takes up residence in the brain's gray matter, from whence signs of the disease are produced.

Incubation ranges from a few days to several months. As with rabies (see page 10), the incubation period of tetanus depends on the point of entry of the organism; the closer the point of entry to the CNS, the sooner clinical signs of disease will become apparent. Also important in the incubation period are the initial amount of bacteria introduced and the condition of the wound itself; a clean, open wound is much less likely to be the source of a case of tetanus than is a contaminated, closed one.

Clinical Signs

The clinical signs are several and include rigid, erect ears; flared nostrils; retracted eyelids; prolapse of the third eyelid; difficulty swallowing (or inability to swallow, hence the term *lockjaw*); and rigid extension of the legs ("sawhorse" stance), which makes walking difficult. Also, there may be cessation of urination and defecation. The animal has an anxious look and even minimal external stimuli (sudden sights or sounds) may cause lengthy muscle spasms. If startled, the horse may fall onto its side and be unable to rise.

Tetanus itself will not kill the horse, but death will occur as the result of several complications: respiratory paralysis, starvation or dehydration (swallowing isn't possible), or pneumonia resulting from aspiration of feed or water into the lungs as swallowing is attempted.

Diagnosis

Diagnosis is made according to the clinical signs and history, although there is often no known injury whereby the organism could have gained entry. Many times small punctures go unnoticed. Culturing the organism from a lesion is difficult and frequently not rewarding, yet the inability to grow *C. tetani* in the laboratory in no way eliminates the disease from a *differential diagnosis* (a list of possible diseases that could cause the signs seen).

History is important in the diagnosis of any disease, but it's especially helpful in tetanus. A nonexistent or incorrect immunization program, coupled with a puncture wound or other laceration in the horse's past, leads to a fairly conclusive diagnosis of tetanus when accompanied by the physical signs.

Treatment

Treatment is prolonged, can be difficult and expensive, and fails as much as 80 percent of the time, but it must be attempted. Tetanus antitoxin (TAT) is routinely administered, but it does *not* affect toxin that has already reached nerves or the CNS. Rather, it functions to neutralize toxin in the circulatory system that hasn't yet reached the nervous system, making it most effective when given to a nonvaccinated horse at the time a laceration or puncture wound occurs.

There is a potential risk in the use of TAT, however. In certain instances, Theiler's disease, known also as *serum hepatitis*, will develop in horses that have received it. This risk may even be a better reason than the threat of tetanus itself for the implementation of a proper vaccination program. (See the discussion of Theiler's disease on page 59.)

Also, a tetanus toxoid injection should be given as part of the treatment. Toxoids create antibodies within the animal that will combat the disease if the animal is exposed to it in the future.

Penicillin will do nothing to combat the toxin already produced, but it will kill any vegetative *C. tetani* organisms that may still be present, so high levels of the antibiotic should be given.

The horse should be housed in a dark, quiet, isolated (if possible) stall to lessen or eliminate external stimuli, and any people who must work with or around the animal should do so slowly and silently. Plugging the horse's ears with cotton is helpful in reducing the impact of auditory stimuli.

Tranquilizers, sedatives, and/or muscle relaxants should be used to control muscle spasms and convulsions. Your veterinarian will instruct as to what, when, and how much. Phenylbutazone (commonly called "bute"), a nonsteroidal anti-inflammatory drug, can be used to control fever and pain.

Nutrition and hydration must be maintained. If the horse can't swallow, it must be fed and watered via stomach tube. Also, the end products of metabolism need to be addressed; if the horse can't urinate and defecate, these functions must be done for it. Manual emptying of the rectum two or three times a day is necessary, as well as catheterization of the bladder.

Prognosis, Recovery, and Prevention

Prognosis varies. A horse that can eat, drink, and eliminate will usually come along well; one that can't, and especially one that goes down, isn't a promising patient.

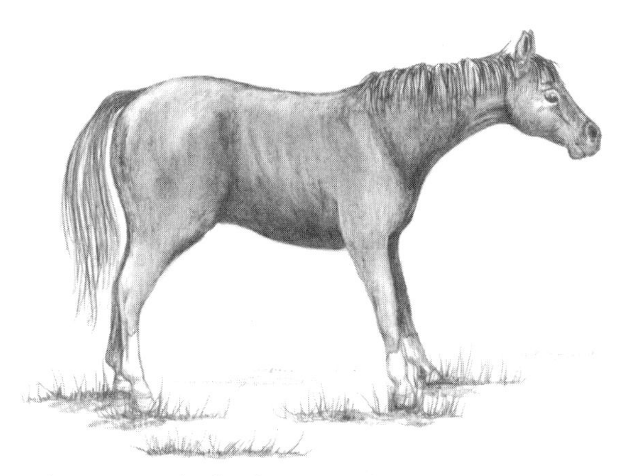

This rigid attitude is typical of a horse with tetanus.

Tetanus has a mortality rate of 30 to 80 percent, depending on which study you read, but recent work with a sixteenth-century Chinese herbal remedy has shown promise in reducing the mortality rate to below 20 percent. This remedy is not yet available in North America, however.

Recovery is slow. Full return to normalcy may take months, but once recovered there are usually no residual effects. Likewise, there is no immunity acquired from having the disease; the next rusty nail can start it all over again.

Prevention is easy: properly vaccinate with tetanus toxoid. After a two-shot initial vaccination, vaccinate pregnant mares one to two months before foaling, and should they not concieve during the subsequent year after foaling, give an annual booster each year. The foal receives initial passive protection via its dam's late-gestation booster, but it must be given a booster at ninety days of age and then annually. (See the box on page 241 for more information.)

If a horse receives a tetanus-susceptible injury (i.e., almost any break in the skin) more than three months after its most recent booster, another booster should be given at that time. If a horse suffers a puncture wound or laceration and it's known that the animal hasn't been vaccinated, or if the vaccination history is unknown, TAT must be given, despite the risks. Also, TAT must be administered if the tetanus toxoid vaccination program hasn't been completed. It's also of extreme importance to cleanse the wound thoroughly; a peroxide flush for a puncture wound is recommended. Pouring peroxide over the wound or infusing it with peroxide will cause any contamination to bubble to the surface.

Some people balk at the nominal cost of the vaccination program, and others don't keep proper records so they don't know when boosters are needed. The cost, length, and inconvenience of treating a horse with tetanus, not to mention the real possibility of the animal dying, should make those considerations inconsequential.

Rhinopneumonitis (Virus Abortion)

MANY YEARS AGO IN A TV COMMERCIAL FOR OIL FILTERS, a mechanic told the audience that cars' oil filters should be changed or eventually the cars would have problems. "Pay me now or pay me later," he told the viewers, clearly insinuating that it would be cheaper to pay him now to change the filter than it would be to pay him later for major engine repairs. So it is with virus abortion.

Farms fire veterinarians and hire them. It's the way of the world. I have been on both ends, as I suspect most equine practitioners have. Sometimes the firing is justified, sometimes not, but when a new guy is hired by an established farm, it rarely crosses his mind that the last guy had to leave for some reason.

I was both hired and fired by one farm within a month. I had met the owner once several months before and then forgot him, until one day in late December he called and asked if I'd stop by his office. I did, and he said he was considering changing veterinarians; did I want to handle his farm? It had two dozen mares and a stallion. Heck yes, I wanted to. I didn't ask why he was changing veterinarians. He introduced me to his farm manager, but, as nothing was going on, I did not meet, or even see, any of his horses.

I heard from him two weeks later. Would I go to the sale and palpate (manually check for pregnancy) a mare he just bought? I did, she was in foal, and he shipped her to his farm. I still hadn't seen any of his other horses, but that soon changed.

About ten days later, he called. A mare had slipped (aborted). I went there right away.

The farm manager showed me to a stall that contained a mare and a roughly eight-month-old fetus, covered by and still attached to the placenta.

And looking at us through the bars from the next stall was a mare with a hip number still on, the new mare from the sale. Unfortunately, I knew what had happened.

"Have these mares been vaccinated?" I asked the manager.

"For what?" he replied.

"Virus abortion. This is what this is." The postmortem later verified it.

"I dunno. Ask Mr. Tolleson." I did. He didn't know, either. He showed me the previous vet's tickets for services rendered over the past six or seven months, and I found no record of vaccination.

I explained that the new mare should not have been put in the barn with the in-foal mares until it was obvious that she wasn't carrying any diseases. "Why didn't you tell me?" he asked.

Good question. Never assume anything.

"I guess our only hope is to get her out of here and vaccinate the rest, then cross our fingers," I said. We did.

The next day, another mare in the barn aborted. Three days later, two more lost their foals. Before it was over, eleven of the twelve mares that been stabled in that barn when the new mare had moved in had slipped, as did the new mare. The vaccinations we gave hadn't helped, which was no surprise (exposure had occurred and the vaccine had insufficient time to work), and I was fired. (I later learned that, although they had moved the new mare to a different barn, she was still being turned out in the same field with the aborting mares. I assumed that was my fault; I hadn't told them not to.)

Another client, one who spent as little money as possible on health care for his animals, once bought a weanling at a sale. Not wishing to expose the three weanlings he already had on the farm to anything the new one might bring in, he put this baby in his broodmare barn. As a result, he went four for four: four pregnant mares, four abortions.

There is a very simple lesson here, of course: vaccinate. And be sure to isolate new arrivals, no matter their age.

What Is Rhinopneumonitis?

The preceding stories concern virus abortion, which is one form — in this case equine herpesvirus 1 (EHV1) — of the disease rhinopneumonitis, caused by the equine herpesvirus. The various forms of rhinopneumonitis can affect all ages and sexes in various manners (respiratory disease, abortion, paralysis, foal death); the name depends on whether it occurs as a respiratory disease or a reproductive disease. Spread of the disease is by aerosol (inhalation) or by direct contact with contaminated drinking water or infected secretions. A possible serious consequence of the respiratory form is secondary bacterial pneumonia. The respiratory form is manifested as flulike symptoms in horses younger than three years old.

Any gathering of horses — at sales, shows, racetracks, or on trail rides — can be potentially disastrous. Horses come from everywhere to a central location and share whatever viruses or bacteria they may have. Stress and exposure: what more could a healthy virus want?

Sales are the worst culprits for spreading viruses. It's probably the most stressful experience any horse goes through. First, the horse is shipped, perhaps only a mile or two or maybe across the country, but any time a horse steps into a van or a plane, stress begins. Then it's put in a strange stall next to other horses it doesn't know. Next, it's taken in and out of that stall maybe dozens of times in front of unfamiliar people who gawk and poke at it. Then it's led through a maze of barns and people into a strange building where yet more people gawk and poke before it's led through a doorway into a small, roped-off area surrounded by even more gawkers. Then some person above it starts babbling wildly and banging a hammer. Finally, the poor horse is shipped again to another new location and placed with a bunch of animals it has never seen before. It's hard to understand why *all* sales horses don't get sick.

Other types of horse population concentration are also stressful, but at least at a racetrack the horses will be there awhile and be placed in a routine, which reduces the stress. Exposure to other animals continues, however.

Fortunately, most horsemen vaccinate against virus abortion or rhinopneumonitis, as you prefer, but there are some who never do and never will, preferring to "save" those few dollars. Most pay for it in time, however.

Prevention

I'm not going to provide a specific vaccination schedule here; your veterinarian may not exactly agree with the one I use, but it probably doesn't matter as long as a schedule is maintained. (See page 376 for a general guideline for vaccination schedules.) I'm sure all equine veterinarians recommend that their clients vaccinate, but that's all we can do. We can't sneak onto a farm at night and vaccinate all the horses on it if the owner refuses to let us vaccinate.

And we can recommend that a new horse or a horse returning from the track or show or wherever be isolated — quarantined, if you will — for two to four weeks to observe for sickness, but we can't do it for them. Some clients will vaccinate their pregnant mares but then tell me, "I'm not gonna vaccinate the yearlings and the teaser. They're not gonna slip." Or, "I'm selling this mare. Don't vaccinate her." But what if the guy selling the mare or the yearling that this client intends to buy says the same thing? And the teaser is probably the most important animal on the farm to vaccinate; he has contact with every mare. (For more on teasing, see page 180.)

We'll never eliminate virus abortion, but we can certainly reduce the incidence of it. The few dollars it will cost to vaccinate against rhinopneumonitis is nothing compared to the potential loss of life from an abortion, not to mention the disappointment of losing an anticipated foal.

Potomac Horse Fever

A NUMBER OF YEARS AGO, I received a board mare from a farm in Maryland. After she had been with me for five or six days, she began to show signs of mild colic manifested as abdominal discomfort. She was depressed and wouldn't eat, and her intestinal sounds were greatly reduced. I thought perhaps she was preparing to have an impaction. I took her temperature; it was elevated.

I treated her for colic with pain reliever and mineral oil. She seemed to feel better, but the next morning the signs returned and she broke with diarrhea, which lasted for two days. I realized then that if this was a case of colic, it wasn't typical.

Fortunately, I remembered reading about Potomac horse fever in a recent veterinary journal. I looked up the article, and the description of the disease fit the signs that this mare was showing. The article said the causative organism was sensitive to tetracycline, so I treated her with the drug for a week, and she responded.

What Is Potomac Horse Fever?

Potomac horse fever is officially called *equine monocytic ehrlichiosis* and is caused by *Ehrlichia risticii.* Most cases occur from June through September in horses boarding near large waterways, but it can occur at any time in any area. All ages and both sexes are susceptible. Sporadic cases and outbreaks occur, and there are endemic areas. The mare previously described was from one of those endemic areas.

Diagnosis is usually based on signs and history, but laboratory tests can be performed to give a definitive diagnosis.

The diarrhea associated with Potomac horse fever can become severe and watery, and a horse can dehydrate. Fluids and supportive therapy are important in these cases. Some horses develop a severe toxemia, and death can result.

A serious consequence of Potomac horse fever is laminitis, or founder (see page 108). It has been estimated that as many as 25 percent of affected horses founder.

Treatment and Prevention

Ehrlichia risticii is sensitive to several antibiotics, especially tetracycline. Response is quick if treatment is begun early, but in longer-established cases it may be necessary to continue therapy for as many as two weeks. There is no natural immunity, and recurrence is common.

Prevention is achieved by vaccination. The products available are technically called *bacterins,* and the protection they give is short-lived, so repeated boosters are necessary.

Because the signs of the disease are relatively nonspecific, it has been estimated that 50 percent or more of cases go undiagnosed. I have often wondered how that figure was arrived at if the cases aren't diagnosed. I do know that I have never seen another case.

Strangles

I HAVE A CLIENT WHO SHOWS, BREEDS, AND BOARDS Mountain Pleasure Horses. It's an uncommonly placid and gentle breed (at least his are; I have never known any others), and consequently these horses are very easy to work with.

This client called one time. "Doc, three or four of my horses are snottin' pretty good. And a couple of 'em's swelled up under their jaws," he said.

I was pretty sure I knew what it was before I went to the farm. These horses are always being hauled off somewhere — to shows, to trail rides, to parades — and therefore come in contact with horses that have likewise been hauled in from all points of the compass.

When I got there, I saw I was right. The swelling under the jaws of the two horses were abscesses. One was just about ready to pop, so I stuck a needle in it and cultured the pus that oozed forth.

The result was a pure growth of *Streptococcus equi.* The horses had strangles, so named because some affected horses have difficulty swallowing. Another name for the condition is *shipping fever* because it often appears after a horse has undergone the stress of vanning a long distance.

We examined all sixteen horses on the farm. They ranged in age from eight months to ten years. The four he had called about were all showing early signs. I told him there was a chance that with vaccination we might lessen the severity in the ones not yet obviously infected. Maybe we could even prevent one or two from getting sick at all but probably not.

"What do you think?" he asked.

"I think all of your horses will come down with it, vaccination or not," I replied.

He chose not to vaccinate, and over the next two weeks all sixteen horses became ill, then slowly began improving as one by one the abscesses popped.

One yearling developed pneumonia. His abscesses apparently opened internally and the pus was aspirated into his lungs. This does not happen often, but it does occur with enough frequency that it's not surprising.

He was placed on antibiotics and recovered just fine. A couple of the others had more serious bouts of the disease, but they, too, returned to normal in a few weeks.

I told my client that the horses probably picked up the disease when he took one of them to a show or some other gathering, but he

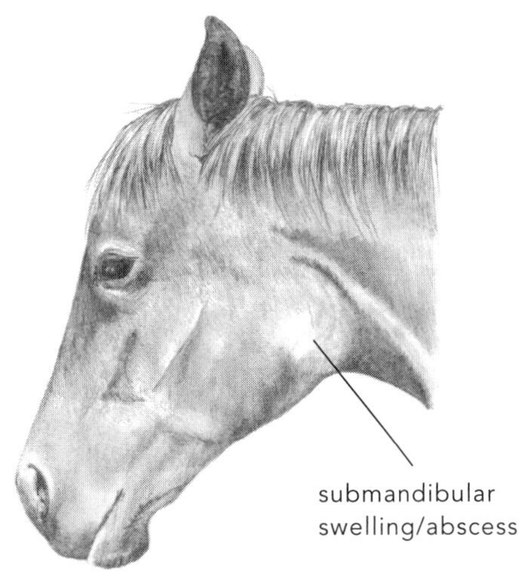

Within three or four days, the submandibular lymph nodes and sometimes the retropharyngeal nodes swell and abscess.

said he hadn't taken any of them anywhere for several weeks, nor had any new horses arrived at his farm.

The farm adjacent to his is a small Thoroughbred operation. There are a few mares and a few horses in training that came and went from the farm to the track or training center. There is one paddock where the Mountain Pleasure Horses can make nose-to-nose contact with the Thoroughbreds. Neither my client nor I knew for certain whether the neighbor's horses had the problem, but I think that we can safely assume they did; there really wasn't any other source.

On the remote chance that the strangles didn't come from the neighbor's horses, my client removed his horses from the suspect paddock so there would be no more contact, canceled all of his show plans for the summer, and closed his farm to visitors. He disinfected his barn and sheds right away and repeated this process after all of the horses were well again.

What Is Strangles?

Strangles is an acute, extremely contagious upper respiratory disease. The cause is the bacterium *Streptococcus equi.* Although most horses on a farm will get sick during an outbreak, mortality is low. When death does occur, it usually results from spread of the disease to other organs of the body.

There is only a brief natural immunity, and horses may get strangles repeatedly. Horses are capable of spreading the disease for several weeks after they appear to have recovered.

The disease is acquired when a horse inhales or ingests the bacterium. Nose-to-nose contact and shared drinking water are the usual sources of infection. All ages are susceptible, but young horses (up to four or five years old) are most susceptible.

Within a week of contact, but often within only a day or two, infected horses run a high fever (up to 105°F) and become depressed. They usually go off their feed. A mild cough and nasal discharge follow shortly, and within three or four days the submandibular lymph nodes under the jaw, and sometimes the retropharyngeal nodes behind the pharynx as well, swell and abscess. The abscesses rupture in one to two weeks, drainage occurs, and the horse feels markedly better; full recovery may take a month or more.

Normally, the course of strangles runs uneventfully, but complications, although uncommon, do occur. The infection can spread to other parts of the body, and the signs of spread, of course, depend on which part or parts are affected. When strangles spreads, it spreads most frequently to the lungs, resulting in pneumonia.

Another serious but rare complication is purpura hemorrhagica, which can follow acute strangles by several weeks. It may also occur in reinfected or vaccinated animals in a matter of days. Signs vary, but those that occur consistently are edema and petechial hemorrhages of the mucous membranes. (See page 45 for more on purpura hemorrhagica.)

Diagnosis

Diagnosis of strangles is pretty easy: the signs and history strongly suggest it, and a culture of the material from an abscessed lymph node confirms it.

Treatment

Penicillin is the best antibiotic for combating strangles, but it should be used early in the course of the disease (after nasal discharge and fever), before the lymph nodes abscess. Once the abscess occurs, there is really little need for treatment unless there are complications. In fact, antibiotic therapy once the abscess begins to form actually slows the course of the disease, thereby prolonging it. Because lymph node involvement may be so mild initially that swelling is not obvious, it is probably best not to treat it and to let the disease run its course.

An infected horse should be isolated, if possible, but usually by the time the disease is diagnosed, other horses have already been exposed. If strangles is caught early, before other horses are exposed, strict hygiene must be observed. Ideally, one person should care for the sick horse and have no contact with other horses. Because that approach is rarely an option, always handle the sick horse last, and carefully disinfect shoes, hands, and anything else that comes in contact with the ill horse before handling other horses. Careful disposal of the sick horse's bedding — burning is best — is essential to avoid further contamination.

Prevention

To prevent strangles, a two- to four-week period of quarantine should be instituted for all new arrivals, although this is rarely possible.

The vaccines on the market have not been successful in my experience, but they are available. Check with your veterinarian if you are considering a vaccination program. But be forewarned: the strangles vaccine is one of the least effective.

The organism is a survivor and can exist in a barn or shed for prolonged periods. (At a few barns here in central Kentucky, strangles outbreaks occur every few years.) *Streptococcus equi* lasts longer in moist conditions and can persist in feed or bedding for weeks or longer, so, following an outbreak, all contaminated materials must be disposed of and all buildings disinfected, preferably two or three times. Disinfecting at least twice with Nolvasan is effective. A horse that has recovered from uncomplicated strangles is none the worse for the experience and will be able to resume normal activity in two to six weeks.

No one ever wants strangles, but if your farm must be plagued by a highly contagious communicable disease, this may be the least of possible evils.

Botulism (Shaker Foal)

Horses are a good idea, but they will never work. There are just too many potential problems, and the natural culling process should have eradicated the species way back around the dawn of time.

First, they are on the menu of many carnivores, not to mention our omnivorous French friends (who also eat snails, so all in all that is a kitchen to stay out of). Then, there are those spindly little legs supporting that big old body. Totally impractical. And there is the intestinal tract. Not only does it narrow to points where solid matter has difficulty passing, it does this narrowing where it makes U-turns, making it even more difficult for digested food to pass through.

And their pain response! A stomachache that would cause us to pass on our second helping of dessert will make horses fling themselves into stone walls or go into shock.

Add to this their susceptibility to certain diseases, and it becomes obvious that their extinction should have come about aeons ago. The *Clostridium* genus and the diseases it causes, alone, should have done them in. This fun family of diseases includes tetanus and botulism — diseases that occur in all mammals and to which horses are particularly susceptible.

I think everyone, or almost everyone, who has horses vaccinates against tetanus now, but botulism is another story. Few horses are vaccinated against botulism, largely due to lack of knowledge and the associated expense.

Taking these points in order, most horse owners are probably unaware that a vaccine exists or, for that matter, that the disease exists.

The expense dissuades many people who are informed from giving the vaccine, however. It is not a cheap vaccine, and because the disease is rarely an epidemic, many folks choose to take their chances. In my opinion, if one foal is saved, even after ten years of vaccinating, it is money well spent. Which presents another quandary for some people: the disease is never seen if a horse is properly vaccinated, which may give a false sense of security and inspire some to discontinue the booster program.

What Is Botulism?

Botulism is a flaccid neuromuscular paralysis that affects both adult horses and foals. The cause is the release of a highly potent neurotoxin by the bacterium *Clostridium botulinum*. In foals the disease is called *shaker foal syndrome*, and in adults it's called *forage poisoning*.

The organism grows and produces toxin in an oxygen-free environment, particularly in certain soils, decaying plant matter, and stagnant water. Type B toxin is the most common cause of botulism in the United States and is typically found in the soils of central Kentucky and the mid-Atlantic states. Type C toxin is most common in Europe but is also found in California and Florida and was responsible for outbreaks in those states in recent years.

Although the disease incidence is generally isolated, outbreaks do occur and usually result from contaminated feed, specifically spoiled feed and feed contaminated with animal parts.

There appear to be three routes of infection: ingestion of the toxin, ingestion of spores that then grow in the intestinal tract and produce toxin, and wound contamination, which includes infected umbilical cords and contaminated castration sites.

Clinical Signs

Clinical signs range from mild to severe, depending on the amount of toxin present, and are related to flaccid neuromuscular paralysis. The central nervous system is not involved, and an infected horse is usually alert, though it may be unable to rise.

In foals, the disease occurs after two weeks of age, and in severe cases the foal may be found dead or so profoundly paralyzed that it is unable to stand. In mild cases, there is muscle weakness, dribbling of milk from the mouth or nose, and an excessive amount of lying down. The muscle weakness at first may appear to be a stilted or stiff gait but will progress to muscle tremors (hence the name *shaker foal syndrome*). As the disease advances, the foal finds it difficult to eat and nurse because of tongue paralysis. Death occurs due to respiratory paralysis and is the expected outcome unless vigorous early treatment is initiated.

The physical signs in adult horses are pretty much the same, but the first signs are loss of tone in the tongue, eyelids, and tail; progression occurs as described for foals. Again, death results from respiratory paralysis.

Diagnosis is made from clinical signs, because laboratory tests are slow or inconclusive or both.

Treatment and Prevention

Treatment consists of botulism antitoxin administration and tender loving care (including nutritional support); the sooner treatment is started, the better the prognosis.

Prevention is achieved through a proper vaccination program. Mares should receive an initial three-dose series, the last in the final month of pregnancy (which protects the foal through the dam's colostrum). A single booster is given in the last month of subsequent pregnancies (or in spring, if barren). Horses not used for breeding should also receive the initial three-dose series followed by an annual booster.

Horses residing outside endemic areas probably don't require vaccinations, but if they are to be shipped to areas where the organisms are prevalent, the vaccinations should be administered. It is extremely important to complete the series and give the annual boosters, even if a horse is not traveling to an endemic area each year.

Remember: just because the clinical disease never occurs in a vaccinated herd, it doesn't mean that the organism hasn't been present many times.

One client didn't vaccinate and operated for many years without a problem, but finally one year a five-week-old foal showed signs of botulism. We did what we were supposed to do, but the little guy needed to be hospitalized and given around-the-clock care. Just as he was improving, another foal, this one three weeks old, began showing signs. Before it was over, a total of eight foals came down with botulism and one died. That farm vaccinated faithfully after that and to date (about six years later) has had no additional cases.

Equine Viral Arteritis

When we learned about equine viral arteritis (EVA) in school, we were told that it was uncommon. That was true; not only did I not see any cases of it, I never even heard of any cases.

But a few years ago, there were some curious abortions here in

Kentucky. In an area where horse reproduction is among the leading industries, quick diagnosis of the cause was essential. The pathologists at the University of Kentucky identified the cause; it was EVA.

Clinical Signs

The signs of the disease are variable, with respiratory signs sometimes occurring. Other signs include fever, depression, loss of appetite, edema of the legs, conjunctivitis, diarrhea, and abortion, although it may be carried without any symptoms. Young horses are especially susceptible.

EVA is commonly carried by stallions, which are usually asymptomatic. It is most common in Standardbred stallions.

Treatment and Prevention

There is no treatment for EVA other than supportive therapy and removal of stress. When the outbreak occurred here, there was no vaccine and there was talk of halting the breeding season. Fortunately, this didn't happen, and a vaccine was developed. There was a suggestion that carriers be identified, which can be done by a viral neutralization test on blood, but a complication existed in that vaccinated horses tested positive.

The outbreak passed, and widespread EVA vaccination never caught on, but it's a cheap precaution. A preventable disease should be prevented.

2

Common Diseases and Conditions

Infections and Antimicrobial Therapy

"I GAVE HER TEN MILLILITERS OF PENICILLIN two or three days ago, Doc, and she's still sick. Should I give her another shot?"

Clients have asked me that question, or something very similar, many, many times, and each time I try to explain that their suggestion is not the proper approach to antimicrobial therapy.

One time a trainer had a two-year-old gelding with a bad cough. "Give him ten milliliters of gentamicin, Doc. That'll take care of that cough," he directed.

"That's possibly not the proper antibiotic or dosage and, even if it is, a one-time administration won't do any good and may be detrimental," I told him.

He told the owner that I refused to treat the horse. The owner called me at home and told me, in no uncertain terms, that if I did not give his horse ten milliliters of "whatever the trainer told you to give him," he would find a veterinarian who would.

I didn't and he probably did.

In both cases, both the antibiotic and the dosage were possibly wrong. (Ten is a great number — Big Ten, top ten, perfect ten, ten fingers — but it rarely is the proper dosage for anything.) Casual treatments such as these accomplish nothing beneficial and may very well be harmful. Any organism present may become sensitized to the drug and develop resistance, so that future proper use of the drug will be rendered ineffective.

The use of antibiotics or other antibacterials in the horse is tricky. There are several reasons for this.

- There are many antimicrobial agents but only a small percentage is approved for use in horses.
- Oral absorption is poor in the horse, necessitating the use of injections in most cases.
- The disposition of many horses, especially after the sixth day of three-times-a-day intramuscular injections, is unapproving.
- The propensity for bacteria to develop resistance is great.
- More and more bacteria are being found that can cause disease in horses.
- Many diseases are caused by viruses, and we have no systemic antiviral agents.

Modes of Transmission

So how does a horse get a bacterial infection? Well, there are several ways, some of which we contribute to.

- Stress — probably the root cause of everything from broken legs to broken wind to broken marriages
- Invasive actions, which can include anything that breaks the skin, from puncture wounds to surgical procedures
- Immune system dysfunction
- Improper use or overuse of corticosteroids
- Improper use or overuse of antimicrobials
- Bacterial exposure

Once the bacteria enter the body, they can produce infection in two ways: multiplication and invasion of the tissues, or production of toxins. Antimicrobial therapy is aimed at killing the invading bacteria (bactericidal) or stopping its growth until the body's own defenses can defeat it (bacteriostatic), but antimicrobial agents alone cannot do the job. Supportive therapy is needed. This includes proper nutrition, fluid maintenance, stress reduction or cessation, and stimulation of the immune system.

Drug and Dosage

Selection of the correct antimicrobial agent and the correct dosage are of prime importance and depend on several factors.

• **Specific organism and its sensitivity.** In many cases the organism can be determined by the disease, history, or by previous knowledge. If Horse A has an already-identified bacterial pneumonia, for instance, and Horse B in the adjacent stall becomes ill with the same clinical signs, go with the antibacterial agent that Horse A's culture and sensitivity indicated. If, however, Horse B develops diarrhea instead of pneumonia, it would be wise to take a culture to determine the organism causing the infection.

In the case of viral infections, they can probably be classified under "stress." Because the body is compromised by exposure to viruses, secondary bacterial infections often follow viral infections. Although antibacterial agents will do nothing against the virus, they are needed to combat the secondary bacterial invaders.

• **Location of the infection.** Location of the infection is important because all antibacterial agents will not reach therapeutic levels in all body systems; that is, a urinary tract infection cannot be treated by a drug that does not enter the urinary tract.

• **Route of administration.** The route of administration matters for the sake of the horse. An antibiotic that must be given by intramuscular injection every six hours is far less preferable than one that can be given intravenously every twelve hours.

• **Frequency of administration and ability to administer the drug at the proper intervals.** The frequency of administration is of great concern if the horse being treated remains on the farm or some other

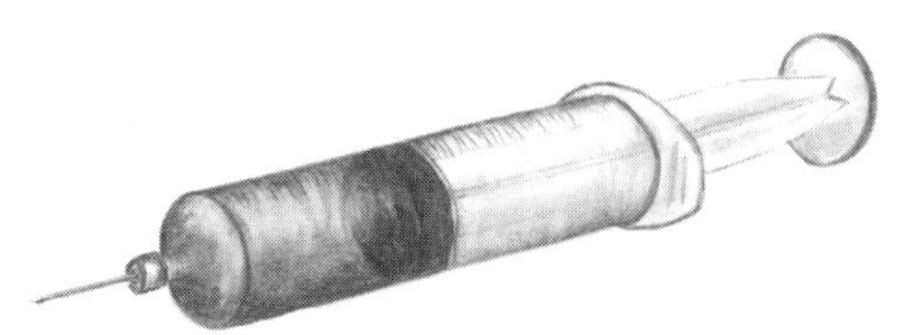

It's critical that drugs be administered at the proper dose and within the specified time frame.

"outpatient" facility. If it's hospitalized, of course, the clinic staff will arrange for treatment at the proper times but in many cases the drug is dispensed to an owner, trainer, or farm manager with instructions. If the treatment times are inconvenient, they are often "adjusted."

For instance, if a horse is to receive an antibiotic every eight hours, ideally that should be at something like 6 A.M., 2 P.M., and 10 P.M. Frequently, reality is more like 7 A.M., 4 P.M., and 8 P.M. Twice-a-day medications are often given when the caretaker arrives (7 A.M.) and again when he leaves for the day (4 P.M.), rather than at the proper twelve-hour intervals. Even once-a-day doses can be messed up if they are given one day at 6 A.M. and the next at 9 P.M.

- **Size of the horse.** The size of the horse determines, in most cases, the dose of the antibacterial agent. A 900-pound, two-year-old filly does not receive the same dose as the 1,200-pound, five-year-old gelding in the next stall.
- **Disposition of the horse.** The disposition of some horses is such that the less often they are treated, the better off everyone concerned, including the horses, will be.
- **Cost.** And cost is important simply because cost is important. It is generally preferable to use the least-expensive product to which a sensitivity is found.

Duration

The duration of antimicrobial therapy is also important. A client had some pills acquired in some manner. He called and said he had had a weanling on them for "over two weeks and she's still sick." There's a lot wrong with that, not the least of which was that the drug insert clearly stated to limit administration to seven days.

When to stop treatment is another tough question. If the horse doesn't show improvement in two to four days, the choice of the drug being used should be reevaluated. If, however, improvement is shown to the point where the horse appears to be normal again, a rule of thumb is to continue therapy for forty-eight to seventy-two hours beyond the time when no further clinical signs are shown.

I guess what this all boils down to is this: let your veterinarian prescribe antimicrobial therapy, agents, and duration, and follow her instructions. After all, you're paying for and relying on professional knowledge and advice.

Equine Protozoal Myeloencephalitis (EPM)

My client owned five producing broodmares and, for the most part, sold their offspring, but he raced one of the fillies occasionally so he could use her to replace a mare every now and then, when one got older or stopped producing foals. He also had one mare, Mattie, that was out of production; I'm sure she had a longer registered name, but I never knew her by anything other than Mattie. She was aged (in her upper twenties), and she had produced some awfully good racehorses through the years, one of which was now one of his broodmares. The old girl had a home for life for that reason alone, but also he liked her. No, he loved her.

I was at his farm to check a mare that had been bred the previous day. He said, "Doc, I need you to look at Mattie. I think maybe her time has come."

He brought her out of her stall and walked her for me. She was noticeably off in her rear and possibly also in her right fore. It wasn't lameness per se; she was just wobbly.

"I see what you mean," I said. "She's awfully old. Maybe she's trying to tell us something."

"She almost fell yesterday. I hate to put her down, but if she's not gonna be able to get around I guess I'll have to. I'll have to think about it, though."

Then he said, "That three-year-old filly I was racing is back here. She's not been training well, and the trainer says she's losing condition. Check her over."

He brought out the filly. She had been a nice racehorse at two years old, winning three races and placing in a stakes race, but she had finished up the track in her first two races at age three. He told me he brought her home when the trainer had said that she was losing condition.

Her gluteal muscles were smaller than they should have been and smaller than they had been the last time I had seen her, which was about five months earlier, when I watched her work out at the local training center.

"Let me see her walk," I said. He walked her for me, then I said, "Trot her." He did. She was slightly off in her rear end, not a lot, but the coordination just wasn't what it should have been.

"I think she has EPM," I told him. "And maybe that's Mattie's problem, too."

What Is Equine Protozoal Myeloencephalitis?

Equine protozoal myeloencephalitis (EPM) is a neurological disease of horses caused by the protozoa *Sarcocystis neurona* or *Sarcocystis falcutula*. The normal life cycle of these organisms involves two hosts: the opossum and certain birds. Horses are not involved in the life cycle but are aberrant, or atypical, intermediate hosts.

Horses ingest the organism through contaminated feed. The contamination typically occurs when opossums are allowed access to stored feed and hay areas. Once in the horse, the organisms migrate through the blood to the horse's central nervous system (CNS), where they reproduce in cells of the nervous system. Horses, therefore, can't transmit the organisms to other animals.

It takes at least four weeks from ingestion to the onset of clinical signs, but it may take as long as two years for signs to become obvious. They may be subtle and fail to progress, so the precise incidence of the disease isn't known. EPM has been diagnosed in all horse breeds, but the incidence seems noticeably higher in Thoroughbreds and

Standardbreds. At least two books suggest that ponies may be resistant to EPM, but I have seen the disease in two ponies, so I disagree. It has been suggested that some horses generate an immune response and shed the organism before it can infect the CNS, although their blood will test positive for antibodies.

Clinical Signs

Typical signs are referred to as the three A's: asymmetric ataxia (stumbling and unsteadiness) and atrophy (wasting tissue). The signs, however, depend on the site the organism reaches, and because it's carried in the blood, that site may be anywhere throughout the CNS. These signs are the results of both direct damage to neurons and indirect damage by edema and inflammation.

The most common signs are ataxia and weakness, usually worse in the hind limbs than in the forelimbs. Atrophy is most often apparent in the gluteal muscles, simply because it's easier to see changes in this area. Falling often occurs as the condition advances.

Early signs of EPM are usually detected by observing the horse during exercise. Head tossing, high head carriage, and bucking are common. Short, choppy strides, inability to maintain a lead, and forelimb lameness (resulting from hind limb weakness) are also typical.

Diagnosis

Diagnosis can't be made based on clinical signs alone, but they can be suggestive. A definitive diagnosis can be made only by cerebrospinal fluid (CSF) analysis. Often when the disease is suspected, treatment is begun without CSF analysis and response to treatment is considered diagnostic. It's foolish, however, to treat without a specific diagnosis, because if you're treating for the wrong thing, you're wasting money and endangering the horse.

Treatment

Presently there are three treatment regimens: an older, prolonged, and expensive course; a newer, shorter, and expensive course; and a brand-spanking-new paste that isn't even available in the United States at this writing. All three treatments are oral.

The older treatment consists of pyrimethamine and trimethoprim for three months. The newer one uses a product (Baycox) that is not yet licensed in the United States but that can be legally obtained by a U.S. veterinarian through the manufacturer in Canada. In personal experience, I have seen some horses thought to be cured by the older drug regimen have relapses. In using the newer product a few times, the horses got better and didn't relapse. The brand-new paste sounds too good to be true; I hope it's effective.

Prevention

Prevention is easy: tightly cover all feed and garbage containers. Trapping opossums and moving them to other areas will definitely reduce the possibility of EPM. Humane traps are available at reasonable cost, and once an opossum is captured, simply take it for a ride far away from horses and turn it loose. Don't kill it.

Preventing hay contamination is slightly more of a problem, but covering the hay with a tarp or otherwise eliminating access is wise.

The prognosis depends on the severity of the signs. Mildly affected horses usually return to full use, while severely affected horses may improve but never return to normal. Exceptions do occur in both extremes. As with most conditions, the sooner the problem is recognized and treated, the better the chances for recovery.

Back to Mattie and the three-year-old filly. I suggested that we take CSF samples and check for EPM. This is a good client; he's concerned with the costs involved, but he's more concerned with his horses' welfare and never refuses to do anything if I assure him that it is for the good of his horses.

On CSF examination, we found that both horses had EPM. We used the newer expensive treatment, and both responded. The three-year-old returned to the races later that year and won twice more for him; then he retired her and she joined his broodmares. Mattie also got better, but at her age she still didn't exactly prance around. She's still there, now about thirty years old. It will be a sad day when she finally goes.

Equine Infectious Anemia

A negative blood test for equine infectious anemia (EIA or *swamp fever*) is required of all equines prior to interstate and international shipment, as well as for most intrastate movement. This state-mandated law is designed to identify horses infected with the disease and to protect those that are not. The required blood test is called a Coggins test.

What Is Equine Infectious Anemia?

EIA is an incurable viral disease that has defied the development of a vaccine. Some horses don't show signs but are carriers and can spread the disease to others. The only protection against EIA is the identification and destruction of those animals that carry it.

Spread is by biting insects, especially horseflies. In the 1948 outbreak that brought national attention to the disease, horses at a racetrack were all vaccinated using the same needle, which subsequently infected dozens of animals. *Never* use a needle more than once.

Clinical Signs

The signs of EIA are fever, anorexia, and petechial hemorrhages that appear as tiny red spots on the mucous membranes in acute episodes. Then there are recurring cycles of fever, edema, jaundice, depression, and progressive weight loss. Pregnant mares may abort. Death is eventual, except in asymptomatic carriers. In horses that are asymptomatic carriers, the initial acute signs are all that may be seen, but the virus remains in the blood.

Prevention

Good record-keeping is important here. If your records are kept properly, you will know when your horses' Coggins tests expire (they're good for a year in most areas). A couple of weeks before they expire, have your veterinarian take new tests. It's the law that Coggins tests be current, for your protection as well as for the protection, health, and welfare of all horses.

WHEN I WAS FIRST OUT OF VETERINARY SCHOOL I worked in a practice in an area where EIA was a serious problem. I once took the required Coggins tests on all eleven horses on a small Quarter Horse farm, and all eleven were positive. That was absolutely heartbreaking; in addition to bringing about the deaths of the horses, the disease put a young couple out of business.

Yet some people try to bypass the law that requires Coggins tests. A client who boards many mares from all over the United States during the breeding season once received two mares — Thoroughbred mares — via a private carrier from a state in which EIA occurs at a higher-than-average rate. The horses were accompanied by the required health certificates and paperwork for negative Coggins tests. One Coggins was for a Morgan and the other for an Appaloosa, which is how the Thoroughbred mares were described on the health certificates.

Some veterinarian, of course, issued those health certificates. This guy is a poor reflection on the veterinary profession. Either he's pretty stupid for not being able to distinguish Morgans and Appaloosas from Thoroughbreds, or he's dishonest. The owner of the mares was obviously both dishonest and stupid.

Many years ago, a new client for whom I'd been doing work for only a few weeks was shipping several yearlings to Florida to be broken. One morning his secretary called me: "The van will be here this afternoon. Please come by and give us health certificates."

I got there and the farm manager showed me the yearlings. I checked them over and said, "Okay, let me see their Coggins."

"I don't have them," he replied. "They must be in the office. Just fill out the health certificates, and I'll put the papers together."

I must look dumber than I actually am. "I'll stop by the office and look at them there," I told him.

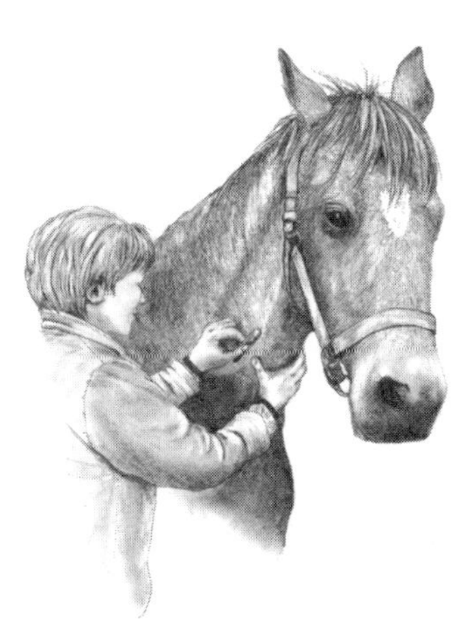

The law requiring a Coggins test is for your protection as well as for the protection of all horses.

At the office, I told the secretary, "I need to see the Coggins tests on these yearlings."

"The what?" she asked innocently.

I explained, and I suspected that she wasn't as dumb or naive as she was acting.

"I'll have to call the boss," she said, and she did. "He'll be right here," she told me.

In a few minutes, the farm owner (the boss) bustled in. "What the hell's the problem here?" he demanded.

"Dr. Kelley says he needs Coggins tests on the yearlings," explained the secretary.

"Well, then, give him some!" he snapped. "Come with me."

She followed him into his office and emerged in about five minutes carrying a handful of Coggins forms. "Here you are." She smiled and handed them to me.

I thanked her and sat down to finish filling out the needed information on the health certificates.

The first Coggins paper I looked at was for a three-year-old filly. The next was for a five-year-old mare. The third was for a two-year-old colt. That was the closest to a yearling in the group. I said, "Something's wrong. These aren't for those yearlings."

She smiled and stepped into her boss's office. A second later he exploded through the door.

"Kelley, what's wrong with you?!"

"These Coggins aren't for the horses you're shipping." I tend to be naive; I still thought it was an inadvertent error.

The discussion continued and escalated. He yelled that he *must* have those health certificates. I tried to explain that I couldn't issue them without valid Coggins. Then, all of a sudden, he stopped ranting. Calmly, smoothly, he laid a hand on my shoulder. "Brent, look," he said sweetly, "I don't have the Coggins on the yearlings, but the van is on its way, and these horses need to be on it. My former vet always did this for me. I'll have Coggins drawn on them as soon as they get to Florida." He smiled. "I promise."

I pointed out that his former veterinarian had been fired or quit. I don't know if those yearlings left that day or not. I also don't know if I quit or was fired. I do know that he never paid his final bill.

I don't think that anyone has ever had a surprise vanning. Everyone knows — or should know — ahead of time that a horse is going somewhere. But if it does happen that a horse has to go somewhere *today,* there's now an enzyme-linked immunosorbent assay (ELISA) test for EIA. It's not accepted for international shipping, but it's fine for interstate and intrastate use. It can be run in two hours compared to the twenty-four hours required to obtain results for the Coggins test. Not all laboratories have the facilities to evaluate an ELISA, however, so it's best to be prepared with current Coggins in advance of shipping dates.

Bacterial Pneumonia

A PERFECTLY INTELLIGENT CLIENT WOULD NOT VACCINATE his young horses. I must have told him a jillion times how important it was. I showed him articles and statistics on it. His argument was always the same: "These horses will get sick when they go to the track anyhow. Why should I waste money on vaccinations?" Well, maybe he wasn't so intelligent.

He was right, of course. They all do get sick, or so it seems. But vaccinated horses can withstand the challenge of exposure so much better, and they don't get *as* sick as horses that have never been vaccinated.

The vaccinations protect against viral diseases. We're talking about influenza and rhinopneumonitis mainly, two viral respiratory conditions that seem to be almost inevitable when large numbers of young horses are brought together. They can knock an unvaccinated horse out of training for weeks, but if the horse has been vaccinated properly, infection may cause a minor setback of only a few days, if that.

One of the major dangers of a serious viral infection is the lowering of the horse's resistance to other dangers. Bacteria don't usually cause primary disease in horses (though it certainly happens), but in its compromised state a horse debilitated by a viral disease is just waiting for a secondary bacterial infection to set up housekeeping. And a viral respiratory disease weakens the body's ability to withstand the challenge of even the standard bacteria in a horse's environment. Bacterial pneumonia is often the result.

This particular client put three to five two-year-olds in training every year and usually had three to five cases of pneumonia. One would think he would learn, but he never did. His veterinary bills were outrageous (but he paid, so I'm not complaining; I'm just sorry his horses had to suffer from his ignorance), and his training bills were much higher than they should have been because his horses stayed in his trainer's care while they were being treated. But he had, and still has, lots of money, and if he wants me to have a bunch of it, so be it. I'd rather get a little less of it by vaccinating his horses, though.

What Is Bacterial Pneumonia?

Several factors contribute to bacterial pneumonia: viral respiratory infection, stress, ventilation, and cleanliness. Stress, as I always say, weakens the immune system and contributes to disease. Poorly ventilated stalls and unclean conditions, in addition to stress, invariably lead to respiratory problems.

Add to this the fact that a racetrack or show ground, or any place where horses from all levels of management mingle, is a marvelous incubator of all diseases known and unknown to veterinary science.

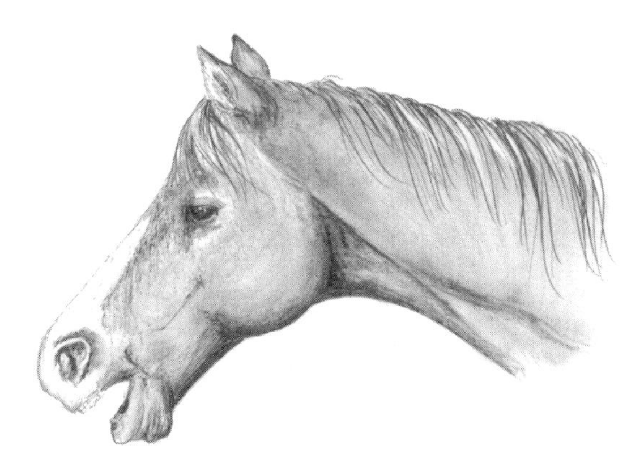

Coughing is a common sign of bacterial pneumonia.

Also, if horses are raised in a closed environment — one in which there are few horses and no outside contact with others — their exposure is limited and they therefore may be more susceptible to potential pathogens simply because they have never been exposed to them before.

Clinical Signs

The signs of bacterial pneumonia are pretty much the same as for influenza and rhinopneumonitis: cough, snotty nose, depression, fever, and anorexia.

Treatment

Bacterial pneumonia requires antibiotic therapy. Most of the time, a horse is given a good broad-spectrum drug, assuming that it will take care of whatever the causative organism is. And most of the time this works, although sometimes a culture is needed. Culturing organisms from the lungs is not as easy as culturing them from most other infected areas of the body, but your veterinarian can do it. That way the exact bacterium can be identified, the proper antibiotic can be used, and the condition resolved. Sometimes, to attain the proper effect from the drug, it must be placed directly within the lungs. Again, this is something your veterinarian can do.

Bacterial pneumonia is going to happen, but incidences can be minimized by properly vaccinating against the viral respiratory diseases that increase vulnerability.

Purpura Hemorrhagica

A LOT OF PEOPLE ARE DONE IN BY DISEASE. I was almost done in twice by the same one.

I'm going to make a confession here: I was *not* at the top of my class in veterinary school. Far from it — I was pretty well buried in the middle.

Maybe I could have had a higher grade point average, but I didn't really apply myself in subjects I had no future plans for. For instance, Poultry Medicine was considered to be a very easy course; show up and stay awake and you got an A. The only plans I ever had concerning poultry centered on Colonel Sanders and his ilk. Out of more than sixty students, there were just two Bs in the class. I got one.

Ruminant Medicine was a tougher course. I never liked cows anyhow, and I sure as heck had no plans ever to work on an uncooked one. I got a C.

I tried to apply myself on dog and cat stuff for two reasons. First, I like dogs and cats, and, second, there was always a chance that I would someday have to work on small animals. But I entered veterinary school to learn about horses, and I studied hard in Equine Medicine. *Real* hard. Of the sixty-some students in our class, I was the only one planning to go into equine practice, so I *had* to learn more than anyone else.

And it went well for the first couple of exams. They were multiple-choice, true/false, and short-answer tests, each with eighty to one hundred questions, and I aced them. Then came the third test; our teacher must have been in a hurry when he made it out, because it had only four questions on it: list the cause, clinical signs, laboratory findings, diagnosis, treatment, and prognosis for the following, and four conditions were listed: Monday morning disease, founder, equine infectious anemia (EIA), and purpura hemorrhagica.

Purpura hemorrhagica? Holy cow! Sure, he had mentioned it in class. Sure, I had read about it in the textbook. Why, then, did I know nothing about it? My mind was a blank — a total blank.

I got a 68 on that test: 24 on Monday morning disease, 22 on founder, 22 on EIA, and 0 (as in zero) on purpura hemorrhagica. Only one person got a lower score (67), and the class average was 81. It was embarrassing.

Purpura hemorrhagica was not going to catch me again, though. I read and reread the book until I could quote it forward and backward. That was nearly thirty years ago. Unfortunately, even though I knew all there was to know about purpura hemorrhagica, once I entered the real world I never saw a case. Not one. Until . . .

What Is Purpura Hemorrhagica?

Purpura hemorrhagica seems to appear as a sequel to an infection, respiratory usually, and frequently a beta-hemolytic streptococcus. It also is known to follow strangles vaccination, but in some cases there is no history of infection or vaccination. The actual cause is unknown, but it's believed to be a hypersensitivity reaction to an immune-mediated disease.

Clinical Signs

In the mild form of purpura, there is muscle stiffness and a reluctance to walk and bend the neck. There is mild edema of the legs and lower abdomen, and urticaria. Temperature, pulse, respiration, and red blood cell count are all normal.

In the severe form, the edema is pronounced and may involve the head; the swollen legs may ooze serum. Petechial hemorrhages appear on the mucous membranes and tongue. Respiratory distress results from edema (swelling) of the nasal passages and lungs. The temperature may be 104° to 105°F, and the red cell count drops to fewer than 4 million cells/mL. After a few days, there is an increase in neutrophil blood cell count.

To show how devious our teacher was way back when, the differential diagnosis of purpura hemorrhagica includes tying up (Monday morning disease), founder, and EIA, so the purpura question was almost a gift — to those who had studied properly. Equine viral arteritis (EVA) should also be included in the differential.

Treatment

Treatment consists of penicillin, corticosteroids, and tender loving care, with blood transfusions necessary in extremely severe cases. Bandaging the edematous legs is helpful to keep the swelling down.

The prognosis is good in mild cases, with recovery generally occurring in ten days to two weeks, but is guarded in severe cases, where there may be a mortality rate as high as 50 percent.

Okay, as I said, I learned that nearly thirty years ago, and it was unused knowledge for, lo, those many years.

But a client called one day. A three-year-old filly just off the track was having trouble moving and her legs were a little swollen. I went to see her. She was walking as if she was foundered, but she wasn't.

"Let's watch her for a day or two," I suggested, and told him to wrap her legs.

The next day my client asked, "Could she be tying up? She's walking like she is."

I said no. He said, "Well, then, what is it?"

She was breathing a little roughly. I took a blood count. The red cells were slightly low, but that isn't unusual in a horse just out of training, and her Coggins test from the track was negative so it wasn't EIA. She also had a negative EVA test, albeit from two years earlier when he purchased her as a yearling.

The next day my client said, "Look here," and raised the filly's upper lip. There were little red spots (petechiae) on the gums.

The edema in her legs was worsening, and another blood count showed fewer red cells and a slight elevation in the number of neutrophils.

My client was extremely worried and so was I. He is a good-paying client, and one doesn't want to lose a horse or a good-paying client, and I feared I could easily lose both if I did not do something for his filly soon.

After receiving the results of the second blood count, I decided to put her on antibiotics. On the way to his farm that afternoon to do so, I stopped by the local veterinary supply house, and a veterinarian acquaintance was also there. In passing the time while our orders were being filled, he said he had been seeing a horse that was not responding to treatment and that it was frustrating him.

I told him about my client's filly. Without so much as blinking, he said, "Sounds like purpura."

Lights flashed! Bells rang! Obviously!

So once again — twenty-five-plus years later — I got a zero on purpura hemorrhagica. I put the filly on penicillin and steroids and she responded. She recovered, and I still have my client.

Purpura will not get me again. I doubt I will be around in another twenty-five years, so I'm not even going to mark my calendar.

Leptospirosis

A FORMER CLIENT HAD LOTS OF PROBLEMS, not the least of which was his horse operation. There were also marital problems, money problems, kid problems, and several other problems, but as this book is about horses, we won't go into them.

He had a pleasant but poorly designed little farm. In front of the only barn were two small paddocks: one about a half acre and the other about a quarter acre. Behind the barn lay a *huge* field of maybe twenty-five acres. And at the front of the farm, a good quarter mile or more from the barn, was another big field, probably ten acres.

The only thing the two little paddocks were used for was to turn out mares and just-born foals. The front field was used for weanlings and yearlings together. The great big field was used for pregnant mares, empty mares, mares with foals older than two weeks, all at the same time. It was a horrible method of management because mares without foals sometimes injure or try to "adopt" foals, not to mention the risk for disease.

All the horses in the big field were put in the barn at night, and his teaser, which was kept in the barn all day, was then turned out in that same field for the night.

In all my years of practice, I have seen just three cases of equine recurrent uveitis (ERU; also known as *moon blindness*, or *periodic ophthalmia*), and two of them were on this farm. I blamed it on bad luck, but I should have known better, considering his management practices.

This fellow also had more than his share of mares that had been in foal come up empty. In most cases, the aborted fetuses were not discovered, because it's difficult to search a field that size and find a small body. One day, however, a mare conveniently aborted right near the gate. It was a late-term foal, about nine months along, and I took it to the local diagnostic lab for a postmortem examination to determine the cause.

The diagnosis came back as "Fetal death caused by *Leptospira gryppotyphosa*." A note was added by the pathologist, "Brent, call me." I did.

He asked, "Do you know how this happened? We don't see many lepto abortions."

I told the farm owner what was found and asked him if I could take blood samples from his horses to determine if any of them had leptospirosis. Ten of twelve mares were positive, and nine of twelve young horses (foals and yearlings) were also positive. He didn't want to pay for the teaser to be tested, but I told him I wouldn't charge for him. The teaser's titer was almost off the scale.

To make an already long story a little shorter, we eventually determined that the teaser was a carrier for leptospirosis. Because he was turned out in the communal field, every time he urinated he shared the virus with every other horse that used the field, which at one time or another was each horse on the farm.

What Is Leptospirosis?

Comparatively little is known about the effect of *Leptospira* species. In horses, it causes ERU and abortion and has also been implicated in kidney disease. ERU has been reported in up to 12 percent of horses and is the leading cause of blindness in horses worldwide. Factors other than *Leptospira* have also been implicated, but *Leptospira* is generally accepted as the main culprit. There are breed predilections to the disease: Appaloosas are high on the list, with Standardbreds less frequently affected. Until a few years ago, moon blindness was believed to be the primary condition, but more and more we're seeing abortions. Personally, I don't think abortion from leptospirosis has become a problem all of a sudden; for a time I think that it just wasn't considered by practitioners or looked for by pathologists.

Whether or not that's true, the genus *Leptospira* is made up of many subgroupings, called *serovars,* that can infect almost anything, including humans, although certain species seem to be particularly susceptible. In horses, *Leptospira interrogans* has been implicated in ocular problems, whereas *L. pomona, L. gryppotyphosa, L. hardjo, L. bratislava,* and *L. icterohemorrhagiae* have, at various times, been associated with abortion. Attempts at perfecting a vaccine for use in horses have failed.

In dogs, the two main culprits — for which there is a satisfactory vaccine — are *L. canicola* and *L. icterohemorrhagiae.* In cattle, *L. hardjo* is number one, and in rats — a problem in any farming operation — it's *L. icterohemorrhagiae. Leptospira* can transmit from species to species.

Spread is by contact with the urine or placental fluids of infected animals, either by ingestion or by contamination of cuts or abrasions.

Clinical Signs

Signs are short-term flulike symptoms, including mild fever, depression, anorexia, and possibly jaundice, which are often overlooked by observers; abortion follows weeks to months later. Occasionally, infected foals are born, but they are sickly and usually die.

In the acute stage of ERU, blepharospasm and lacrimation (involuntary winking and tear production) and usually photophobia are evident. The eyelids are swollen. Repeated bouts of inflammation follow and cataracts develop; ERU is the leading cause of equine cataracts. The first recurrence after the initial acute phase is usually within a year, and subsequent recurrences occur progressively sooner. Blindness is the final outcome.

Diagnosis

Diagnosis of ERU is made by ophthalmic examination and by blood tests or by isolating the bacterium, although this is difficult and often unsuccessful, in systemic cases.

Treatment

Anti-inflammatory therapy, topical and systemic, is the usual course of action, but in recent years several vitrectomies (surgical removal of the vitreous humor in the eye) have been performed with excellent results. Blind, painful eyes should be removed. Penicillin, streptomycin, and tetracycline are effective treatments for leptospirosis but have little efficacy in ERU.

Prevention

Proper hygiene is the best preventative, though it's difficult to convince a rat not to urinate wherever it wants to. For this reason, sealed feed storage bins and automatic waterers are strongly recommended.

The farm owner didn't get rid of his teaser, though I strongly urged him to do so. Instead, he put him in the half-acre paddock and allowed no other horses in there at any time. About a year later, after two more mares came up empty, he and I parted company, so I don't know whether the problem continued.

Vesicular Stomatitis

Some diseases that occur in horses may also affect food-producing animals and sometimes people. Although they are not plentiful in number, their threat to public health makes them of greater overall concern than some plain old, horses-only conditions. Vesicular stomatitis (VS) is one of them. It is a reportable disease, which means that it is reported when it occurs and the government steps in and "helps." I have several thoughts concerning the efficacy of this approach, but this is a veterinary forum, not a political one, so my editorialization will end here.

A few years back, there was a problem in the Southwest with VS, a viral disease that affects not only horses, but also pigs, cattle, certain wild ruminants, and people. The chief restriction we faced was the shipment of horses to and from certain areas. This confinement, while inconvenient, helped control and contain the outbreak.

What Is Vesicular Stomatitis?

There are several types of the VS virus, and all affect horses. The disease doesn't seem to be spread by contact but is believed to be transmitted by sand flies and possibly other biting insects. Ninety percent of the cases occur in August and September, and most seem to be associated with moist environments; wetlands or pastures with streams or ponds seem to produce increased incidence. Incubation is short, one to three days.

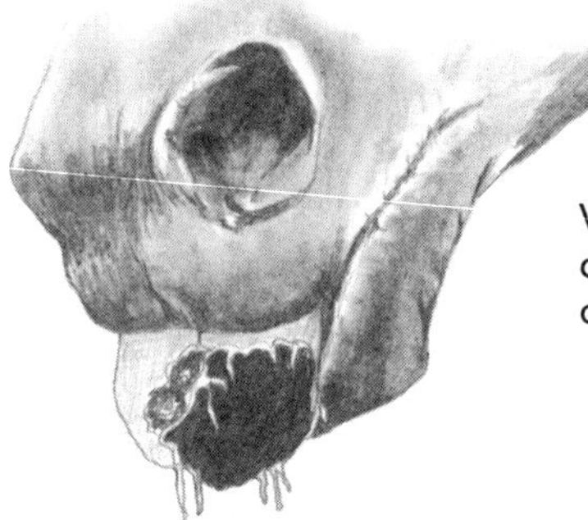

Vesicles coalesce and rupture, denuding as much as 50 percent of the tongue.

Clinical Signs

In horses, the main sign is inflammation of the tongue and oral mucosa. Vesicles (fluid-filled bubbles), ranging from one to three millimeters in diameter, form, coalesce, and then rupture, denuding as much as 50 percent of the tongue. Severely infected animals may refuse to eat or be unable to eat. (Any time a horse refuses to eat for no apparent reason, the tongue should be checked.) The denuded area is red and raw and has strands of tissue hanging from its edges. There may be frothy, blood-tinged saliva. Water intake may be greatly increased or reduced, and fever, depression, and excessive salivation are the usual symptoms.

In some cases, vesicles may also appear on the feet (usually around the coronary band), the sheath of males, and the mammary glands of females. Because of discomfort, an infected lactating mare may not allow her foal to nurse.

Diagnosis

The clinical signs are sufficient for a diagnosis, but to satisfy epidemiologists, viral isolation, a complement fixation test, or a serum neutralization test is definitive.

Treatment

VS runs its course in a week to ten days, and there is no mortality from the disease itself, although supportive therapy, including tube feeding and watering in severe cases, may be necessary. There is always the possibility of secondary bacterial infection of the ruptured vesicles, so antibiotic therapy should be considered: systemic for the mouth and tongue and topical for the external areas.

Because it is a reportable disease, infected horses must be quarantined. Strict isolation and sanitation procedures must also be implemented. It's a pain and an inconvenience, but it's the only way to properly control what could become a disastrous disease for food animal–producing farmers and ranchers. It is recommended that food animals with VS be destroyed.

Prevention

Prevention is difficult, especially because the disease may occur in a wild population near your horses' grazing areas. Insect control is your best bet.

Sinusitis

Sinusitis is a bear to treat. No veterinarian looks forward to seeing a case. The treatment is prolonged, and all too often the response isn't what we want. Also, the horse thinks little of it. And the cost of treatment can exceed the value of the horse, increasing the horse's value out of proportion.

Clinical Signs

The signs of sinusitis in a horse are pretty much the same as the signs in a person: snotty nose and difficulty breathing. The discharge is usually thick and colored (yellowish or greenish), has a very bad odor, and may be present in one or both nostrils.

There are several causes of sinusitis. In decreasing order of frequency, they are:

1. Dental disease
2. Primary bacterial infection
3. Trauma to the sinuses
4. Sinus cysts
5. Neoplasia (cancerous tumor)
6. Ethmoid hematoma
7. Fungal infection

The first three are far and away the most common. The last three are rare; I've never seen neoplasia or fungal infection. I have seen two cases of ethmoid hematoma; even so, it's rare. And I've also never seen sinus cysts, although I've read that they occur semi-commonly. Given all of this, we'll address only the first three: they account for at least 75 percent of the cases of sinusitis.

Dental Disease

By a wide margin, dental disease is the most common cause. It's certainly the main cause of chronic sinusitis in mature horses, although it's uncommon in horses younger than three years old. Problems of the cheek teeth, such as fractures and displaced or malpositioned teeth, can result in sinusitis. Treatment consists of removing the affected tooth or teeth, establishing proper drainage, and administering the proper systemic antibiotic(s) at proper levels for the proper length of time. Also, the socket from which the tooth was extracted must granulate in and heal; otherwise, reinfection will occur because food particles will enter through the socket and infect the sinus. (See page 348 on dental care for more information about teeth.)

Primary Bacterial Infection

Primary bacterial infection of a sinus is treated by irrigation and systemic antibiotics, which is typically effective, but it must be emphasized that treatment is often lengthy. Irrigation must occur daily for at least two weeks, and antibiotics must be continued for at least that long. Culturing the mucous discharge to determine the proper antibiotic or combination of drugs is critical. Broad-spectrum antibiotics often do more harm than good, as they can lead to resistant strains, particularly due to the chronic nature of the disease.

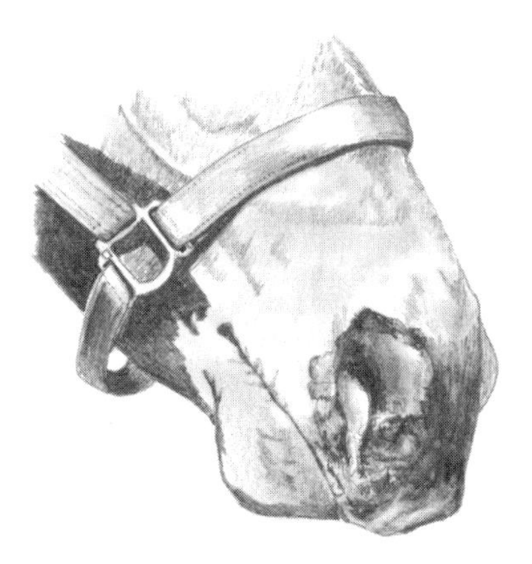

Sinusitis can result from several causes, and there is usually a foul-smelling nasal discharge.

Trauma

Trauma is usually fairly obvious: the facial bones are fractured. I imagine a kick is the typical cause. I saw one case in which the skin wasn't broken, therefore the fracture wasn't obvious, but I don't think that happens often. Fractures usually heal, but sometimes the sinus is blocked. In such cases, the bones must be repositioned, which is easier said than done. Any skin lacerations must be sutured, and the horse is treated with antibiotics.

Prognosis

The prognosis for dental disease is fair, for primary bacterial infection good, and for trauma at least good. All are challenging to deal with and expensive to treat.

Guttural Pouch Problems

There are aspects of equine health that have given me repeated problems over the years. Obscure (and some not so obscure) muscle strains and sprains have always been difficult for me to diagnose. I comfort myself, however, in the belief that they are difficult for other veterinarians to diagnose, too.

Eye problems are a real bear. How can you tell the difference between a normally visioned horse (bearing in mind that in a horse "normal vision" is lousy at best) and one that sees very poorly (even for a horse)? Fortunately, there are equine eye specialists around and I don't hesitate to call them if I encounter an eye problem I can't solve, which isn't all of them but sure is a bunch.

Guttural pouch problems used to be difficult for me. However, with time and experience (Nature's two greatest teachers), I have become proficient at diagnosing and treating them.

The first guttural pouch case I saw was way back in the beginning, about one month A.G. (After Graduation; veterinarians have two time divisions: B.G. and A.G.). A horse presented with a bilateral nasal discharge that was blood-tinged. "Aha!" I exclaimed. "Sinusitis, or perhaps just a bad case of the flu." But it was neither, because further diagnostic work eliminated both. I had my employer look at the gelding.

"Did you notice this swelling?" he asked after about thirty seconds of examination.

"What swelling?" I replied, which pretty well answered his question.

The Viborg's triangles under the throat were both swollen. The problem was an infection of the guttural pouches. Once the obvious was pointed out to me, I was able to treat it.

Since that time, I have seen several similar cases. Early on I still wasn't as sharp as I should have been in spotting them, but now I'm a whiz at guttural pouch infections. I defy anyone, human or horse, to try to sneak one by me.

What Are Guttural Pouches?

Guttural pouches are unique to the equine family. Each horse has two of these sacs, which are located in the walls of the Eustachian tube below the base of the skull and first vertebra and above the nose and throat area.

In a full-sized horse, each guttural pouch has a capacity of about 300 milliliters and is divided into two portions by the larger protuberance of the hyoid bone at the base of the tongue The pouches

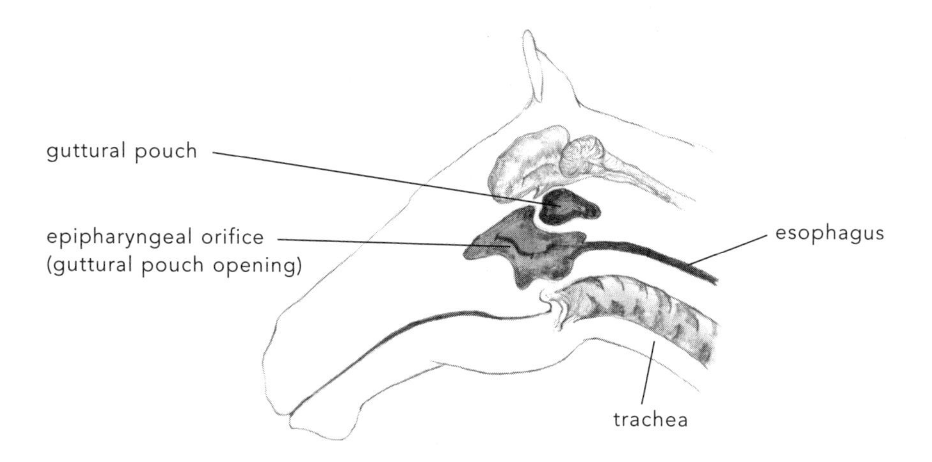

The guttural pouches are located in the walls of the Eustachian tube.

communicate with the nasal passages and throat through an opening (the epipharyngeal orifice) in the Eustachian tube.

The function of the guttural pouches remains an equine mystery, as far as I can tell. One theory says that they help to equalize pressure across the eardrum. Another theory says no one knows. Yet a third theory holds that they evolved millennia ago in anticipation of the invention of the endoscope.

Whatever their function, their location allows them to become infected, although not as often as one might think, considering that the neighboring epipharyngeal orifices open into the pouches during swallowing. The general signs of guttural pouch problems, which occur more or less simultaneously, are:

- Nasal discharge
- Nose bleeding
- Swelling in the area of Viborg's triangle in the throatlatch region; access to the guttural pouches and lymph nodes of the region is through this area

The three main problems occurring with the guttural pouches are guttural pouch empyema, guttural pouch mycosis, and guttural pouch tympany.

Guttural Pouch Empyema

Guttural pouch empyema is a bacterial infection accompanied by pus that fills one or both pouches. It frequently occurs as a result of an upper respiratory infection, especially strangles.

The chief signs are a persistent discharge from one or both nostrils that increases when the horse lowers its head and a decrease in performance. Diagnosis is made by endoscopic examination or radiography.

The pus may be removed and cultured to determine treatment, which consists of antibiotics and irrigation of the pouch through a catheter passed through the nose and the epipharyngeal orifice. Occasionally surgical drainage of the pouch is required. Prognosis is typically good.

Guttural Pouch Mycosis

Fungi can invade the guttural pouches and set up housekeeping. Fungal infection can cause damage to the other structures in the area, such as the carotid artery and cranial nerves. Common clinical signs are nosebleed and difficulty eating or refusal to eat. Nasal discharge is common.

Diagnosis is made using an endoscope, a fiberoptic device that is passed through a nostril so the guttural pouches can be examined, and treatment is difficult. Systemic treatment is usually unsatisfactory, and the drugs used in these treatments have potentially serious side effects. Topical treatment is difficult because the fungi are often limited to the upper areas of the pouch. Daily infusions of medication, using the same route as for irrigation of the pouch, must be continued for a month or more. And if the internal carotid artery is involved, it must be repaired surgically to prevent potentially fatal hemorrhage. Prognosis is only fair because of the difficulty of treatment.

Guttural Pouch Tympany

The precise cause of guttural pouch tympany is not known, but because it occurs primarily in foals some have suggested that it's a developmental defect in the formation of the epipharyngeal orifice that allows air to enter the guttural pouches. It may occur on one side or both sides.

The chief sign is swelling in the area of Viborg's triangle; the foal may have difficulty breathing and may make a snoring noise while nursing. Finger pressure in the area will usually give temporary relief, but the pouches refill with air in a short time. Treatment consists of surgery, and the prognosis is good in most cases.

Theiler's Disease (Serum Hepatitis)

When I entered the world of equine practice, I encountered things that I had never heard of, including Theiler's disease, or serum hepatitis. I really don't think it was taught to us in school.

I had been out of school only a few months when I was called to look at a pony that was "acting crazy." When I got there, I was told that this little guy was normally as gentle as a lamb. What I saw was a four-legged maniac. He was running in an uncoordinated manner, bellowing, and bouncing off trees. I was not sure what they wanted me to do because he couldn't be caught — or even approached. I learned that he had been acting this way for several days.

But then he made diagnosis easy. He dropped dead. The necropsy report said "serum hepatitis (Theiler's disease)." Having never heard of it, I got out my textbooks and looked it up.

What Is Theiler's Disease?

Theiler's disease, or serum hepatitis, is a subacute hepatic necrosis (liver death) resulting in liver failure and acute encephalopathy (brain damage) in horses. The history usually includes an injection of tetanus antitoxin (TAT) one to three months before the onset of signs. (The pony in the above case had received TAT after cutting his fetlock several weeks before his demise, I subsequently learned.) Occasional cases have been reported in horses that had not received TAT but had been in contact with a horse that had, which baffles me.

Clinical Signs

The usual signs are central nervous system (CNS) problems, jaundice, and dark urine (brown or reddish brown in color). The CNS signs may be manifested either as in the case of the maniacal pony or as depression. Ataxia (stumbling or unsteady gait) is common, and blindness may occur.

Diagnosis

Diagnosis is based on history (TAT within the previous 12 to 14 weeks), clinical signs, and lab tests indicating liver damage or failure.

The lab tests that indicate liver disease measure serum or plasma levels of certain enzymes. Gamma glutamyl transaminopeptidase (GGT) is always elevated in cases of serum hepatitis. Aspartate aminotranferase (AST) is also elevated but decreases in a few days if the horse is to recover, so it should be measured two or three times over a period of a few days. Sorbitol dehydrogenase (SDH), initially increased, decreases rapidly in improving horses. Total bilirubin is elevated in serum hepatitis and this is the cause of the discolored urine. Prothrombin time (PT) is very high. (My spellcheck is panting.)

A definitive diagnosis may be made by liver biopsy, but with history, signs, and lab results indicating serum hepatitis, a biopsy is not necessary. (If it looks like a duck, acts like a duck, and quacks like a duck, you don't need to toss it in a lake to see if it swims.)

Treatment

Supportive therapy is all that can be done. Intravenous fluids supplemented with potassium and vitamins are indicated. Sedation is important in the case of out-of-control behavior. Stress should be avoided.

Oral neomycin should be given to decrease ammonia production in the gastrointestinal tract. Also, decrease the total protein in the feed for the same reason. Feed only cracked corn and grass hay until recovery is complete.

Because the eyes are dilated, the horse should be kept in a dark stall, as excessive light can damage them.

Prognosis

Affected horses that continue to eat usually make it. PT and SDH decreases, accompanied by an improving appetite, are good indicators of a horse that will pull through. One that is exhibiting severe CNS signs that cannot be controlled by sedation has a very poor prognosis.

Recovery will occur in one to two weeks in most cases that are going to recover, and there are rarely any residual problems.

Prevention

To prevent Theiler's disease in your horses, maintain a proper tetanus vaccination program, consisting of an initial series of two tetanus toxoid injections one month apart, followed by annual boosters. If a broken-skin lesion occurs more than three months after a booster, boost again with tetanus toxoid at that time. Use TAT *only* if a horse contracts tetanus or if the tetanus toxoid vaccination history is not known in a horse that has a lesion.

After my first case of Theiler's disease, when I did not know what it was and could not have done anything about it even if I did, I saw two more cases.

The next was not long after the first one and it, too, was a pony. This filly was very depressed and did nothing but stand in one spot. She had received TAT a month before, after graveling (see page 121). Her gums and sclera were bright yellow (jaundiced), indicative of liver problems. With much pushing and pulling we managed to get her to a stall. She ate and drank a little when it was offered. All of her liver enzymes were elevated, but with the previously described treatment she was near normal within ten days or so and went on to recover.

The other case, and the last one I have seen to date, was a long time later. I guess it was in the early 1990s. Another veterinarian had sutured a race mare after a wound and gave her TAT at that time. She became depressed about two months later, when he was out of town, so I was called. The trainer kept excellent records, and he had recorded "TAT" in her file. She, too, was jaundiced and her enzymes were very high, as was her PT. Both AST and PT counts were very slow to decrease, but both started to go down in about a week. Supportive therapy sustained her, although she did not eat well. She eventually came around and was sent to the farm to become a broodmare.

Internal Abscesses

WAY BACK WHEN I HAD BEEN OUT OF SCHOOL for only about six months, my employer asked me to go see a horse that the owner said was "doing bad." It was a farm I had never been to before, and I said so.

"And you may never go there again, either," my boss said. "He only uses me as an emergency service when his regular vet is unavailable."

When I got to the farm, the owner showed me a three-year-old gelding that appeared to be about two hundred pounds underweight. "He's been losing weight for a month or so, and now he hardly eats," he told me. "Doc's on vacation, so I had to call you." It was apparent that he didn't like the idea of using another veterinarian.

This was an area where equine infectious anemia was fairly common, so I drew blood for a Coggins test and a blood count. The Coggins was negative, but the blood count showed a low red cell count and a slightly elevated white cell count. The horse's temperature was between 101° and 102°F, perhaps a little high but not alarmingly so.

Other than that, I couldn't find anything wrong with the animal. I started him on antibiotics for the sake of doing something, but four days later he was visibly worse and not eating at all. A second blood count was almost the same as the first, and his temperature remained about the same.

I switched antibiotics and asked my employer to come see him. He didn't know what was wrong, either, and he suggested that we give him an anabolic steroid, which we did.

Four more days later there had been no response to the second antibiotic, and the horse had reached a point where I was afraid he was a goner. The owner wasn't pleased. "Boy, this is a rotten time for Doc to be gone. He'd have straightened him out by now," he told me.

That made me a little angry. "He'll be back in two days. He can have a chance then," I replied.

But his regular veterinarian didn't get the chance. The gelding died that night, a fact that I learned early the next morning when the owner called and chewed me out.

Fortunately, he was willing to have a postmortem examination performed. Three good-sized internal abscesses were discovered, probably resulting from his castration, which had been done three months earlier.

The abscesses possibly could have been detected by a rectal examination, which I had not done. In retrospect, I probably should have asked when the horse had been gelded, but outward healing had taken place and I had assumed something that I possibly shouldn't have.

Be that as it may, the horse was beyond hope and veterinary medicine by the time I saw him, if indeed he had ever been savable. His owner blamed me and never called us again in the time I remained there.

That was aeons ago, and it was the first case of internal abscesses that I had seen, I think. (Another horse before that had been mysteriously ill but had responded to treatment with antibiotics; I'll never know whether he had abscesses.) Since the gelding and the disagreeable owner, I've seen a few horses that I suspected had internal abscesses. Two have died and my diagnoses were confirmed by autopsy, which is little consolation. One died that I felt certain had abscesses but didn't. Of course, I have no idea if the horses that lived actually had abscesses.

What Are Internal Abscesses?

Internal abscesses can occur in either the abdominal cavity or the chest cavity and may be a sequel to several conditions: castration, abdominal surgery, penetrating lesions, rectal or vaginal perforations, penetration of the gut wall by a foreign body (nails, staples, pieces of

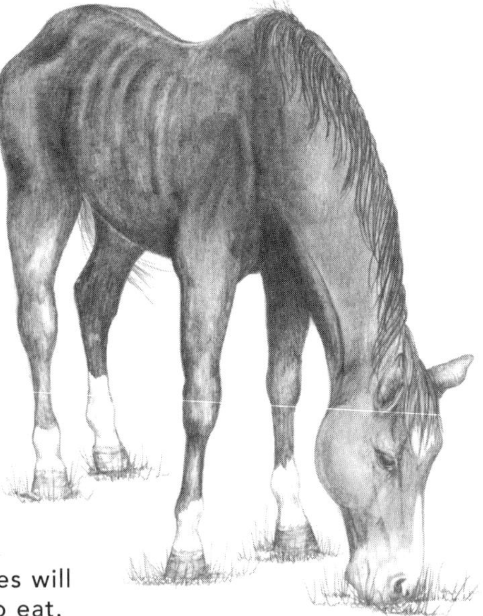

A horse with internal abscesses will lose weight and may refuse to eat.

wire), bacterial infection, or migrating parasite larvae. Additionally, pulmonary abscesses may result from improper use of antibiotics, either incorrect dose or duration.

Clinical Signs

The most apparent outward sign of internal abscesses is a horse that's not doing well. Depression and weight loss may or may not be accompanied by a refusal to eat. A mild fever may be present, and abdominal abscesses may produce occasional colic. There also may be edema toward the belly, and nasal discharge in the case of pulmonary abscesses.

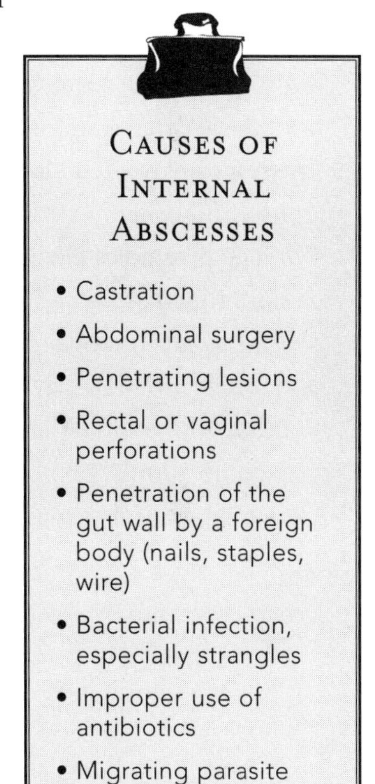

Causes of Internal Abscesses

- Castration
- Abdominal surgery
- Penetrating lesions
- Rectal or vaginal perforations
- Penetration of the gut wall by a foreign body (nails, staples, wire)
- Bacterial infection, especially strangles
- Improper use of antibiotics
- Migrating parasite larvae

Diagnosis

Blood work may or may not reveal anything. On a blood count, the red cells are decreased and the white cells are elevated, but neither may be remarkable, although the white cell count sometimes may be as high as 40,000 cells/mL or more, which *is* very remarkable. A blood chemistry analysis will show that the globulin is up and the albumin is down, but again, the changes may be minute. The abscess can cause peritonitis. The key to diagnosis is a good history, which is often hard to come by. If the horse is doing poorly (see Clinical Signs above), internal abscesses should be suspected.

A good way to diagnose a thoracic abscess is by chest X-ray, but the growth may not be visible if the abscess is small or has not been present long enough to produce a well-developed capsule. Also, most field X-ray equipment is not powerful enough for use on the chests of adult horses, so this approach is most useful with foals. A person experienced in ultrasound examinations of the chest area may be able to detect something. Abdominal abscesses may or may not be palpable through the rectum; pain may be elicited by rectal palpation. Many internal abscesses, however, are never diagnosed if the animal lives, and response to treatment provides only a tentative diagnosis.

A postmortem examination is the most reliable way to diagnose internal abscesses, although the diagnosis matters little at that point.

Treatment

Crossed fingers and long-term, vigorous antibiotic therapy are the only hopes for successful treatment. The organism that caused the abscess is usually unknown, so a broad-spectrum antibiotic should be used. Unfortunately, long-term, high-dose antibiotic use can result in colitis and other gut complications.

The prognosis is guarded to poor, especially if response to therapy is not immediate.

So what it boils down to is this: if a horse develops internal abscesses, no definitive diagnosis is likely to be made until death occurs, which has at least a fifty-fifty likelihood. Veterinary medicine has come a long way, but some conditions, such as internal abscesses, defy a quick and easy fix.

Chronic Diarrhea

WAY BACK WHEN I FIRST GOT OUT OF SCHOOL, my employer had a breeder of Tennessee Walking Horses as a client. This man also bred hogs and made the best sausage I ever tasted.

As we were driving to the farm about a week after I had gotten out of school, my employer asked me, "What did they teach you in school about chronic diarrhea?"

"That it happens," I honestly replied.

"That's about all anybody knows," he said.

On this farm was a young Walker, a yearling or two-year-old, I don't remember which now, that had chronic diarrhea. It wasn't the shooting, brown-water type of diarrhea; he would have dehydrated if that had been the case. It was the runny cow-pile type of diarrhea, and he had had it for several months.

I asked my boss what he had done for the colt. He had wormed him and done a fecal check and found him to be as free of parasites as was attainable. He had cultured the feces and found nothing that wouldn't be found in any normal horse.

"Why don't we ask another vet to see if he has any ideas?" I suggested. He had already had *two* other vets look at him. Okay, then, why don't we refer him to a university clinic? Okay, we'd do that.

He was sent to the nearest vet school and everything was checked. Nothing was discovered. He returned home. Over the next few months he lost condition, and I was afraid he would have to be put down, but all of a sudden — for no reason that we could see — the diarrhea stopped. He had had it for nearly a year.

From this you can see that chronic diarrhea is very frustrating to attempt to treat, and treatment is too often unsuccessful.

Causes

One thing that I have learned about chronic diarrhea along the way is that sometimes horses on sandy soil have it a little more often than horses on other types of soil. Sand accumulation in the gastrointestinal tract often causes signs of colic, though not always. The sand causes inflammation and the inflammation causes diarrhea. Diagnosis is tough, but sometimes sand can be felt on rectal palpation and in some cases there is sand in the feces.

There are many other known causes of chronic diarrhea, in addition to unknown causes, which may number in the hundreds. Among the known causes are salmonella, aseptic peritonitis, chronic liver disease, trichomona infestation, granulomatous enteritis, and gastrointestinal neoplasia. In most cases, however, the cause is never determined and therapy, therefore, is only supportive and frequently to no avail. Some horses seem to go on forever with the diarrhea, while others return to normal, and still others die. There is no way to predict which is which, but young and old horses (under two years old and over eighteen years old, respectively) seem to be the leading candidates for death.

Treatment

If sand ingestion is suspected, treatment is best accomplished by altering the feeding method. If the horse is being fed on the ground (hay *or* grain) in an area of sandy soil, stop feeding there. (If grain is being fed on the ground anywhere, stop the practice.) Unfortunately, if there is no lush grazing in the area and the soil happens to be sandy, a horse will continue to ingest sand. Also, try adding a psyllium fiber product to the feed until the diarrhea lessens or abates. But if the horse is allowed to continue to ingest sand, the problem will recur.

One treatment I've found to be useful in some of the cases where there is no apparent reason for diarrhea is the use of mineral oil. A gallon of oil delivered via a nasogastric tube will help to move anything along that may be irritating the intestinal wall, and quite often after the oiling the horse is improved. This is also moderately effective in the case of sand ingestion.

Prognosis

Most horses with chronic diarrhea lose body condition and in time may need to be euthanized, but be patient. Good grazing and maintaining electrolyte balance (there are many products available for this purpose) frequently work wonders. And sometimes, as we see from the young Walking Horse above, the problem resolves by itself.

Colic

I DON'T KNOW HOW IT IS IN OTHER VETERINARIANS' PRACTICES, but I know that in mine, colic is the bane of my existence.

First, a colic is an emergency. True, most cases are minor and many rectify themselves, but you don't know that when colic is first apparent.

Second, a colic never occurs at a good time. At least, not for me.

Rarely does a relaxing holiday pass without at least one case. Easter,

Memorial Day, and July Fourth don't count; those occur during the breeding season so it's already ensured that I can't relax. But Labor Day, Thanksgiving, Christmas, and New Year's Day — days when I might sit back and do nothing — are colic days. The horses seem to know. "He's not doing anything," they say to themselves or maybe to each other. "We can give him something to do." And at least one of them colics.

They also somehow sense when I'm relaxing late at night or on a lazy Sunday in the late summer or fall.

Also, they know when I'm very busy and well behind schedule, when I have more calls than I can possibly fit into one day. Somewhere there will be a colic. And if I'm *extremely* busy and *way* behind, there'll be two or three.

What Is Colic?

Colic is not a disease in itself. Rather, it's a collection of signs that indicate pain or discomfort, usually abdominal in origin.

I once read an old veterinary textbook. In the section on colic it said, "Before therapy begins, it is imperative to determine the cause of the colic." Well, more than seventy causes have been identified so far. The patient would die of old age before I could possibly go through all seventy-plus. Other books recommend that we record our findings on a long form when examining a colic case. That's swell, but most of the time the horse needs to be attended to rather than written about.

Evaluation and Treatment

The first thing to do when evaluating a colic is to take the horse's pulse. Pulse rates will vary with the age, breed, and disposition of the patient, but the pulse should be no higher than 30-something per minute. Forty to 45 indicates mild discomfort (usually), 55 to 60 indicates considerable pain, 60 to 80 means serious pain, and greater than 80 is *bad* pain. The higher the pulse, the worse the pain, and the worse the prognosis.

Next, gut sounds should be determined. Intestinal sounds can best be evaluated by using a stethoscope. Normally, mild abdominal

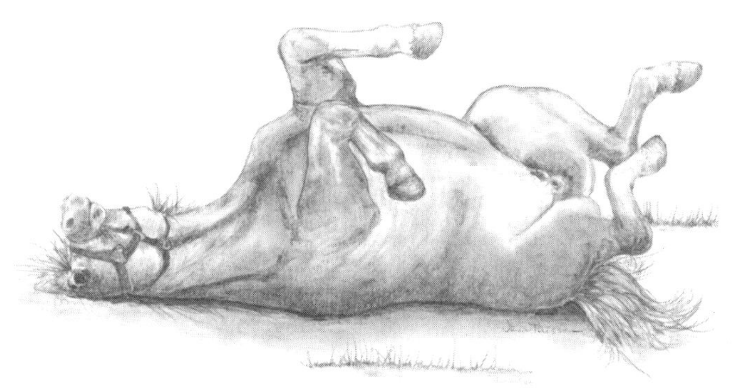

Horses often roll when colicking.

gurgling is present, but in colic the sounds may be magnified or speeded up, or there may be none at all. None is real bad. It means a blockage of some sort (volvulus, torsion, strangulation, impaction).

If there are gut sounds and the pain level is not too great, treatment is usually simple and response is favorable. Flunixin meglumine and xylazine given intravenously for sedation and mineral oil and/or dioctyl sodium sulfosuccinate given via stomach tube will usually handle these. If there are no gut sounds and/or if the level of pain is great,

Overview of Colic

Signs and Symptoms

- General pain and discomfort
- Pawing
- Rolling
- Lying down and getting up
- Looking at or biting the flanks
- Refusal to eat
- Raising the upper lip

Causes

- Tympany (excessive gas production in the intestinal tract)
- Spasmodic (hypermotility of the gut)
- Volvulus (rotation or twisting of the small intestine)
- Torsion (twisting of the large intestine)
- Strangulation (interrupted blood flow, often accompanying volvulus, torsion, or intussusception)
- Intussusception (telescoping of the intestine into itself)

Sand in the intestinal tract

- Impaction

Contributing Factors

- Changing feed or feeding time
- Moving to a new field or paddock
- Sandy soil
- Change in routine (training schedule, shipping)
- Parasites
- Medications

it's likely the intestine has twisted and the horse probably needs surgery. Surgical cases are few because most colics are rather easily resolved, but your veterinarian will determine if surgery is needed and whether sedation is indicated. Oiling is not indicated if there are no gut sounds, but it may be helpful in other cases.

Where I am we're lucky to have some of the finest equine surgical facilities and equine surgeons in the world, but many places are not blessed in this way. There may be a university or a surgical facility within hauling distance. On veterinary recommendation, get the horse there ASAP.

Certainly, this is an overly simplified discussion of colic, but remember: colic is an emergency. If a horse acts colicky, call your veterinarian and tell him to step on it.

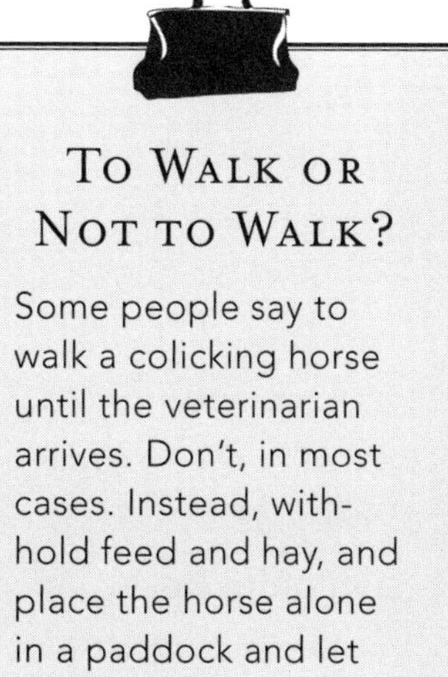

To Walk or Not to Walk?

Some people say to walk a colicking horse until the veterinarian arrives. Don't, in most cases. Instead, withhold feed and hay, and place the horse alone in a paddock and let him roll, unless he's abusing himself: throwing himself down, beating his head on the ground, and so on. In that case, you can try to walk him.

Gastroduodenal Ulcers

I once naively thought that the abuse of nonsteroidal anti-inflammatory drugs, especially bute (phenylbutazone), was prevalent only in racehorses, but then for a while I did veterinary work for a trainer of Tennessee Walking Horses. This guy had fourteen head in training and I eventually learned that he gave each one ten milliliters of phenylbutazone daily, even though there was no need in most cases. This is one of the real problems with bute and its relatives; trainers often give it "just in case" a horse is sore.

The reason this trainer called me in the first place was because one of the horses was colicking. He reported that the horse, a six-year-old gelding, wasn't "doing well" and had lost weight. He had colicked mildly about three or four weeks earlier, also.

The same horse colicked again two weeks later and again in another two weeks. By this time I had learned about the daily bute. I suggested that the horse's stomach be scoped and he agreed to it. I didn't have the proper instrument so I referred the horse to a local clinic, where several ulcers were found in the stomach. More and more we find that horses under stress are developing ulcers. (Ulcers are uncommon in horses not in training, though they do occur.) Stress is usually a by-product of training, and nonsteroidal anti-inflammatory drugs add to the problem. These drugs promote gastric ulceration by inhibiting local mucoprotective mechanisms, so the combination of stress and overuse of nonsteroidal anti-inflammatory drugs is a quick route to ulcers.

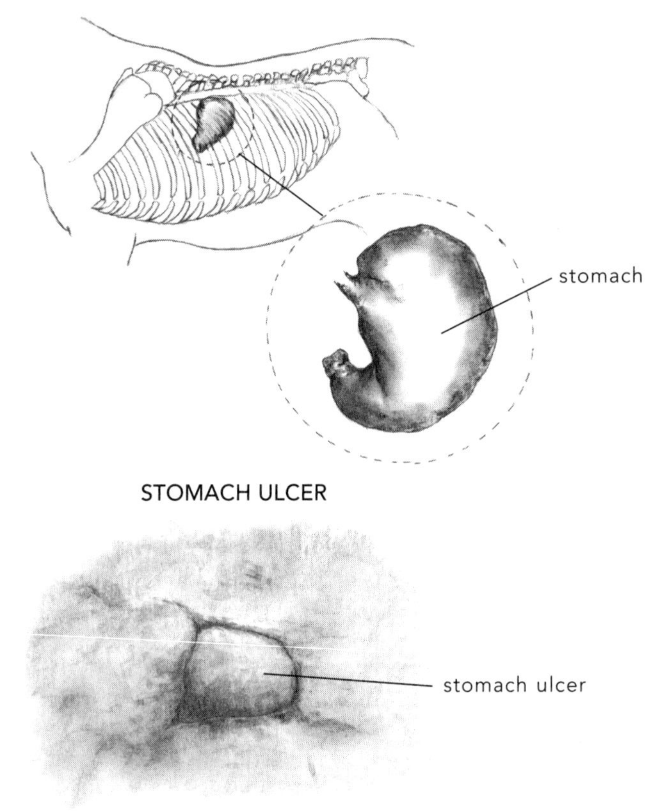

The appearance of deep red patches in the stomach's normally pink lining indicates bleeding.

Clinical Signs

This Walking Horse gelding showed typical symptoms (recurrent colic, doing poorly, weight loss; diarrhea and loss of appetite are other common signs). Depression is seen often, and in horses less than two years of age teeth grinding is likely, but mild, recurrent colic is the principal sign.

Many cases of ulcers are "silent," however, showing no outward signs until an ulcer perforates the stomach wall and peritonitis develops. Extremely high fever and a rapid decrease in condition follow. This is about as serious a problem as a horse can have. Death is the usual result unless surgery is performed quickly, and even then death may ensue.

Intelligent use of nonsteroidal anti-inflammatory drugs will greatly reduce the occurrence and the severity of ulcers. Also, stress is a contributing factor, if not an outright cause, of every bad thing in this world, and here we see it again. The artificial environment of training and the work required of many horses are great stresses.

Treatment

Oral cimetidine or ranitidine for three weeks is the treatment of choice. Some veterinarians use large doses of Mylanta II three times a day, but I've never tried it. Success is best achieved if the stress is reduced and the nonsteroidal anti-inflammatory drugs are stopped. Depending on the number and severity of the ulcers, the prognosis is good to guarded.

Ulcers in Foals

In foals, the cause of gastroduodenal ulcers isn't known. Rotavirus, a cause of severe foal diarrhea, has been implicated.

The signs in foals are grinding of the teeth, excessive salivation, pain (a foal will often lie on its back and groan), loss of appetite, and cramping after feeding. In severe cases, the stomach may rupture. Severe colic and shock will follow and the foal's condition deteriorates rapidly.

Oral cimetidine and ranitidine are the drugs used for treatment, but the prognosis is guarded. Some farms seem to have outbreaks of ulcers in foals, adding to the likelihood that an infectious agent is involved.

Moldy Corn Poisoning (Mycotoxic Encephalomalacia)

ONE EARLY SPRING AFTERNOON MANY YEARS AGO, a client called. "Doc, come quick!" he said. "We have a bad colic!" This was a client not given to exaggeration.

As is usually the case (in my experience, at least) when an emergency arises, I am as far away as I can be and still be in my practice area. I headed toward his farm right away, but with distance and traffic it took more than half an hour to get there.

I arrived just in time to watch the horse (a four-year-old Thoroughbred gelding that had been laid up for the winter after racing all spring and summer) break through the closed lower half of his stall door and plow right through a cement block wall some fifteen or twenty feet away. I don't mean he hit the wall; I mean he crashed *through* it! About ten or fifteen feet beyond the demolished wall, he fell. I don't know if he died before he fell, as he fell, or after he fell, but he was definitely dead in the few seconds that it took me to get to him.

"That's the damnedest colic I ever saw," my client said.

"I don't think this was colic," I said. "What was he doing when you called?"

"He was walking his stall, going in circles. Sweating. He didn't want his feed."

The horse was taken to the university laboratory for a postmortem exam. The next morning the pathologist called. "Brent, I don't see how this horse was alive as recently as yesterday. More than half of his cerebrum was rotten," he told me.

His tentative diagnosis at that point was mycotoxic encephalomalacia, also called *moldy corn poisoning* and *blind staggers.* On histological exam, he was proved correct.

What Is Mycotoxic Encephalomalacia?

Mycotoxic encephalomalacia is a condition caused by a toxin produced by *Fusarium moniliforme,* a mold that grows on cereal grains, most notably corn. In overwhelming doses, the toxin causes severe liver damage (resulting in death), but in milder doses it causes brain damage (also resulting in death most of the time).

It occurs most commonly from late fall to early spring (i.e., when grazing is poor and grain feeding is at its highest) in horses on a feed ration containing (or composed of) corn. Several horses on a farm may be affected, and the mold must be ingested for at least two to four weeks before signs appear.

Clinical Signs

Sometimes the only symptom a horse shows is sudden death, but more commonly the animal loses interest in feed and begins to act "weird," as one client described a mare he had that died quickly.

"Weird" is manifested by any or all of several signs: depression, blindness, circling, ataxia, frenzy, inability to get up, coma, and seizures.

Diagnosis and Treatment

Diagnosis in the live animal is very difficult, but liver enzymes in the plasma are usually elevated and this, along with the physical signs, gives a pretty good idea of what's going on. Analysis of the cerebrospinal fluid doesn't always show anything, but most of the time there will be increased total protein and neutrophils (a type of white blood cell). Examination of the feed will show large numbers of *F. moniliforme* spores and this, while not conclusive, is a pretty good indication of what the problem is. As noted above, postmortem examination of the brain is really the only certain way to diagnose mycotoxic encephalomalacia. The cerebrum, or a portion thereof, is necrotic (composed of dead and decaying tissue) and liquefying.

There is no specific treatment, but several regimens have been suggested to decrease the clinical signs, including nonsteroidal anti-inflammatory drugs, steroids, and intravenous dimethyl sulfoxide (DMSO). Tender loving care is also useful: be quiet and gentle and avoid stress.

I have seen only three cases in more than twenty-five years of practice (and none in the last fifteen years or so) and only one was "treatable" (i.e., alive) when I got to the horse. I used a little bit of everything described in the preceding paragraph, but she died in three days. The prognosis is always poor.

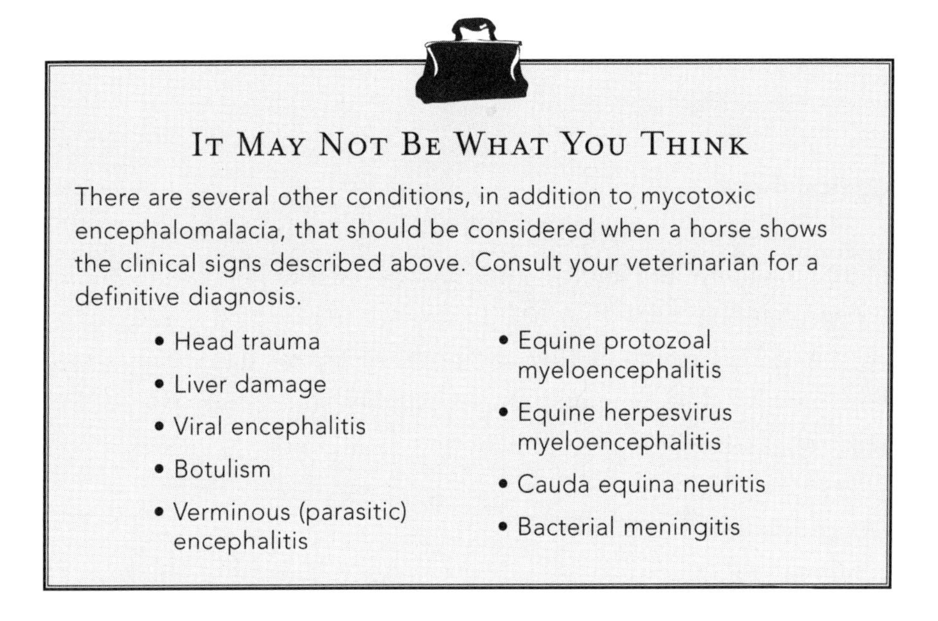

It May Not Be What You Think

There are several other conditions, in addition to mycotoxic encephalomalacia, that should be considered when a horse shows the clinical signs described above. Consult your veterinarian for a definitive diagnosis.

- Head trauma
- Liver damage
- Viral encephalitis
- Botulism
- Verminous (parasitic) encephalitis
- Equine protozoal myeloencephalitis
- Equine herpesvirus myeloencephalitis
- Cauda equina neuritis
- Bacterial meningitis

Prevention

Around here (central Kentucky) we do not see mycotoxic encephalomalacia often, but I suspect in other areas, those in which horses are not such a major part of the economy, it is more common.

Prevention is easy.

- Know your feed and/or feed dealer
- Do not store corn or feed containing corn for prolonged periods (throw away any feed not used within sixty days)
- Examine the feed (do not just throw it in front of the horses)
- Clean feed tubs, buckets, and other implements often (at least weekly)

Hyperlipemia

That fat mare out there in the paddock seems to grow fatter on air. It's getting to the point where you're not sure she'll fit through her stall door, and now she's barren for no apparent reason. The last time the veterinarian was out he told you a good part of her problem — maybe all of it — was her weight. "Put her on a diet," he prescribed.

She looks as if she could go indefinitely without food and still be a blimp, so the temptation is great to just stop feeding her grain or cut her ration back to a handful.

I once owned a mare with a really good pedigree; she had been a pretty fair racehorse. She had the potential to produce some quality foals, but she was like the mare I just described. She gained weight by looking at grain, or so it seemed. She was very difficult to get in foal, and a broodmare that won't produce foals is not much of a broodmare.

As I said, the temptation may be great to just turn off the feed supply until she gets her figure back. But don't: you run the risk of inducing hyperlipemia. Although primarily a problem in ponies, it can occur in horses, especially overweight ones, and is extremely serious when it does occur. The recovery rate is low and the death rate is high.

What Is Hyperlipemia?

Hyperlipemia is the term for elevated blood lipids, often accompanied by fatty infiltration of the liver. Moderately elevated levels of serum lipids, known as *hyperlipidemia,* generally occur in horses that are off their feed due to illness or injury. Unlike hyperlipemia, that condition is of only minor concern, although it does indicate the necessity for nutritional support.

A quick look at lipid metabolism will aid in understanding the cause of hyperlipemia. Adipose tissue (fat) is broken down into fatty acids and triglycerides during periods of feed deprivation or severe reduction. A large portion of the fatty acids is deposited in the liver, where they may be used to provide energy or be released back into the circulatory system; some may be retained in the liver. Therefore, from lengthy fasting or starvation, lipids continue to increase in the plasma, resulting in lipemia, and in the liver, resulting in fatty liver.

Clinical Signs

Signs of hyperlipemia are related to liver dysfunction and none is specific, but general signs may include weakness, depression, ataxia, diarrhea, jaundice, ventral edema, a grayish coating on the tongue, and rank, malodorous breath. Death may occur, prior to which the horse goes down on its side and is unable to rise.

Diagnosis

A blood sample must be taken and the serum (or plasma) examined. Normally this should be clear, but in hyperlipemia it is yellowish or creamy, and opaque. The color is due to an increase in bilirubin, which occurs in anorexia, and the opacity is the result of the excessive circulating lipids.

If this is found, the degree of lipemia may be determined by triglyceride assay of the serum. To determine the level of liver damage, liver function tests must be done. Acidosis is also a frequent finding; bicarbonate levels should be checked. And there is often an associated azotemia (accumulation of nitrogenous waste products in the blood) resulting from reduced renal filtration.

There are several changes found on necropsy, both grossly and histologically, but we need not go into them because correction of the condition by then is a real challenge.

Treatment

Because the cause of hyperlipemia is lack of feed intake (for whatever reason), the treatment is to get the horse to eat. Obviously, if the horse isn't eating because it's ill, the causative disease must be addressed. Nonsteroidal anti-inflammatory drugs may help, but tube and/or intravenous feeding may become necessary. If these conditions are the result of a crash diet, just increase the grain ration a little.

The acidosis and azotemia must be corrected, also. Administration of sodium bicarbonate will correct the acidosis, but the azotemia may be more of a challenge. The administration of glucose is very helpful.

An attempt must be made to remove excess lipid from the blood. Insulin therapy is probably the course of choice. Bear in mind, though, that the prognosis is guarded to poor.

If the liver is severely damaged, as determined by liver function tests, correcting the condition may not be possible.

Prevention

Prevention is pretty simple: maintain adequate feed levels. This makes getting that extra weight off Miss Roly-Poly a slow process, but slow it must be. It's much better not to let her get fat in the first place.

It took nearly a year to get my mare down to a respectable weight, but one day I turned my back on her and she became a blimp again. I sold her and let someone else have the challenge of maintaining her at a decent weight.

Hypothyroidism

Thyroid hormones affect every organ system in the body by helping to regulate growth, cell differentiation, and metabolism. There are those who say that thyroid disease doesn't exist in horses. These same people probably also doubt death and taxes. The evidence is strong for all three.

There are others who reluctantly admit that thyroid disease *does* occur but they say it's rare. I'm not saying that it's seen every day, but it's a long way from rare.

The books do say that *hyper*thyroidism doesn't occur. According to those books, there has never been a case reported, but that has been said of other conditions and has been found to be wrong. I know I have never seen a case, so for now I will just say that hyperthyroidism has not yet been recognized in horses.

Hypothyroidism, or reduced hormone production, however, is widespread. I have no statistics to back this up, but I would hazard a guess that it may occur in as much as 5 percent of the horse population. I think this has always been the case and it's only recently that veterinarians have started looking for it and, more important, only recently that laboratories have been set up to test for it.

Back in the 1970s, when we suspected a thyroid deficiency in a horse, we had to send the serum sample off to a distant lab. Then a local human lab agreed to do the testing (the lab personnel were nice enough to modify the normal procedure to accurately test horses). Eventually, a lab was set up in Kentucky, mainly for the purpose of doing hormonal assays in horses. Also, there are now labs around the country with the ability to determine equine thyroid levels.

A SOMETIME CLIENT USED ME AS AN EMERGENCY SERVICE. I was slow to realize that, and I really didn't appreciate it. I gladly tend to emergencies at any hour for regular clients but I react unfavorably when people call me late at night because they can't get their regular vets out.

The first time she called it was around 10 P.M. She had a colic and "didn't have a regular vet." I went, of course.

The second time was about three months later. It was earlier — about 8:30 A.M. — and a horse had a cut on its face. I suspected then that I was being used, but I went anyhow.

Then, one day at the local lab, I saw her name on a Coggins test submission. The veterinarian who signed it was a fellow here in town.

Several weeks later, early on a Sunday morning, she called. A horse was down. "Why don't you call your regular vet?" I asked and mentioned his name.

There was a pause. Finally, she said, "He's out of town."

I went. It was the same horse that I saw the first time I went there. He was down in the field with a touch of colic. It was easily treated, but while doing so I saw a chestnut mare in an adjacent paddock. Her head was down, she was walking slower than a turtle, her legs were swollen below the knees and hocks, and her coat was long, matted, and dull.

"Good grief," I said. "That mare's in bad shape."

"Oh, she's just slow to shed out," the woman said.

"Slow!" I exclaimed. "It's August! No horse is that slow."

"She is. She's that way every year."

"Lady, that mare is hypothyroid. Super hypothyroid."

She wouldn't believe me. Finally, we made a deal: I would take a serum sample and if the mare was *not* hypothyroid I wouldn't charge her. If she was, she would pay for the test.

She paid. The mare had the lowest thyroid levels I had ever seen.

I told her and said the mare had to be treated. She said she would talk to her regular veterinarian when he returned, and I never heard from her again.

Clinical Signs

As was evident in the chestnut mare, signs of hypothyroidism are lethargy, depression, edema of the lower limbs (not always), reproductive inefficiency, and a long, rough coat. Another problem seen in performance horses is a general, nonspecific myopathy. Other signs are decreased stamina, a stiff or stilted gait, a variable appetite (failure to "clean up" at times), and a general depressed demeanor.

Diagnosis

Diagnosis is made by analyzing serum samples for the thyroid hormones T_4 (thyroxine) and T_3 (triiodothyronine). There are age (younger is higher) and sex (males are higher) distinctions in values, so correct interpretation is important. There is also a thyroid-stimulating hormone test that is quite accurate in providing a valid assessment of thyroid function, but I have always found the measurements of T_3 and T_4 to be diagnostic.

Treatment

Treatment consists of adding sodium levothyroxine powder to the feed, although some books suggest dosing the horse with the powder mixed in corn syrup. In the few horses I have found that were reluctant to eat it, I have poured a little corn oil on top of the feed and powder and they all took it well. Periodic serum samples should be taken to

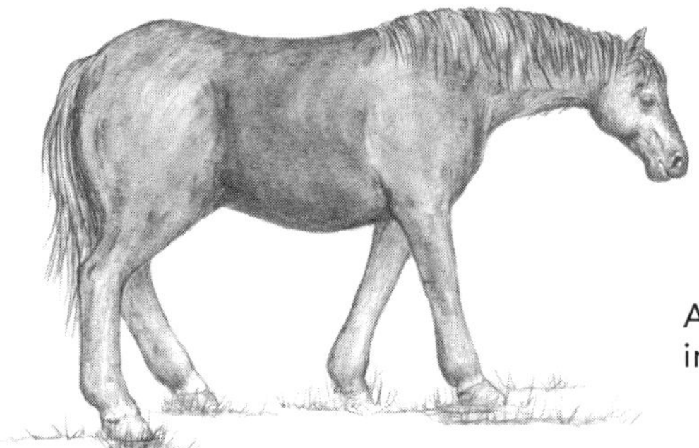

A depressed attitude is typical in the hypothyroid horse.

make sure you're not over- or under-doing it; adjust the amount of powder accordingly.

Also, iodinated casein may be given orally instead of the sodium levothyroxine powder. Again, monitoring the serum is important.

Foals may be born hypothyroid or develop the condition at an early age. Signs include either rapid or delayed growth, contracted tendons, degenerative changes (and possibly collapse) of the tarsal bones, abnormal respiration, lethargy, and inability to stand and nurse. Because growth may be permanently affected, a hypothyroid foal is almost always a losing situation. To those who say hypothyroidism does not occur in horses, I say, "Wake up and pay your taxes before death claims you."

Lymphoid Hyperplasia

ONE OF MY FEW RACETRACK CLIENTS told another trainer to ask me about a three-year-old colt he had that made unusual noises when he exercised heavily. Most things make noises when they exercise heavily — I know that I sure do — and I have heard many horses make lots of noise when running. Most trainers are familiar with roaring (see page 342), and this guy said it wasn't that, so I told him that I'd watch the colt work out and see what I heard. He also said that the colt had become unable to run even a half mile without being exhausted.

The colt did make unusual noises. It's hard to describe; it was sort of like he was trying to breathe through a space that wasn't intended to be breathed through. I had never heard breathing like it before in a horse in training. The trainer asked me if I knew what it was. I told him I had no idea, but if he wanted me to I would scope his colt. *Scoping* means using an endoscope, a tool made for visualizing internal areas normally unable to be seen; a scope is a fiberoptic device that, in this case, is passed through a nostril so the throat can be seen.

It was a condition I had never encountered before: lymphoid hyperplasia. The colt's pharyngeal tonsil was about twice as large as it should have been. It was partially blocking the airway so the colt truly was breathing through a space far too small to be breathed through normally.

What Is Lymphoid Hyperplasia?

The lymphoid system is responsible for the production and destruction of blood elements. It consists of primary lymphoid organs (bone marrow and thymus), secondary lymphoid organs (spleen, lymph nodes, liver, kidneys, stomach, intestines), and the reticuloendothelial system, responsible for destroying foreign cells.

Hyperplasia is defined as an increase in the number of individual tissue elements whereby the bulk of the part or organ is increased. *Lymphoid hyperplasia,* therefore, is basically a swelling of lymphoid tissue. When lymphoid hyperplasia is mentioned in conjunction with horses, it usually concerns the pharynx, and more specifically the pharyngeal tonsil.

Diagnosis and Treatment

Pharyngeal lymphoid hyperplasia seems to be a more or less normal occurrence in young horses, probably as a result of an immune response to pollutants and respiratory viruses. Signs are breathing noises, especially during exercise, and an intolerance for strenuous exercise. Regular vaccinations for rhinopneumonitis and flu at sixty- to ninety-day intervals appear to aid in prevention, but this program must be adhered to at least through a horse's three-year-old year. Diagnosis is made by endoscopic examination.

Once the condition occurs and persists, treatment may be begun, but there is no agreement on the best approach. Systemic penicillin, sulfa drugs, or both have been used with varying degrees of success, as have topical nasal sprays consisting of DMSO (dimethyl sulfoxide), a steroid, and antibacterial agents. Surgical curettage has been used in severe cases.

I asked this colt's trainer about his vaccination program. "I figure they're gonna get sick anyhow so all I ever give 'em is tetanus," he said.

We treated the colt with penicillin and I also gave him some systemic corticosteroids. He was slow to respond, but he did respond and got back to the races in about six weeks. I recommended to the trainer that he vaccinate for flu and rhinopneumonitis in the future, but he and his horses shipped out to the Chicago area and I never saw him again, so I don't know if he did.

Selenium Deficiency and Toxicity

Quite some time ago, mares around here were aborting for no apparent reason. This is not an unusual happening; it seems that we are cursed with this every few years, but most of the time we have an idea what the problem is or the researchers at the university come up with an explanation in a short time.

This time, however, the cause couldn't be found. Someone, I don't remember who, suggested that we check the mineral balance of the feed rations. That was a good idea, but there were almost as many different rations being fed as there were farms.

But some of us did. We found nothing amiss.

Okay, someone else said, check the mineral levels in the horses themselves. Take blood samples. Some of us did that, too, and we found that the level of selenium in the serum was low in almost all of the samples that we submitted. The various feeds had selenium listed as an ingredient but for some reason, even though the horses were ingesting it, it was not being utilized. We (or at least I) never learned why it wasn't, but we found that when we supplemented the feed rations with selenium the problems stopped, and the serum levels of selenium were back in the normal range.

What Is Selenium?

Selenium is a trace mineral important in muscle function. It is a component of glutathione peroxidase, an antioxidant enzyme that catalyzes the conversion of peroxidases to alcohols in tissues. Selenium-dependent glutathione peroxidase activity occurs in cardiac and striated muscle, but lung and liver glutathione peroxidase is not dependent on selenium. Vitamin E also has antioxidant properties and can partially replace selenium in the diet, but vitamin E prevents oxidation of membranes, while selenium functions intracellularly.

Selenium Deficiency

Selenium is deficient in the soils of the Great Lakes region, as well as those of the East, Northwest, and Gulf Coasts; young horses in these areas are in danger of developing white muscle disease, a condition characterized by muscle weakness, due to this deficiency. (The disease is so named because on necropsy the muscles are very pale.) Foals younger than one month are in greatest peril, but the condition may also occur in horses up to a year of age. Older animals are usually not affected. A diet containing less than 0.1 part per million (ppm) of selenium is the usual culprit.

Clinical Signs

The main sign of white muscle disease is muscular weakness exacerbated by physical exertion. Muscle stiffness, myalgia, and dysphagia, or difficulty eating or swallowing, are evident. In younger foals, there may be extreme myocardial, respiratory, and diaphragmatic muscle involvement. There is evidence of protein in the urine (proteinuria), myoglobin in the urine (myoglobinuria), and also blood in the urine (hematuria). In severe cases death may occur within two to three days following the onset of clinical signs. Increased muscle enzyme activity and decreased glutathione peroxidase are diagnostic.

The reason for abortion is fetal death. Postmortem findings include steatitis (inflammation of fatty tissues) and coagulative necrosis of the muscles, especially those of the hind legs, neck, and heart. On histological examination, calcification of muscle is apparent.

Treatment

Treatment is by administration of a vitamin E–selenium injection and supportive therapy. Prevention can be achieved by feeding a ration containing 0.5 ppm selenium (on a dry matter basis) or by providing trace mineral salt containing 15 to 30 ppm selenium.

Prevention

Foals are sometimes born or aborted with evidence of selenium deficiency, making it imperative that broodmares in selenium-deficient areas receive selenium during the last four to six weeks of gestation. In areas of severe selenium deficiency, it is probably advisable to administer vitamin E–selenium at birth and then periodically to the age of six or eight months.

In mature horses, selenium deficiency may be associated with exertional rhabdomyelitis ("tying up"), although there is evidence that this condition occurs in "myopathy-prone" individuals rather than in cases of selenium deficiency (see page 318 for more on tying up). Nevertheless, there appears to be a favorable response to the administration of vitamin E–selenium.

Selenium Toxicity

Acute selenium toxicity (too much selenium) can result from excessive selenium administration and is manifested by neurological and gastrointestinal signs. Neonates born to mares fed a prolonged ration high in selenium have deformed hooves.

Chronic selenium toxicity affects mainly adult horses and is most likely to naturally occur in the Rocky Mountains and Great Plains.

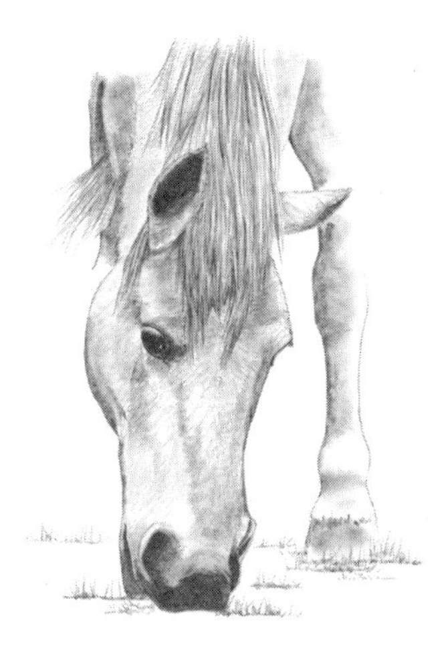

Selenium levels, both low and high, are affected by the levels in forage.

Clinical signs include lameness; hair loss; brittle, coarse mane and tail hair; swollen coronary bands; and transverse grooves in the hooves, which are often mistaken as evidence of past laminitis.

Diagnosis is best made from hoof wall samples (greater than 5 ppm selenium), but feed, water, hair, or blood samples may also be tested. Treatment consists of removing the source of the excess selenium. If the source is pasture, a low selenium concentrate should be fed, which probably necessitates bringing in grain that was grown in a low selenium area. Supportive hoof care, such as frequent, proper trimming, is also important.

There haven't been any abortions in recent years that we could blame on selenium levels: that would be too easy. We have learned how to handle that.

Melanoma

DR. HOFFMAN TOLD US IN VETERINARY SCHOOL, "Melanomas will kill all gray horses if they live long enough."

The worst case of melanoma I ever saw was on an old gray mare owned by a new client. The mare was twenty-three, and she had tumors in abundance. They were around her anus and around her vulva. She had them around both eyes, on her ears, and on her neck. She had them on her legs; I had never seen them on legs before. There were probably thirty of them altogether, ranging in size from a quarter-inch in diameter to as large as a golf ball.

But the owner wasn't concerned, and treating a twenty-three-year-old mare seemed to be an unnecessary expense, so we just let it go. She died at twenty-six; we assumed that it was due to old age but it may have been the melanomas that did her in. The owner didn't want a postmortem examination done.

What Is Melanoma?

Melanoma is usually a malignant skin tumor that metastasizes, or spreads, to the lymph nodes and then to other parts of the body. (They aren't all malignant, though most are.) I have heard of them occurring in bay, brown, and black horses, but I've never seen them on anything but grays.

Clinical Signs

The most common sites for the tumors to occur are around the anus and vulva, but they also occur *in* the eyes and on the penis of males, as well as the other areas where the old mare had them. They appear as hard, round, black nodules. Occasionally, a tumor appears as a subcutaneous lump rather than as a distinct nodule.

I have read that 80 percent of gray horses older than fifteen have

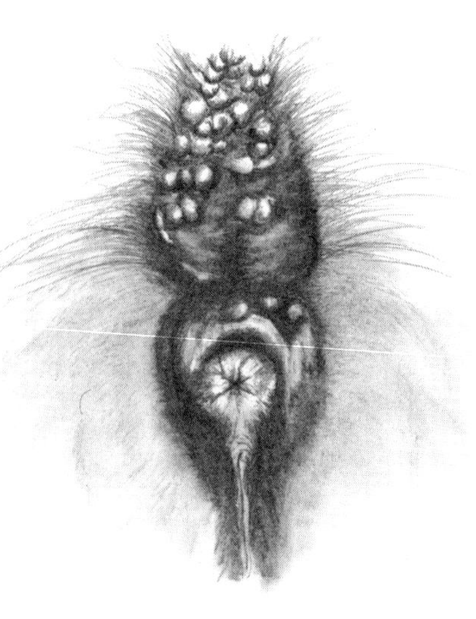

Melanomas typically form under the tail (as shown) and around the muzzle.

melanomas. I say it's at least 90 percent. The highest incidence is probably in Arabians because that breed has so many grays.

Treatment

Surgical excision has been tried and is sometimes successful with single tumors, but because so often they are multiple, the procedure is generally impractical. Also, many of the tumors grow back after being excised.

The best treatment that I've found is one that is amazingly unlikely (to me): oral cimetidine (Tagamet). It's expensive and treatment is prolonged but effective, although I have read that in some cases it hasn't been successful. I've used it on eight horses and there has been a reduction in the number of tumors in seven of them. Two cleared up completely.

Prognosis

Some horses go on for years with melanomas with seemingly no ill effects, but I've seen two grays die in their mid-teens, and postmortem exams indicated that they died from metastasized tumors. A few others have died earlier than expected (eighteen to twenty or so) and no postmortems were performed. I think the tumors were probably responsible in those cases, too.

Rain Scald Versus Ringworm

Dermatophilosis and dermatophytosis are two somewhat similar and all too common skin conditions seen in horses. Dermatophilosis is rain scald; dermatophytosis is ringworm.

Rain Scald

Rain scald is caused by a microorganism called an actinomycete, and though it occurs in a variety of species, I'll describe it as it affects the horse. It is usually seen in fall and winter and is most often associated with times of increased rainfall. Stress (prolonged exposure to

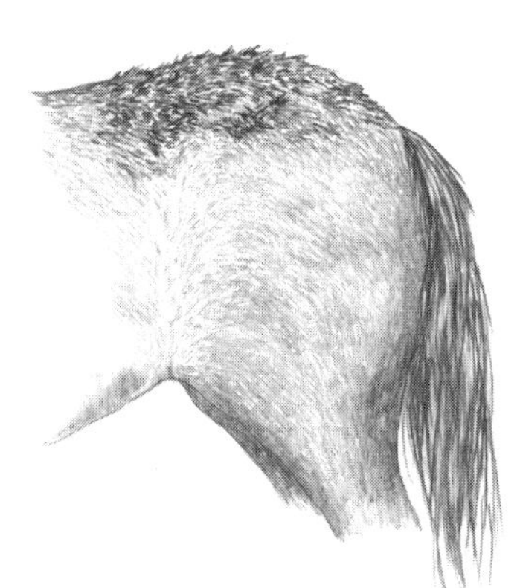
The main sign of rain scald is clumps of matted hair.

cold and wet) and ectoparasites (houseflies, stable flies) are also involved. Stress reduces resistance, and ectoparasites provide a means of access for the infective organisms via bites in the skin. Stabled, non-stressed horses may also contract the condition by way of contaminated clippers, grooming materials, or tack.

Clinical Signs

The chief signs of rain scald are variously sized clumps of matted hair, under which are scabs. The undersides of these scabs hold pockets of yellowish to grayish pus, and the areas may be painful to the touch. The appearance and history are usually diagnostic, but the causative organism may be grown in cultures for a positive diagnosis.

Treatment

Rain scald is self-limiting; that is, if you leave it alone it will eventually go away. This is not fair to the horse, though, so something needs to be done. The most important part of the treatment is the removal of the scabs. As the areas are often painful, the horse may not fully appreciate your efforts in this regard, so soaking them (the scabs, not the horses) in a warm, iodine-based shampoo accomplishes two things: (1) the scabs and matted hair soften and are more easily removed, and (2) the iodine shampoo kills the causative organism. Once the scabs are gone, the iodine shampoos should be continued for several days, or until there are no "wet" spots remaining where the scabs were.

Some cases of rain scald are extremely severe, however, and for these the use of systemic antibiotics or fungicides is indicated, even though the organism is neither a bacterium nor a fungus. Your veterinarian will determine the drug of choice.

Possibly more important than any of the above, though, is the need to keep the animal dry and free from stress and ectoparasites until full recovery has occurred. This is also the key to prevention in the future.

Ringworm

Ringworm is caused by any one of several species of fungi, and there is a wide range of susceptibility among horses. Some can seemingly wallow in a vat of the organisms and never have a problem, while others suffer extensive hair loss if a single fungus wafts through the county.

Dirty, damp, and warm conditions are predisposing factors. Ringworm, like rain scald, can be spread by contaminated clippers, brushes, saddle pads, and so on, as well as by direct contact with other infected animals or people.

Clinical Signs

The signs are diagnostic: several affected areas or alopecia (hair loss) radiating outward from a central point, along with scaliness of the area and, in some cases, pruritus (itching). Unlike rain scald, where the organisms are under the scabs in the middle, the ringworm organisms are most abundant at the periphery of the lesions. If a culture is desired, it should be taken from these areas.

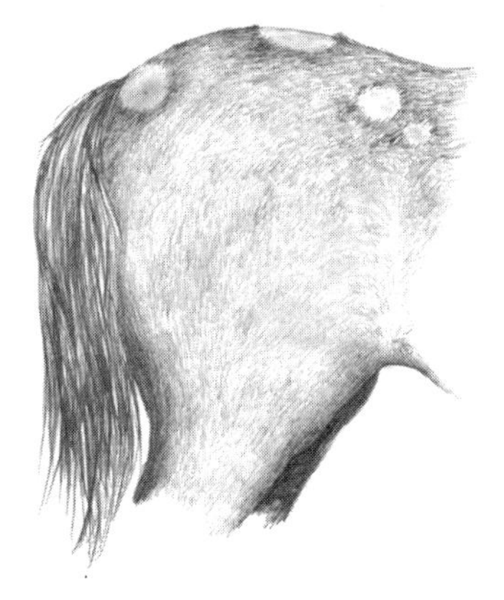

Ringworm causes circular areas of hair loss.

RINGWORM VS. RAIN SCALD*		
	RINGWORM	RAIN SCALD
Appearance	Radiating alopecia; no pus	Scab clumps, matted hair; pus
Agent	Fungus	Actinomycete
Contributing Factors	Warm, moist, dirty conditions; stress	Cold, wet conditions; stress, break in skin, ectoparasites
Season	Spring, summer	Fall, winter
Mode of Transmission	Direct contact	Bite; contaminated grooming tools
Site of Organism	Periphery of lesion	Center of lesion
Treatment	*Topical:* clip, iodine shampoo *Systemic:* antifungals	*Topical:* remove scabs, iodine shampoo *Systemic:* antibiotics, antifungals

*Both conditions are self-limiting.

Treatment

As with rain scald, ringworm is self-limiting. It will run its course in six to twelve weeks, but during this time the horse is contagious, so it's important to try to shorten this natural course. This can be done easily: (1) clip the affected areas (disinfect the clippers both before *and* after use); (2) bathe the horse with an iodine-based shampoo and let the shampoo remain on the skin for twenty to thirty minutes before rinsing *thoroughly;* and (3) repeat the baths daily for four or five days and then twice a week until the infected areas are healed. Systemic antifungal agents that cover wide areas may be used for extensive cases. Sunlight and fresh air are important in the control of ringworm.

Prevention

A major factor in controlling the spread of ringworm and rain scald and preventing future problems is the disinfection of all equipment: clippers, brushes, halters, blankets, pads, saddles, and stalls — whatever your horses come in contact with. Actually, this is a commonsense procedure that should be done on a routine basis anyhow.

The chart above summarizes rain scald and ringworm. Although both conditions are promoted by inattention or neglect, they may happen in spite of the best care. Proper, early action will prevent severity and spread.

Seborrhea

"MY HORSE IS ICKY!" The caller was a girl of about eleven or twelve years old. She had been a horse owner for less than a year and I was seeing her horse because her mother and my wife were friends.

Her horse was a twelve-year-old gelding of indiscriminate lineage. When I got there I saw that she was right. He *was* icky. He was lethargic, and on his back, sides, and chest were white flakes, like overwhelming dandruff. There was a gooey, oozy substance in the area of his throat, and overall his coat felt slimy and smelled bad.

The family had been away for a week and a half and a neighbor had been feeding him, but obviously not looking at him. They had left my phone number with the neighbor so I could be called if anything happened to the horse in their absence, but I hadn't been called.

I had to go to the books to identify it: idiopathic equine generalized seborrhea. I had never seen it before and I've never seen it since, but there are other conditions called seborrhea that appear from time to time.

What Is Seborrhea?

Seborrhea is a flaky, scaly condition that looks like dandruff. Bare patches occur where scabs peel off; it may resemble ringworm.

Other seborrheic conditions in horses are localized in the mane or tail or cannons, but whether it's localized or generalized, the treatment is the same: antiseborrheic shampoos twice a week until the condition is resolved. I don't think there is any specific antiseborrheic shampoo made for horses (there may be several that I don't know about), but human and canine products work well.

I don't know the cause of idiopathic equine generalized seborrhea and I think I'm not alone in that. Other veterinarians I've spoken with and even the reference books seem to be as ignorant as I am. Feed

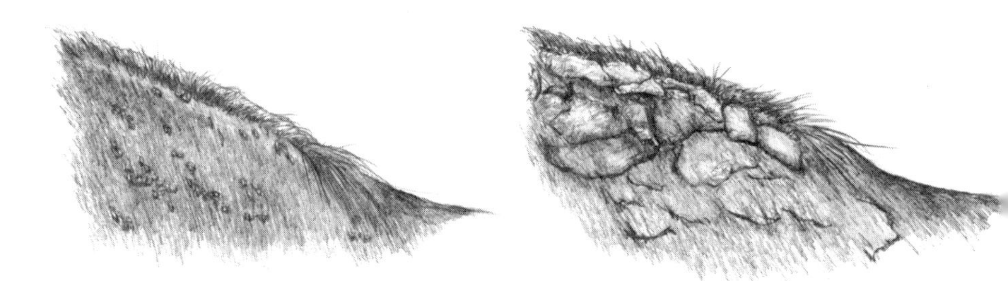

Mild seborrhea *(left)*, and the crusting of chronic seborrhea *(right)*

quality has been implicated in many cases; adding corn oil (two to eight ounces a day) to the grain ration seems to be helpful in prevention and treatment.

The other "seborrheic" conditions aren't really seborrhea; because sebum is not produced, they are actually keratinization disorders. In keratinization disorders there is a decrease in the turnover of cells, usually secondary to other skin disorders.

Clinical Signs

Consistent signs of idiopathic equine generalized seborrhea are scaling, crusting, alopecia (hair loss), and greasy-feeling hair. Other signs that may be present are pruritus (itching), self-inflicted trauma, inflammation, and secondary bacterial infection. There is often a foul odor to the coat. The primary skin condition should be treated, but steroids, systemic or topical, are helpful, along with the baths. Antibiotics are necessary if infection is present.

The girl's horse was given steroids for two weeks and antiseborrheic baths for more than a month. He got better, was fed corn oil, and never had the problem again.

Part II
Lameness

Pain and discomfort and what to do about them

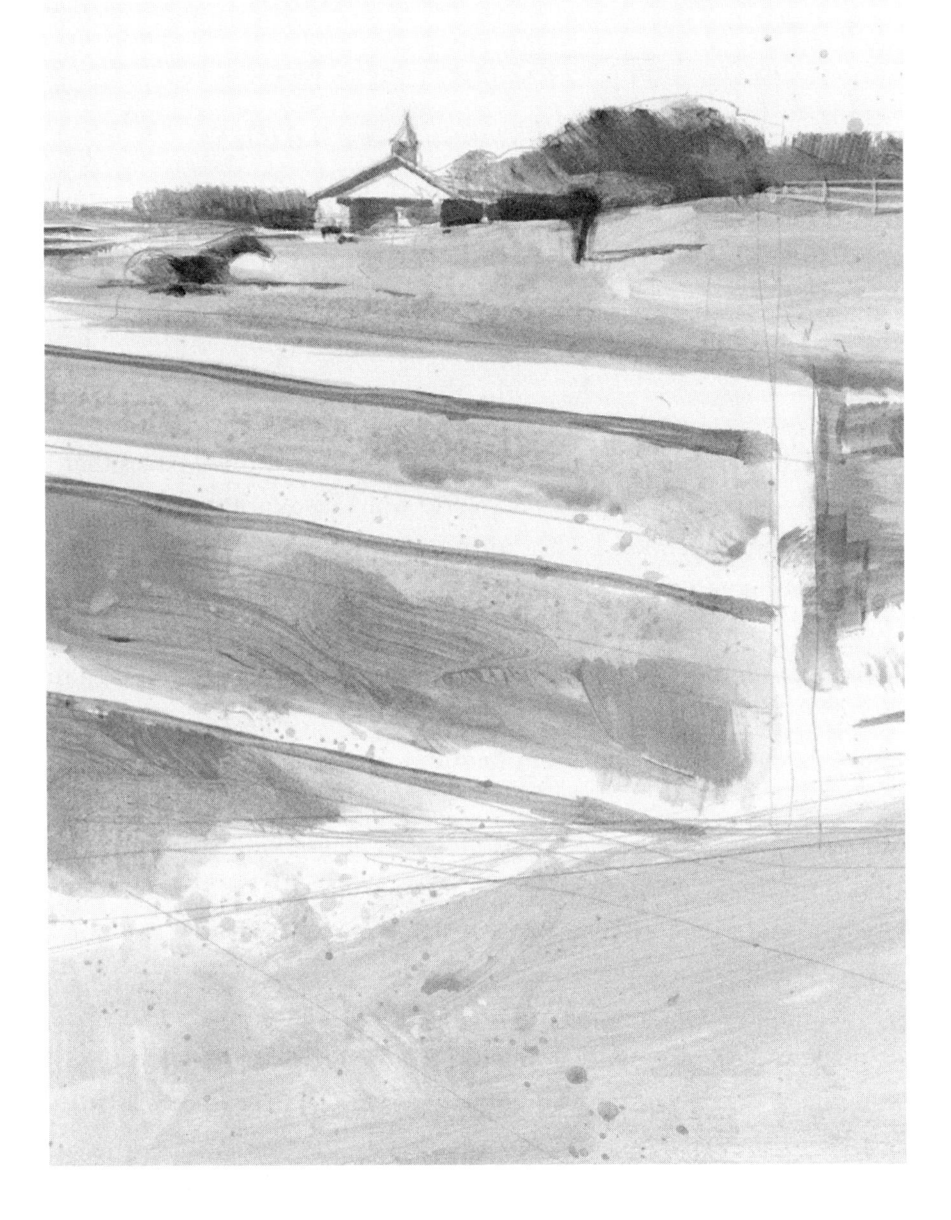

3

Injuries to Muscles, Ligaments, and Tendons

Muscle Strains

THE READER MAY GET THE IDEA from reading some of these pages that I was fairly unprepared for the real world when I was granted my release from veterinary school. I was, but no more so than 99 percent of my fellow graduates around the country each year. The fact is, we just don't see as much in school as we might, especially with horses. It's not the school's fault; we can only be shown the cases that are presented to the school's clinic.

Also, there are a whole lot of conditions that we are told about in class, but there are also many we aren't told about. One of my teachers said, "That diploma you guys have been working so hard for is only a license to learn. You'll learn more veterinary medicine in your first year out of school than you learned in your four years in school." He was right.

With that disclaimer, when I first got out of school I was really bad at diagnosing lameness. If it was broken or bleeding I could usually find where the problem was, but if it was sprained or strained I had a terrible time. To make matters worse, shortly after graduation I met a veterinarian of many years' experience who was unbelievably gifted at recognizing lameness. He would turn his back on the horse and close his eyes and ask the handler to walk and trot the animal on a hard surface; he could tell where the lameness was just by listening. I usually couldn't tell by looking, probing, squeezing, or any other method.

"It's a function of time, Kelley," he told me. "Do it long enough and you'll get it."

He was right, but I'm still not anywhere as good as he was. It's very frustrating. Strains and sprains are still challenging, but I'm in good company. A whole lot of vets have trouble with strains and sprains.

Incidence and Predisposing Factors

Muscle strains can occur in any performance horse and usually occur in the hind limbs. The most common muscle groups involved are the longissimus and gluteal muscles (croup myopathy) and the biceps femoris, semitendinosus, and semimembranosis muscles (caudal thigh myopathy). Strains occur far less often in other muscle groups.

There are many potential factors influencing muscle strains; the main ones are fatigue, lack of sufficient training or conditioning, lack of proper warm-up, and low ambient temperature. Fatigued muscles

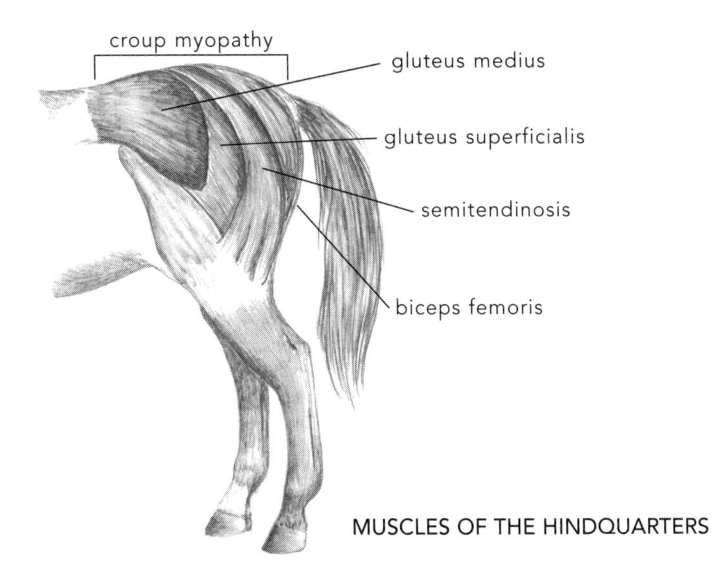

MUSCLES OF THE HINDQUARTERS

lose elasticity and don't function efficiently, therefore increasing the possibility of strain. Insufficient training predisposes a horse to fatigue. Proper warming up is necessary to enhance circulation, thereby increasing the ability to eliminate the muscular waste products (lactic acid) that are produced during exercise. Cold temperatures decrease circulation and increase muscle tension; the combination leads to fatigue.

Muscle strains are classified by severity, from first degree to third degree. A first-degree strain is, in essence, a pulled muscle, and occurs when a muscle has reached its limit of elasticity. Muscle fibers are torn, but not the entire muscle, and it can continue to function, albeit painfully and in limited capacity. A third-degree strain is a complete tear; the function of the muscle is lost.

Clinical Signs

A horse with a muscle strain will show pain on firm hand pressure, but the area showing pain may not be the exact area of the injury. The best method of diagnosis is thermography, but this is often not available in the field.

Lameness associated with muscle strains is highly variable. A croup myopathy is usually much less serious and involves less lameness than a caudal thigh myopathy. A croup myopathy lameness is usually noticeable as an apparent stiffness coupled with a shortened stride on the affected side and is often diagnosed incorrectly as stifle lameness. A flexion test by a veterinarian will differentiate between a croup myopathy and a stifle problem, because the flexion test won't increase the lameness in a horse with croup myopathy. A caudal thigh strain usually presents itself as a heightened hip action accompanied by a hoof slap.

Treatment

A muscle strain needs time to heal, so there is no specific therapy. When I was younger, I played baseball every chance I could and in California, where I grew up, that was year-round. One year I tore a muscle in my side and it took nearly six months to heal to the point where I could throw or swing a bat again. There is no substitute for time.

Nonsteroidal anti-inflammatory drugs will reduce the pain but, depending on the degree of damage, may not correct the altered gait. Except in the case of a complete muscle tear, though, it isn't necessary to stop work. Rather, the intensity of actual work should be reduced and warm-up and cooling-out times should be increased. Therapeutic aids include massage, ultrasound, electrical stimulation, and, if there is toe-dragging, corrective trimming and shoeing.

Prognosis

The prognosis in first- and second-degree muscle strains is good, but time is necessary. Horses with croup myopathy usually return to normal function within ninety days, but caudal thigh injuries may require six months to a year. A third-degree strain offers only a guarded prognosis for return to normal function and, therefore, full training capacity. Damaged muscles are more susceptible to further injury if pushed too hard, so follow the veterinarian's guidelines for exercise.

As with so many things concerning horses, patience is the key.

Ligament Injuries

HAVE YOU EVER BROKEN A BONE? Hurts like the dickens, right? Have you ever done serious damage to a ligament? That makes a broken bone seem like a picnic in the park.

I have suffered both, thanks to my patients, those creatures that I was trying to help. A mare I was palpating kicked me in the shin and cracked the bone. It hurt like the devil, but I continued working. I limped a little, sure, but I made my usual daily rounds and eventually it healed.

But a yearling got me in the side of my knee, forcing it to bend in a manner that Mother Nature never intended for a knee to bend. A ligament was ruptured. I didn't work for three months and I hobbled around for two or three more months when I did go back to work. (I

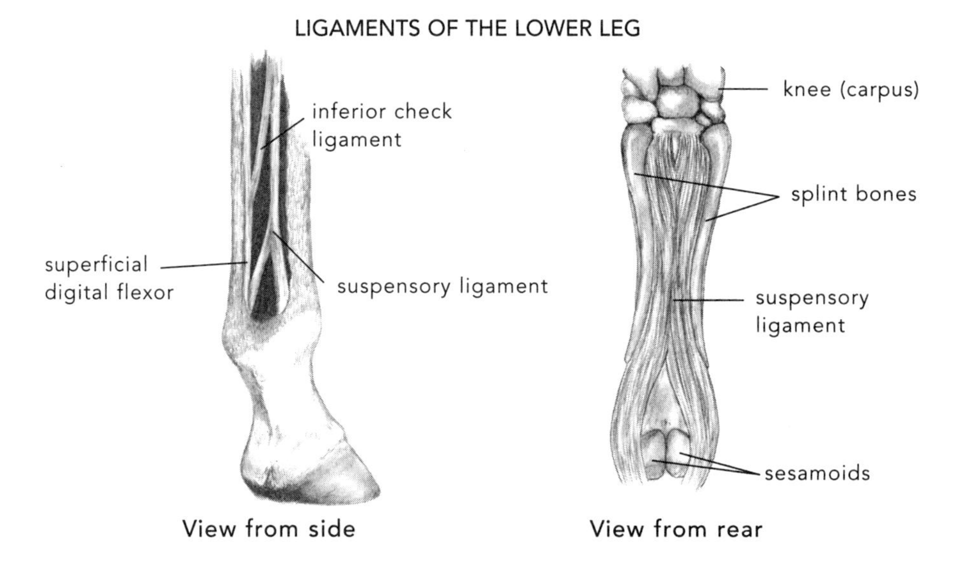

discovered an interesting fact about my disability insurance: I had to be disabled for ninety days before I could collect any benefits. At ninety days I was able to work again, but I still pay my premiums.) There was no comparison between the two pains. That happened years ago, and I still have intermittent pain in that knee.

Before I get started with ligament injuries, it's necessary to understand what a ligament is and how it differs from a tendon. A *ligament* is a band or sheet of fibrous tissue connecting two or more bones, cartilages, or other structures. The ligament serves as support for muscles or fasciae. A *tendon,* however, is a fibrous band or cord that attaches a muscle to a bone.

Most cases of inflamed ligaments (desmitis) have several things in common:

- Treatment consists of early, initial, frequent cold applications (ice, hosing), pressure bandages, and nonsteroidal anti-inflammatory drugs (NSAIDs), such as phenylbutazone.
- There is often an associated avulsion fracture of a bone that may be detected on follow-up X-ray two to three weeks after injury.
- Stall rest, often lengthy, and controlled hand walking, also for quite a while, are necessary.
- X-rays are usually of only limited benefit in a diagnosis.

Ligament injuries are often misdiagnosed, and much X-ray film is wasted in a vain attempt to find a fracture that isn't there. Because the prognosis of desmitis is dependent on early initial treatment, any lost time may prove to be critical down the road. Desmitis often leads to retirement because of misdiagnosis, particularly if insufficient time is given for healing.

Common Sites of Injury

Although I suppose an injury can occur to any ligament, we're primarily concerned with those that lead to lameness.

Stifle and Hock Areas

Ligament injuries commonly occur in the stifle region. Injury can occur to the cruciate, collateral, patellar, or meniscal ligaments. Trauma — usually fairly severe trauma — is the most common cause of injury to these structures. Meniscal ligament injury is often accompanied by damage to the meniscus, the cartilage that separates the ends of the femur and tibia. The onset of lameness is sudden and may be severe. As is usually the case, best results are achieved when treatment is initiated early. If in doubt, immediately ice or hose with cold water the suspected point of injury and call your veterinarian.

Injuries to ligaments of the hock are most commonly seen in steeplechasers and other types of jumpers, especially those that have fallen. Lameness may be mild to severe and seems to improve after ten to fourteen days of rest. Flexing the leg makes it worse. There may or may not be swelling, and X-rays are of little use in diagnosis until about sixty days after the injury occurs, as it takes time for changes to become visible radiographically. Nuclear scintigraphy (see page 159 for more information) and arthroscopy are the best methods for immediate diagnosis.

If the diagnosis is made early, NSAIDs will reduce the inflammation, but six months' stall rest and controlled walking are necessary because the hock and stifle don't lend themselves to supportive pressure bandaging. The prognosis is fair to good. In the case of tarsal ligament damage, there may be small avulsion fractures of the tibia, and these must be removed surgically.

Suspensory Ligament

Signs of suspensory ligament desmitis include swelling over the ligament and pain on palpation and flexion. In some cases, there may be an accompanying fracture of the lower end of one or both splint bones, in which case the swelling is diffuse. X-ray or ultrasound aids in diagnosis.

Initial therapy consists of NSAIDs, cold therapy, and pressure bandages. If a splint bone is fractured, the portion of the bone below the fracture should be removed. Stall rest is mandatory, but recurrence is common. The prognosis depends on the degree of damage to the ligament.

Inferior Check Ligament

One of the more common forelimb ligament injuries occurs to the inferior check ligament, correctly called the accessory ligament of the deep digital flexor tendon. It's usually seen in older jumpers but may occur in all breeds, especially ponies, at any age. The onset of lameness is acute and there is much swelling in the area of the ligament. Ultrasound is the best method to determine the extent of the damage. Inferior check ligament desmitis may become chronic if not treated immediately and is unresponsive when it does.

Treatment consists of NSAIDs, frequent cold applications, and pressure bandages for at least ten days. Ninety days' stall rest is a minimum, followed by controlled hand walking and therapeutic ultrasound, with healing monitored by periodic ultrasound examinations. Recurrence is expected if the horse is returned to work too soon. The prognosis is poor to guarded for the animal to be able to perform at its previous level.

Distal Sesamoidean Ligament

The signs of damage to the distal sesamoidean ligament are similar to those of inferior check ligament desmitis, and many times both conditions are present. Overextension of the fetlock joint is the cause. These ligaments lie on either side of the back of the pastern and severe damage can result in sinking of the fetlock. Treatment is the same as for injury to the inferior check ligament, but horses with sinking of the fetlock should be placed in a cast for six to eight weeks. At best, the prognosis is guarded, and recurrence is common.

Distal Annular Ligament

The only sign of a distal annular ligament injury is a thickening of the ligament, and it's uncertain that this actually causes lameness. If lameness is present, it may be severe and there is probably an avulsion fracture of the long pastern bone associated with the desmitis. Even with an avulsion, the treatment is the same as for an injury to the inferior check or distal sesamoidean ligament, with three to six months' stall rest. The prognosis is good.

In ligament injuries, time is of the essence; initially, there is none to waste and later the horse needs a great deal of it.

Bowed Tendon

Before I entered my teens I fell in love with Thoroughbred horse racing. I would have loved to be a jockey, but I was almost six feet tall and weighed about 170 pounds at age twelve so I decided I'd be a professional baseball player. That didn't work out, either, but I continued to follow both sports as closely as I could.

I came to learn that two problems beset competitors in both endeavors. Baseball players have rotator cuff injuries and racehorses have bowed tendons; coming back from either is difficult. Later, in veterinary school, I learned what bowed tendons are, why they happen, and what can be done about them. (It wasn't until my older son was a college pitcher that I learned the same stuff about rotator cuff injuries.)

I also came to believe that bowed tendons were peculiar to racehorses. I never heard of a bow occurring to any other type of horse, and our teacher stressed that it was a serious problem in racehorses.

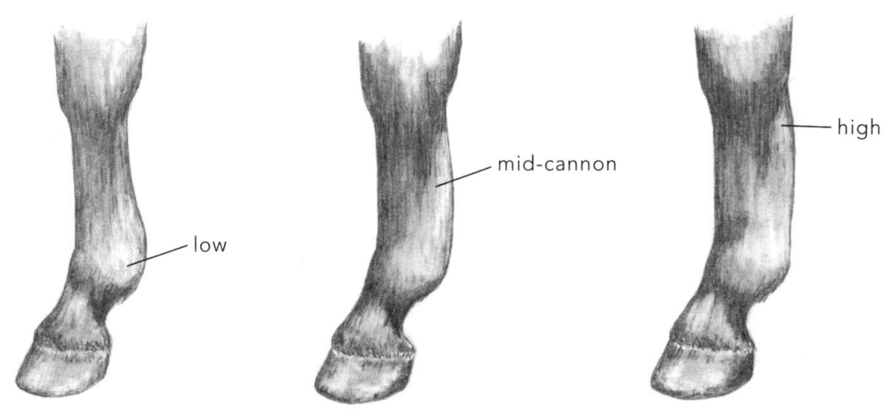

THREE COMMON SITES OF BOWED TENDON

Imagine my surprise, then, when the first three bowed tendons I saw after I left school were in non-racehorses. The first was in a Thoroughbred-cross foxhunter. He apparently took some sort of misstep while doing his job. The second was in a Quarter Horse cow pony. He, too, was injured while working. The third was in a Welsh show pony. She came in one morning with a bow.

I eventually saw many — too many — in racehorses; about half of them raced again, albeit not as well as they had before the bowed tendons. Neither the Quarter Horse nor the Welsh pony returned to its previous work.

In racing breeds in the United States, where races are run counterclockwise, the most common site of a bowed tendon is the left front leg, although bows can occur in any limb. I once worked on a horse that bowed sequentially over a three-year period: first the left fore, then the right fore, then the right hind. (He returned to racing each time and continued to earn money.)

What Is a Bowed Tendon?

A bow usually results from a "bad step." A horse steps in a divot or hole at high speed and something has to give; a tendon is stretched forcefully and farther than nature intended. Bows involve the superficial digital flexor tendon or the deep digital flexor tendon, with the superficial tendon being involved more frequently.

A bowed tendon is actually a torn tendon or, perhaps more correctly, a disruption of the tendon fibers. The visible swelling is a result of both hemorrhage and the protective inflammatory response of the body to the damage. Injury can occur anywhere along the length of the tendon (knee or hock to fetlock), but the most frequently involved area is the region near the middle of the cannon bone, possibly because the tendons are narrowest there.

The term *bow* comes from the appearance of the injured leg: the swelling on the back of the leg resembles an arched bow. As well as the typical mid-cannon bow, there are "high," "low," and "deep" bows.

Clinical Signs

Lameness is often mild or nonexistent initially, but there is heat in the swollen area and pain on digital palpation. Continued exercise only worsens it, and eventually lameness will appear.

One problem is that the initial swelling is often very mild and, when accompanied by no gait alteration, is overlooked or ignored, resulting in more extensive damage when use is continued. There is a lesson here: any outward change, no matter how innocuous it seems to be, should be thoroughly investigated.

Diagnosis and Treatment

Diagnosis is best made by ultrasound, as is monitoring the progression of the bow. Initial treatment — and it can't begin too soon — consists of frequent cold-water hosing or icing of the leg, support bandages, nonsteroidal anti-inflammatory drugs, and stall rest. Follow-up ultrasound reveals when sufficient healing has occurred for the next stage of recovery to begin. At that point (probably sixty to ninety days after the injury occurred), walking by hand can be started, followed by light jogging as the elasticity of the tendon improves. In the presence of heat or additional swelling, resume stall rest; monitor progress with ultrasound until healing is complete.

There are several other treatments that have been tried over the years, but the conservative approach outlined above is the most successful and least traumatic to both horse and wallet. The important thing to remember is: tendons heal slowly.

Prognosis

Prognosis for a horse suffering from a bowed tendon to return to its previous level of performance or work depends on the severity, and to some extent the location, of the injury. Most bowed horses can return to use if the injury is diagnosed early, treated vigorously, and given proper time to heal, although they may not be quite as "good" as they were before. If a bow is allowed to become chronic (that is, if inadequate rest and care are provided), the prognosis for full recovery lowers significantly.

"Big Leg" (Lymphangitis)

I REMEMBER THE FIRST "BIG LEG" I SAW. As I've said, my older brother showed American Saddlebreds and as a little boy I was always around them. One day we were at a trainer's barn and there was a horse in a small dirt pen. It had a huge hind leg and could barely bend it. Walking was evidently very difficult for the poor horse.

I asked the trainer, "Jimmy, what's wrong with that horse's leg?"

"It's swollen," he replied.

Well, duh. I was only about six years old but I thought I deserved a better answer than that.

Maybe three weeks later we were at Jimmy's barn again. The horse with the big leg was still there, and the leg was still big.

"Can't you do something about that horse's leg?" I asked.

"You tell me what," Jimmy answered. I never liked him much.

It was more than twenty years later when I saw the next horse with "big leg." I was just out of veterinary school and a new client asked me what was wrong with his mare's leg. This time, however, I knew what it was and what to do about it. What I didn't know then, however, was that treatment doesn't always work and that sometimes the problem recurs. They didn't tell us that in school.

What Is "Big Leg"?

"Big leg" is lymphangitis, an inflammation of the lymph vessels and peripheral lymph nodes. It usually occurs in one hind leg and may affect the leg from the hock down. The affected leg is stiff and walking is difficult. The horse often keeps weight off the leg, which may lead to problems in the other one. The cause is probably bacterial but that isn't known for sure.

Treatment

Treatment consists of hosing or icing the leg, systemic steroids, and long-term (four to six weeks), broad-spectrum antibiotic therapy. Best results are achieved when treatment is begun early. Satisfactory resolution becomes increasingly difficult to attain the longer that prolonged, aggressive therapy is postponed. Unfortunately, even though the condition may be resolved, recurrence is not uncommon. Treatment is the same for recurring cases.

An old-time remedy that still has some merit is to stand the horse in a pond or creek. This seems to provide the benefits you'd expect from hosing the leg constantly. An old farm employee who had been working with horses for more than sixty years once told me of a horse he cared for that came up with "big leg." It was back in the days before penicillin and the local veterinarian had no idea what to do, so the horse was just ignored.

One day, though, when the old man (who was then a young man) went to bring in the horses, the one with the swollen leg was standing belly-deep in a pond. He couldn't get her to come out and as far as he knew she stayed in the pond day and night for about a week. When she finally did emerge, her leg was normal. Mother Nature works in mysterious ways.

4

Hoof Ailments

Founder (Laminitis)

"SOMEBODY DIDN'T CLOSE THE BARN DOOR, and he got into the pig's corn. I'm afraid he's gonna colic."

That call, in one form or another, is one that I have received numerous times over the years. This particular call, however, came when I had been out of school for only a few weeks. The caller had reason to fear that his horse, a twelve-year-old gelding, would colic, but he had more reason to fear that he would founder, and somehow that situation rarely enters the horse owner's mind.

When I got there (in about twenty minutes), the man had one sick horse. Yes, he had a bellyache, but he also had very sore, hot front feet. I learned that he had probably gotten into the corn overnight; it was nearly noon when the owner called. More on this guy follows later.

What Is Founder?

Founder (laminitis, acute laminar degeneration) is a challenging condition. What basically occurs is this: something causes the blood flow to the foot to decrease, resulting in damage to the interconnecting,

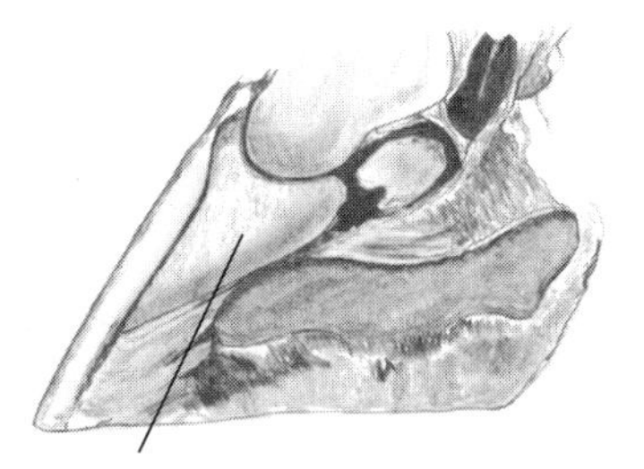

normal position of the coffin bone

rotation of the coffin bone

ROTATION OF THE COFFIN BONE IN LAMINITIS

fingerlike projections (laminae) that hold the hoof wall to the coffin bone. Because of the damage to the laminae, the coffin bone is no longer secured and can rotate and drop, resulting in lameness.

Often there seems to be no identifiable cause, but of course there must be one (as in the case of the horse just mentioned). Several commonly accepted causes, or *predisposing factors,* as they should more correctly be called, have been identified (see the box on page 110). If the cause can be determined, steps must be taken to eliminate it.

Some horses are predisposed to founder. Geldings founder more easily than stallions and mares. One of my teachers in veterinary school told me, "Kelley, always remember: there are two kinds of ponies, those that have foundered and those that will." What he was saying is that ponies are prone to founder and, boy, was he right. A pony gelding is almost doomed from the start. And don't believe this nonsense put out by miniature-horse people that their minis aren't ponies. They are, and they'll founder in a second.

Clinical Signs

Lameness associated with founder can range from extremely mild and hardly noticeable to so severe that the horse cannot stand. Unless properly managed, the mild cases can and will progress. Founder also ranges from acute, which must be treated as an emergency, to chronic. It usually seems to occur in the front feet but can occur in all four feet; occasionally just one foot is involved.

Treatment

Your veterinarian will undertake several management steps if your horse has founder. (See the box for a brief overview.) Carefully follow the veterinarian's care instructions because founder can be life-threatening.

- **Remove the cause and begin treatment.** Determine the cause, if possible, and remove it; give antibiotics, nonsteroidal anti-inflammatory drugs (NSAIDs), intravenous fluids, and oral mineral oil; support the frog; bed the stall deeply; and give blood thinners (aspirin or heparin).
- **Stop or ease the pain.** Administer NSAIDs; bed the stall deeply; and block (inject local anesthetic into the nerves) the feet if pain is severe.
- **Increase blood flow to the feet.** Use blood thinners (aspirin, heparin); administer ace (acepromazine, a vasodilator); and support the frog and sole.
- **Perform corrective trimming.** Enlist the aid of the farrier to trim the involved foot, if necessary. Maintain proper hoof trimming.
- **Prevent coffin bone rotation.** Support the frog and sole, and maintain proper hoof trimming. The veterinarian may perform a deep digital flexor tenotomy or inferior check ligament desmotomy if warranted.
- **Promote healing of hooves and soles.** Maintain proper trimming and shoeing, administer methylsulphonylmethane (MSM; available as a powder in most tack shops under various brand names) or methionine, and apply hoof dressings.
- **Tender loving care.** If the laminitis progresses to the chronic stage, the horse must be kept comfortable through general care if the decision is made to let it live. In most cases, however, the truly humane course is to euthanize because the pain can't be adequately controlled.

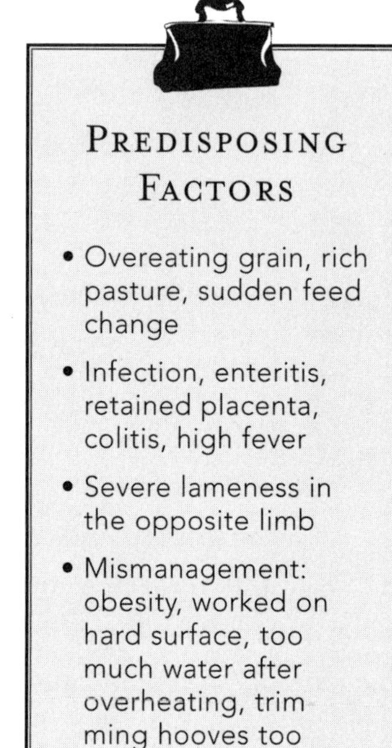

Predisposing Factors

- Overeating grain, rich pasture, sudden feed change
- Infection, enteritis, retained placenta, colitis, high fever
- Severe lameness in the opposite limb
- Mismanagement: obesity, worked on hard surface, too much water after overheating, trimming hooves too closely
- Overuse of steroids
- Hypothyroidism

Prognosis

As with most everything, the sooner that treatment is begun, the better the prognosis. Prognosis actually depends on several things: duration of acute lameness, number of feet involved, response to treatment, and degree of coffin bone rotation (as determined by X-rays).

If caught and treated early, the prognosis is guarded to fair, and these horses may eventually return to their previous activity or use. If not caught early, however, the prognosis deteriorates in relation to time, response to treatment, and other factors.

In the case of the horse we began with, we oiled him, gave him phenylbutazone and ace, took X-rays, put him on penicillin, and had shod him with pads. Initial X-rays showed no coffin bone rotation, but five days later X-rays showed a small amount of rotation. He was kept from then on in a dry lot and shod and trimmed faithfully and was able to continue as a lightly ridden pleasure horse. He was lucky.

Navicular Syndrome

A woman bought a Thoroughbred gelding just off the track. After she paid her money a "friend" told her that the horse probably had navicular problems because "all Thoroughbreds have navicular problems." The woman called me to see whether I could find out if her horse did, indeed, have navicular problems.

Part of the examination of the navicular bone is to have someone trot the horse. After observing the horse in action and then taking X-rays, I decided that the gelding didn't have navicular problems. The young woman's friend told me I was nuts because "all Thoroughbreds have navicular problems."

What Is Navicular Syndrome?

Navicular syndrome has been called the most common cause of forelimb lameness in horses. The navicular bone is a cuboidal rectangular bone within the horse's foot. It is officially a sesamoid bone, but generally when someone refers to the *sesamoids* he means the two bones at the rear of the fetlock. The navicular bone is always called the navicular bone, but in navicular problems more than the navicular bone is involved. Also involved are the bone's suspensory ligaments, the coffin joint, the navicular bursa, the deep digital flexor tendon, and the blood supply of the navicular bone. Hence the term *navicular syndrome* rather than the old term *navicular disease*.

Five changes are visible radiographically in navicular syndrome:

- Marginal osteophytes (spurs)
- Bone remodeling (calcification of the central portion of the navicular suspensory ligament or along the impar ligament; the latter is sometimes misdiagnosed as a bone chip)
- Enlarged synovial fossae
- Cysts within the navicular bone
- Flexor cortical lesions along the median edge

Any or all may be present, but in the absence of clinical signs they are not diagnostic of navicular syndrome.

The highest incidence of navicular syndrome occurs among seven- to fourteen-year-old performance horses. Racing Thoroughbreds and Quarter Horses have a higher frequency than other breeds (thus the friend's insistence). Predisposing factors include contracted heels, small feet, underrun heels, shear heels, improper or mismatched hoof angles, and an incorrect breakover point.

Clinical Signs and Diagnosis

Diagnosis of navicular syndrome is based on history and clinical signs; diagnosis should be made before radiographic examination, which is meant for confirmation. Navicular syndrome is a chronic, bilateral forelimb lameness seen most readily after heavy work and will decrease or disappear with rest. Because the horse will tend to land on its toes, the typical gait is short and choppy. Longeing will worsen the lameness on the inside forefoot.

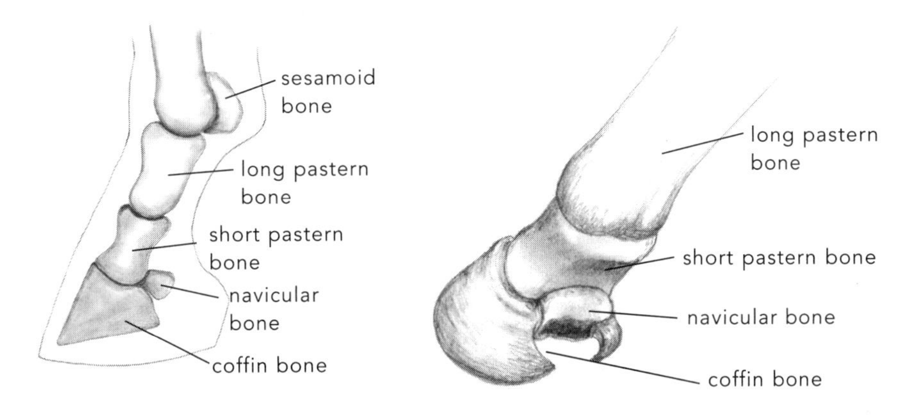

BONES OF THE LOWER LEG AND FOOT

Pain may be elicited when a hoof tester is used across the heels, from the central grooves on either side of the frog (sulcus) to the toe, or from the collateral sulci to the contralateral hoof wall. In some cases of navicular syndrome no response to hoof testers is evident. A thorough examination of the entire forefoot should be made to be certain that the source of the painful response isn't in another area of the foot.

Nerve blocks (injecting local anesthetic into nerves) may be the best diagnostic test. After blocking the medial and lateral palmar digital nerves in the front feet, a horse with navicular syndrome should become essentially sound.

Two other diagnostic tests are helpful: a hyperextension test and a wedge test, in which pressure is placed directly on the navicular bone. The lameness will usually be exacerbated after flexion of the distal limb. After performing the tests, the horse is trotted and the lameness worsens. Again, a negative test here doesn't rule out navicular syndrome.

Treatment

Treatment of navicular syndrome varies with each case. The best is proper shoeing aimed at correction of preexisting problems, accompanied by an allowance for hoof expansion (a larger shoe is used and the nails placed farther forward than normal).

Nonsteroidal anti-inflammatory drugs won't cure anything, but

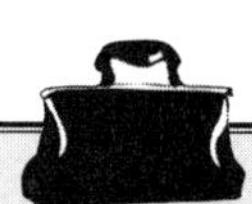

Don't Forget the Prepurchase Exam

Navicular syndrome is common in racehorses, and because racehorses are usually Thoroughbreds and Quarter Horses, these breeds have a higher incidence than others do. There is a better chance of encountering this condition in a former racehorse of these breeds, but remember that many other things are more likely to be wrong if you're considering acquiring a retired racehorse.

A thorough prepurchase examination by a veterinarian proficient in diagnosing lameness will help to ensure that the horse under consideration is free of navicular syndrome, but there is no guarantee that the condition won't develop. This examination will identify other possible problems, too, so from that standpoint it's money well spent.

they will ease the discomfort and allow more proper use of the foot; they work well in combination with proper shoeing. There are vasoactive drugs that show promise, but various problems are associated with them, and none is commonly used.

Surgery may be necessary if proper shoeing and pain relievers fail. The most commonly performed procedure is the palmar digital neurectomy. Soundness is achieved in the majority of cases, but the course of the condition isn't altered; eventually, as the condition progresses, lameness will return.

I have performed palmar digital neurectomies on two horses. One went sound immediately and has remained sound for several years. We keep expecting the lameness to return, but so far so good. The other horse never went completely sound and was as bad as ever within a year. I have no idea why the responses in the two horses were so different.

Canker Versus Thrush

Several conditions in horses are outwardly similar to other ailments, and in some cases it really doesn't matter what the condition is because treatment is the same.

For instance, if you have a filly housed in a barn full of other people's horses and she is depressed, with a snotty nose and a cough, it really doesn't make a difference if she has flu or rhinopneumonitis (see pages 5 and 7, respectively). You're going to respond pretty much the same way in either case. But some conditions that look alike may not be at all similar. That same filly may walk a little off in what appears to be the right fore. It could be a gravel in that foot, but maybe it's a small fracture of the coffin bone in the left rear. Treatment would be very different in each case.

Horses can't tell us where they hurt or with whom they've been sniffing noses. Frequently, two conditions with similar signs require different therapies, so obviously a correct diagnosis is necessary.

Aeons ago, when I was first set free from the halls of academe, I saw several cases of thrush, which I treated as I was taught in school. They all responded as I was taught they would.

Except one. It didn't get better. Instead, it got worse. Finally, I called another veterinarian, one of long experience. He came to see the horse, poked and dug for a minute, then said he had to get something from his car and asked me to accompany him.

Once there, and out of earshot of the horse's owner, he said, "Brent, that's not thrush. It's canker."

Well, that told me why my treatment wasn't effective. I had guessed. I had no idea what canker was or how it was treated. I kept encountering things in my new practice that I didn't remember being taught in school. I also learned a little about finesse from my experienced vet friend that day. Never having been blessed with much tact or diplomacy, if I had been in his place I probably would have said, right in front of the owner, something like "No wonder the foot's not getting better. It's not thrush and you're not treating it right," and I may well have added, "Dummy."

So I learned about canker and how to tell it from thrush, which turned out to be a good, if not overly used, bit of knowledge. In the nearly thirty years since, I have seen roughly a zillion cases of thrush and only two cases of canker. But I recognized them.

What Is Thrush? Canker?

Before we go into the similarities and differences of the two conditions, we need to define what each one is.

Thrush is defined as a moist, exudative (oozing), odoriferous (smelly) dermatitis that specifically involves the central and lateral sulci (grooves) of the frog. A contributing factor in some cases of thrush is chronic lameness, which results in decreased heel expansion from reduced use of the foot. This creates contracted heels, accompanied by deep sulci, making feet much more susceptible to contamination.

Canker is also a moist, oozing dermatitis characterized by a foul-smelling exudate (pus), but the body of the frog is where it occurs, rather than the sulci.

Classically, canker was known as a condition occurring in the hind feet of draft horses, but in recent years, it seems to affect light breeds and front feet as well, whereas thrush has never seemed to care in the slightest about the breed of horse or which foot it attacks.

Both conditions are the result of poor (or no) foot care combined with unsanitary, moist conditions. Anaerobic bacteria, especially *Fusobacterium necrophorus,* are commonly cultured from both conditions, but these are not considered to be the cause of the disorders. Once allowed to gain a foothold, however, they can add to the severity of the conditions and must be controlled.

While thrush is confined to the sulci and can possibly involve the heels if left unattended, canker initially involves the body of the frog and will affect the whole frog and even the sole if allowed to become chronic.

Treatment

In thrush, treatment consists of the veterinarian excising extraneous frog and sole tissue and then packing the sulci with a tamed iodine solution (such as Betadine) and bandaging it. The bandage should be changed daily until the discharge is no longer evident. Healing usually occurs within two weeks and the prognosis is good or better for return to normal use.

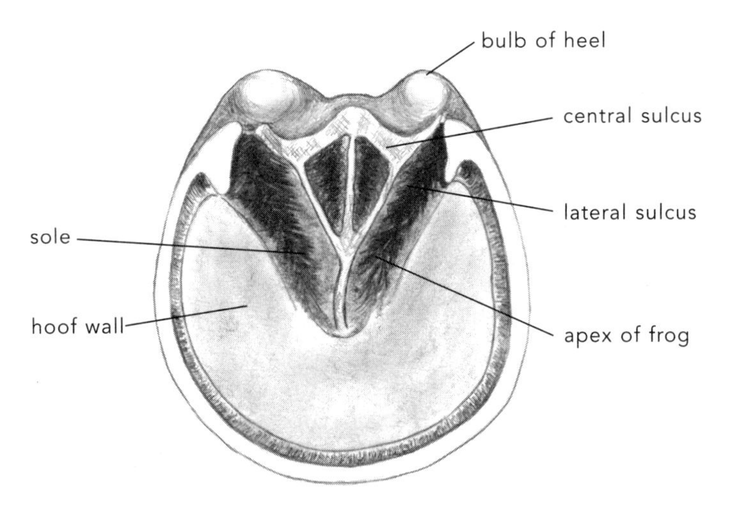

EXTERNAL ANATOMY OF THE EQUINE FOOT

Treatment for canker is far more complicated and prolonged. Early recognition helps greatly. Close debridement (removal of dead or damaged tissue) under general anesthetic is necessary, followed by topical application of metronidazole ointment and daily bandaging.

Most important at this point is a clean, dry environment for the feet. The foot must be cleaned with clear water and dried thoroughly each time the bandage is changed. Complete healing may take a month to six weeks and prognosis is fair for the horse to return to its previous use.

As in most everything, prevention is the best treatment in both cases. With these conditions, proper foot hygiene and care are necessary to avoid these problems in the first place.

Back to my first case of canker. It involved a forefoot (I don't remember which) of a Thoroughbred-cross hunter, and the experienced veterinarian handled the treatment. The foot cleared up in a few weeks, but the horse was never 100 percent sound afterward. He was sold several months later as a pleasure horse, a job he handled well. Earlier recognition might have kept him a hunter.

Hoof Cracks and Acrylic Hoof Repair

WHEN I FIRST GOT OUT OF SCHOOL, the practice I worked in had more pleasure horse clients than any other kind. This is probably representative of most of the U.S. horse-owning population, who have one, two, maybe three backyard horses that are ridden every now and then.

Among the clients were two lawyers and a dentist. As far as I could tell, they really liked their horses and wanted them to have the best care possible. The problem: these three gentlemen worked all day in their respective professions and were unable to be at the barn from 9 A.M. to 5 P.M., during what we have come to call "normal working hours." So they could be there when their horses were being tended to by the veterinarian (my employer or me), they routinely asked that we come later in the evening.

What Are Hoof Cracks?

Hoof cracks are a real problem for any horse. Small cracks can be taken care of by the farrier, but not all cracks are small. Many extend up the hoof wall and approach (or reach) the coronet. Others go deep, all the way through the hoof wall. And they hurt the horse; they are a chief cause of lameness. Healing is slow and a horse cannot be used while the hoof (and crack) is growing out.

Treatment

Most cracks, however, can be repaired using acrylic. While in school I didn't learn about acrylic hoof repair. I don't think it was ever mentioned; at least I never heard it mentioned. It was up to Dr. Springer, my employer in those early days, to teach it to me.

The crack is drilled out and cleaned, and acrylic material is placed in it. This holds the crack together and prevents further spread of the crack; eventually the hoof grows out and the crack is no more. It really works well and the horse can remain in full use in most cases.

Dr. Springer showed me how to do it on a couple of horses, then he said, "You can do the next one."

One of the above-mentioned lawyers had a horse with a pretty bad crack. I told him that we needed to repair it with acrylic and he said to come out at 7 o'clock the next evening and do it then. I didn't want to come out at 7 P.M. and neither did Dr. Springer (he needed to be present in case I had a problem), so he and I decided to go out earlier in the day and do the repair without the lawyer being present. It went well and when I finished you could hardly tell that there had ever been a crack.

That evening, about 6:15, as I was eating dinner, the phone rang. It was the lawyer. "Kelley," he said, "you don't have to come. The hoof fixed itself. Boy, am I glad. Now I won't have to pay another big vet bill."

I told him he *would* have to pay another vet bill (and it wasn't very big) because we had been out that afternoon and done the job. I don't think he believed me but he paid.

Prophylactic Measures and Prognosis

There are potential problems with acrylic repair, though. Until recently, deep and infected cracks were not candidates for acrylic patching, which meant that these horses could not be used during the long healing time.

But several years ago, in an effort to provide a prophylactic measure against infection in human hip replacements, medical researchers added antibiotics to polymethyl methacrylate bone cement, a product that is contained in some of the newer hoof-repair materials.

Veterinary researchers hypothesized that, based on the human medical work with antibiotic-impregnated bone cement, antibiotics could be added to acrylic hoof-repair material to help prevent or control hoof infection after injury.

These researchers performed three studies to test their hypothesis: (1) an impregnation and elution (rinsing) test to determine whether an antibiotic would mix with the acrylic and, if so, whether it would be released in the hoof wall; (2) a clinical trial on normal equine hooves; and (3) use in clinical cases.

In the first test, they added gentamicin powder to hoof acrylic and found that the antibiotic combined with the acrylic and dispersed appropriately in therapeutic concentrations. In the second test, the researchers added metronidazole, which earlier had proved useful in controlling hoof infections, to the hoof acrylic instead of gentamicin. Using a group of normal ponies with hoof resections, they applied this antibiotic-impregnated material to one forefoot of half the group. The remaining ponies were treated with conventional hoof-repair material. The result: repair was successful in those ponies treated with the antibiotic-impregnated material and it failed in half of those treated with the regular acrylic material.

In the third trial, the metronidazole-impregnated material was used on twenty-five hooves with various types of damage. In each case it was left in place until the hoof grew out. Healing occurred in all cases, often faster than the researchers had anticipated. Of course, the lesion, whatever its nature, must be properly prepared by cleaning and debriding it before the medicated acrylic can be applied. Also, because the antibiotic powder slows the curing time of the acrylic, the patch needs extra time to set between applications of the layers of acrylic.

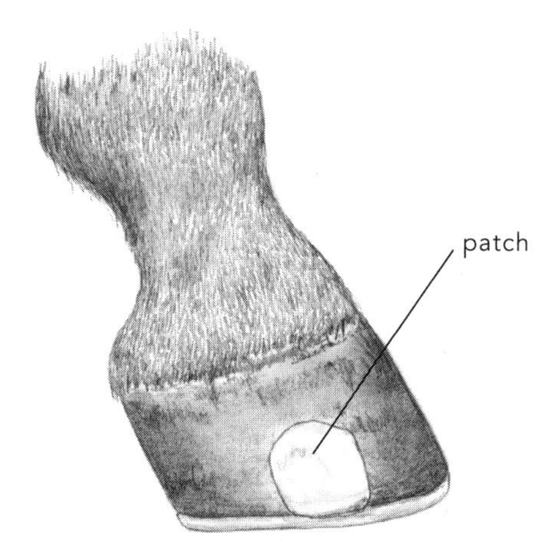

Antibiotic-impregnated patching materials have met with favorable results, though such patches need extra time to set between applications of acrylic.

Since the original work, there have been additional trials conducted with the antibiotic-impregnated patching materials, and favorable results have been reported. With time, patience, and using this method of hoof repair, horses with feet that are severely damaged can return to work more quickly, with fewer complications and greater soundness.

Gravel

THE ADVANCES IN MOBILE COMMUNICATION over the last several years have been phenomenal. When I first got out of school, there were two-way radios. To be of any use, there had to be someone in the office to relay calls. That person was my employer's wife, but when she went shopping or visiting we were without communication.

Then there were mobile phones, but the first ones also required an "operator" in order to make and receive calls, which would then be "patched" through. This worked well, but, as with the two-way radio, other people could listen in.

Mobile communication eventually progressed to today's cellular phones. Easy, convenient, and relatively inexpensive, they are absolutely essential to a person who must spend his life in a car and who has to be reachable in emergencies.

Not all calls are emergencies, however. One day back when we still had to be patched through, my wife called and asked me to stop at the grocery store on my way home to pick up a few things. At least I didn't think it was an emergency; I've never known a milk and hamburger buns crisis.

While in the store I saw a woman who was a fairly new client. She owned a couple of pleasure horses. "Doc Kelley, I was gonna call you; now I won't have to. Can you come see my mare? I think she's pebbled."

"Pebbled?" I responded.

"Yes. You know, she's holding one foot up."

I still wasn't sure what she meant. I said I'd meet her at her place on my way home, but she wasn't going home then, so I said I'd stop by on my way out the next morning.

When I got there, she said, "It's okay. The pebble popped out."

Still not sure what she meant, I asked to see the horse. There, on the front of the right front coronet, was an open sore from which pus was oozing.

"Oh," I said, "it was a gravel."

"Right. That's what I said. A pebble."

What Is Gravel?

Gravel is a condition possibly unique in equine medicine: it doesn't have a fancy, multisyllable name, at least not one that I'm aware of. Textbooks say *gravel* is a lay term but fail to furnish us with any other name, so gravel it remains. The fact that the medical condition has nothing to do with road gravel is secondary.

For those unfamiliar with the term, a gravel is a condition of the horse's foot manifested by a hoof abscess and varying degrees of lameness. It derives its name from the old belief (still held by some) that a piece of gravel enters the bottom of the foot and migrates upward, eventually popping out at or slightly above the coronary band.

What actually happens is an infectious microorganism enters the sole or white line through a puncture wound or crack and multiplies, triggering the body's natural response to any foreign invader: white blood cells gather around the bacteria and pus results. As the white blood cells battle the bacteria, the affected area within the foot enlarges and creates pressure as more pus is produced. The normal course is for the infected area to travel to the nearest outer surface in order to erupt. But because this occurs within a horse's foot, the nearest outer surface is either the sole or the hoof wall, neither of which is amenable to being penetrated by an abscess. Therefore, the pus pocket travels in the direction of least resistance — up — where it eventually meets the soft tissue it seeks, the coronet, and pops.

Predisposing Factors

As stated, the infection enters through the sole or white line via a puncture or crack. Although these can occur at any time, there are three conditions that predispose their occurrence: extremely dry conditions, extremely wet conditions, and founder.

- **Extremely dry conditions.** In extremely dry conditions, the horse's foot dries out. This leads to cracks in the sole and especially in the white line. Times of drought are probably when gravels are most common; bacteria enter these cracks and infection sets in.
- **Extremely wet conditions.** I'm not sure why we see an increase in

gravels during extremely wet times but I have a theory. Let me preface it by saying I don't know if there's a higher incidence of gravels elsewhere in the world in wet weather. I just know I see more here in central Kentucky. My theory is this: in extremely wet weather, a horse may sink one to four inches or more into the mud while moving about. In so doing, his foot encounters buried bits of debris that, in normal or dry times, would remain unreachable. This could be why I see a drastic increase in the number of gravels in really wet weather.

- **Founder.** Gravels are also seen frequently in previously foundered animals because of the "seedy toe" associated with the condition. With seedy toe, the white line in the toe area is never fully sealed and bacteria can enter readily.

Clinical Signs and Treatment

Lameness is the chief sign of gravel, but the lameness may vary from slight to three-legged, depending on the point of entry of the offending organism, amount of pus generated, path traveled by the infection, and proximity to the coronary band. If detected early, the offending crack in the sole can be pared and scraped clean with a hoof knife to facilitate drainage, but if not caught early — and most aren't — opening the sole does no good because the tract of infection will have progressed too far upward.

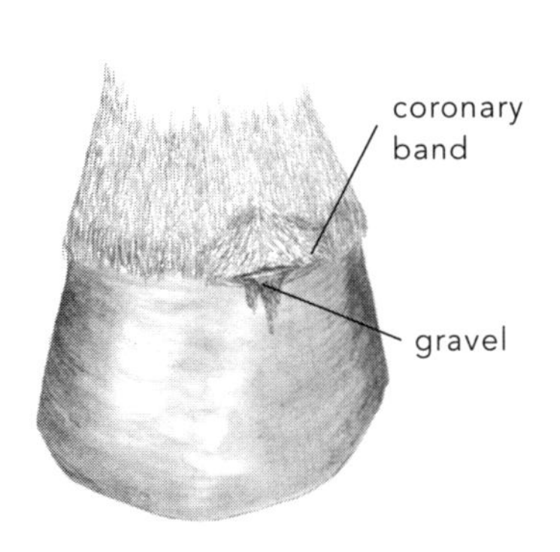

A gravel has erupted just below the coronary band.

If drainage is established through the sole, iodine and a bandage need to be applied and changed daily for three or four days. If it has progressed too far for paring to promote drainage, soaking the foot in Epsom salts will help to bring the infection to the surface. In either case, a tetanus booster should be given. (Reminder: use tetanus antitoxin (TAT) *only* if a horse contracts tetanus or if the tetanus toxoid vaccination history is not known in a horse that has a lesion.)

Some veterinarians recommend the administration of a pain reliever and/or antibiotic before eruption, but because these tend to slow the progression of the infection and thereby prolong the condition, I don't feel either is indicated. Also, stall rest is often recommended. This accomplishes two things: retarding the upward movement of the infectious tract and the creation of more work, in the form of a dirty stall, for whomever performs the task of stall mucking. The animal is better off turned out because the effect of moving about will allow the infection to move up faster and erupt sooner.

Prognosis

Except in severe instances, the prognosis of a gravel case is good. The pus pocket migrates to the region of the coronet, breaks open, drains, and heals, and the horse is none the worse for the experience. In some cases, several areas erupt around the coronet, and these require soaking, antibiotics, and the attention of a farrier.

Prevention

Prevention is difficult, especially in horses at pasture and in previously foundered animals. Keeping the feet moist in times of drought greatly helps in reducing the incidence of the condition.

Dew Poisoning (Equine Pastern Dermatitis)

LIFE NEVER CEASES TO AMAZE ME. When you are a veterinarian, you may have a limited view of life, and when you are an equine veterinarian, it is probably even more limited. So what may not amaze, or even interest, someone in the real world actually stuns me.

A few years ago I was amazed. No, make that stunned.

My wife is a physical therapist now, but previously she was a horse farm manager. It is surprising (or maybe it isn't) how many people who work with horses need physical therapy at one time or another, and her present profession combined with her former one leads to many horse-related conversations while tending to her patients' infirmities.

She came home one evening and asked me if I had ever heard of "greasy or grease heel."

"Sure," I replied. "It's one of several names for dew poisoning or cracked heels. Some people call it 'scratches.' Why?"

She knew what dew poisoning and cracked heels were, and it seemed a patient of hers thought he had a mare with this problem. He had had three veterinarians look at her and none of them had identified the condition or resolved the problem. (The greasy heel diagnosis was made by the owner, not a veterinarian.) Treatment of one kind or another had been going on for four months with no improvement.

Whether this next step is ethical may be in question, but I said, "Tell him to call me."

This was the second time that this had happened. About two years before, a new client had a stallion he showed at halter. This horse had had a dermatitis on his pasterns for several months, and the two previous veterinarians had neither identified nor satisfactorily treated the problem. I wrote that off as poor communication or misunderstanding or something else, because this is a condition that is so common that I thought *everyone* knew about it.

My reasoning was simple: I am no whiz, so if I know what grease heel is and how to treat it, everyone should. Especially veterinarians. But apparently that isn't the case.

What Is Equine Pastern Dermatitis?

This condition usually involves the bulbs of the heels and rear aspects of the pasterns but may sometimes extend up the legs to near the knees or hocks. The signs vary from mild scurfing ("scratches") and hair loss to a heavy exudate (a fluid discharge known as *grease*) and a thick crusting. If allowed to become chronic, granulation tissue called *grapes* (characterized by grape-sized round lumps) develops. This may occur as early as a few weeks but usually doesn't appear for many months.

Books say the condition is precipitated by an injury such as a scratch or small cut. I'm not sure about that because this problem usually occurs on two legs, front or back, or on all four legs, and I can't picture horses acquiring abrasions to several legs at the same time under normal conditions.

Prolonged exposure to moisture is the predisposing factor in most cases. White or heavily haired pasterns are most often affected, and hind legs seem to have a higher incidence than front.

Microorganisms — fungi, bacteria, or both — can usually be cultured from the areas; these may be primary or secondary causes of the dermatitis.

Treatment

The main remedy in the treatment of pastern dermatitis is the elimination of wet conditions. Clipping the pasterns to prevent the hair from retaining moisture is very helpful, but maintaining a dry environment is most important.

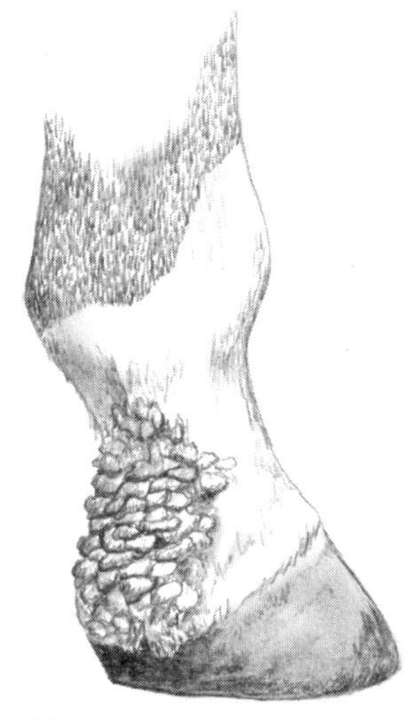

Chronic equine pastern dermatitis ("grapes")

A horse with pastern dermatitis should be kept in a dry, clean stall during periods of wet weather. Even during dry weather, the horse should be kept in a stall overnight and not turned out until the dew has dried each morning. Dry conditions alone will allow many milder cases to heal.

In more severe cases, it's necessary to apply topical medication, but before doing so, any crust or scaling must be removed. The best way to remove dried crust is to soak with warm water until it softens. Then remove the crust and dry the area thoroughly with a clean towel.

When I write about horse health, I make every attempt to avoid recommending or even mentioning products by brand name. That said, Panolog (Schering-Plough) is far and away the best product I have found for treating pastern dermatitis. It comes in both ointment and cream forms, but I think the cream is more effective because it is thicker and gives longer effect.

Apply Panolog twice a day until the dermatitis is healed. This may take three or four days or a few weeks, depending on the severity and the length of time the condition has existed. Alternatively, the medication may be applied under a bandage that is changed every other day, but this does not seem to be as effective in my experience.

In the case of grapes, surgical removal of the granulation tissue is necessary, but shame on you if you have ignored your horse so long that it has reached this point. After surgery, Panolog should be used until healing is complete.

The prognosis is good in cases of pastern dermatitis, even severe ones, but recurrence of the condition is common if the horse is returned to a damp setting.

By the way, both horses mentioned earlier, the mare owned by my wife's patient and the new client's stallion, responded to treatment, which should have been instituted weeks before it was.

5

Bone Problems

Ringbone

The phalanges in humans are the finger bones. In the horse, they are the bones in the pastern (long and short pastern bones) and the foot (coffin bone).

One of the most common problems (perhaps *the* most) associated with the phalanges is ringbone (phalangeal exostosis). Ringbone is classified in two ways: *articular* or *nonarticular,* depending on whether the interphalangeal joints are involved; and *high* or *low,* depending on whether it involves the proximal and middle phalanges or the middle and distal phalanges (the long and short or the short and coffin phalanges, respectively).

Most people say *ringbone* as if they're saying *bubonic plague.* No one wants ringbone, but most of the cases that I've seen over the years are no big deal; the horse isn't lame and the ringbone is hardly even detectable. I have had more than one person call and say, "My horse has ringbone. It wasn't there yesterday." Well, it was. It takes time for exostosis to develop; it doesn't just suddenly appear. These people weren't paying proper attention to their animals; be sure that you do.

Clinical Signs

Ringbone can occur in both the forelimbs and the hind limbs, but it is more common in the forelimbs. It can also be unilateral or bilateral. The cause is trauma. Ringbone occurs most commonly in older horses with straight pasterns, but it can also result from kicks and wire cuts. Outwardly, there is swelling around the fetlock and palpable bony enlargement. X-rays show bone growth on the phalanges and in the interphalangeal joints.

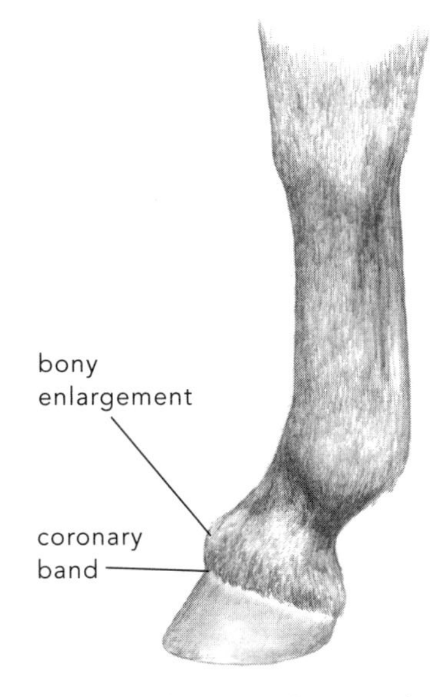

High ringbone with typical enlargement above the coronary band

Lameness is usually not present in nonarticular ringbone (I don't believe I've ever seen lameness in such cases) but is always evident in articular ringbone. When present, lameness is chronic and gets worse with time. If lameness is present in nonarticular ringbone, nonsteroidal anti-inflammatory drugs will make the horse usable.

Treatment

Treatment is difficult. Obviously, if a horse isn't lame nothing needs to be done. The exostosis (bone growth) will probably continue, however, so something needs to be done to control it. I've had luck using a combination of dimethyl sulfoxide (DMSO) and a steroid applied over the area.

If the horse is lame, the problem of treatment increases. In high articular ringbone, fusion of the joint works and the horse can usually return to full use. Low articular ringbone, however, is untreatable. Nonsteroidal anti-inflammatory drugs will help to control the pain, but basically you have an unusable horse. Fortunately, low articular ringbone is the least common type.

Developmental Orthopedic Disease

We have all seen developmental orthopedic disease (DOD) at one time or another, although most of us have never called it by its correct name. DOD is not just one condition; rather, it is a complex of problems (diseases, if you will) in growing horses.

Before I continue, I'll explain the process by which cartilage is converted to bone. Bones are lengthened by the laying down of cartilage in the area of the long bones called the *physis,* the growth plate. Eventually the cartilage turns to bone and growth ceases. (This is a greatly simplified explanation.)

DOD develops when this process of converting cartilage to bone is interfered with or altered. The main sources of interference are nutritional, genetic, and physical problems, such as trauma.

Such interference can produce fissures in articular cartilage, osteochondral fragments, cysts, delayed bone formation in the carpus (knee) or tarsus (hock), or angular limb deformity when growth is uneven. Three main syndromes result: angular limb deformities ("crooked foals"), physeal dysplasia (physitis, commonly but incorrectly called epiphysitis), and osteochondrosis (osteochondritis dessicans).

These are common problems in young horses. Carpal deformity is the one we see most frequently, but it also occurs in the fetlock and the tarsus.

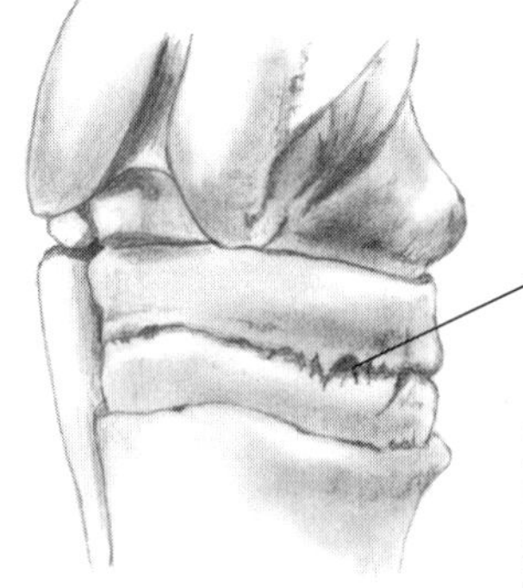

One of the three main syndromes of DOD is osteochondrosis (osteochondritis dessicans, or OCD), shown here in the hock.

Crooked Knees

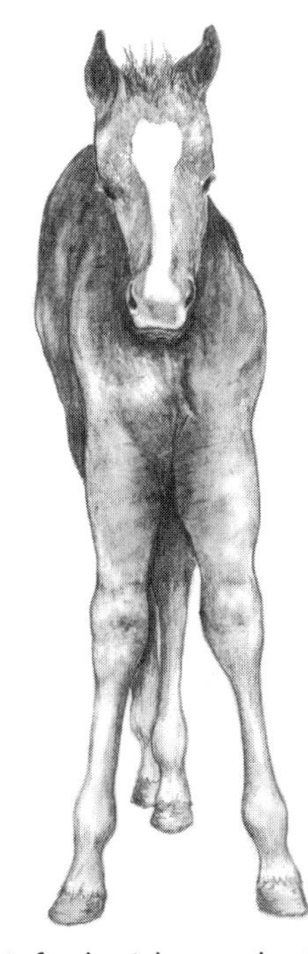

A foal with crooked knees (carpal deviation) is sometimes a candidate for periosteal elevation.

Crooked knees are subject to stresses that horses are not able to withstand, and injuries — even breakdowns — can occur, even among pleasure horses. Crooked legs are also a serious no-no in the conformation of show horses.

Once upon a time, a foal with crooked knees (carpal deviation) was written off as a loss or, at best, a liability. Some were even put down. Some of these crooked-legged foals would eventually straighten and some wouldn't, and no one knew which would be which. And we still don't. Those that didn't straighten, of course, became problems.

Diagnosis and Predisposing Factors

The fact that a foal is crooked is easily seen, but X-rays are necessary to determine the exact area of the problem. It is commonly believed that a "crooked knee" is a result of a problem in the growth area of the radius (the long bone from the shoulder to the knee), but it may well lie in the cuboidal bones of the knee. Only radiographs can reveal this.

Treatment

In carpal deviation, the degree of angulation determines the treatment. Angulation of fewer than five degrees is considered to be mild, between five and fifteen moderate, and greater than fifteen severe. Mild cases frequently resolve themselves with light, controlled exercise.

Because of the angulation of the leg, hoof wear is uneven. It is essential to rasp the feet frequently. *Frequently* does not mean every four to six weeks when the farrier comes; it means as often as twice a week but at least every two weeks.

Fetlock angulation also can often be corrected by frequent corrective trimming or rasping, but periosteal elevation and stapling may also be used (see below). Surgical success rates at the fetlock are lower because the growth plate here closes very early (by about three weeks). For surgical success here, correction must be done almost immediately.

Periosteal elevation. More than two decades ago, someone came up with the idea of hemicircumferential periosteal transection and stripping, more conveniently called *periosteal elevation* (PE). For any degree of angulation involving the radius, the bone just above the knee, periosteal elevation (PE) works wonders if done early, before rapid bone growth ends. (If the deviation is in the carpal bones, PE is of no use.)

This procedure requires general anesthesia and very minor surgery, but usually only once for each limb, and doesn't require placing and

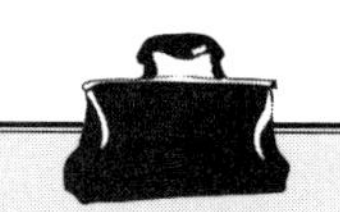

A Little History

Over the years, many corrective measures for crooked knees have been devised and tried. Corrective foot trimming was probably the first attempt to remedy the situation. It may have worked in some cases, but those were probably the ones that were going to straighten anyway. Even today, though, proper foot care is a necessary adjunct in correcting crooked legs.

Braces and splints probably came next, followed by casts. Maybe some of these worked, but those that straightened once again probably did so in spite of the external devices rather than because of them. And these strategies had the disadvantages of weakening the limbs and making it difficult or impossible for the foal to get up or lie down. Additionally, there was the possibility of abrading the prominent areas over the joints; severe ulcerations resulted in many cases.

In time, various surgical procedures were attempted, ranging from the simple and mostly ineffective to the bizarre, complicated, and mostly ineffective. My personal favorite was one that involved the removal of a wedge-shaped section of bone, turning it around, and then replacing it. I never saw it done, but I did see a drawing of it once. I suspect it's much easier to draw than it is actually to do.

leaving, albeit temporarily, any foreign objects within the foal. Unlike stapling (see below), PE is done on the short side of the deviation and on the radius above the growth plate. PE may also be done on crooked ankles, but it's trickier at this location and must be performed at a younger age because the growth plates in the ankles close earlier.

Timing. Timing is important here, too, but then timing is important in everything we do. PE must be done while there is still growth potential, but in the case of mild carpal deviation it can be delayed to see whether Mother Nature will handle it. In severe cases or those that seem to be worsening, surgical intervention should occur early, within the first month, when there is still ample growth potential. Those in between — the wide, gray area considered moderate deviation — require careful consideration and evaluation.

To wait or not to wait, that is the question. A good guideline to action is the degree of deviation. Five degrees or less, wait a while. Twenty-five degrees or more, hop on it as soon as possible. In between, PE will probably be needed, but don't be too hasty. I have successfully done foals as old as sixteen to eighteen weeks, but as a rule I think that's a little long to wait. I prefer about three weeks of age.

Limitations and prognosis. With PE, exercise must be limited because it aggravates and worsens the deviation. Because the deviation causes uneven hoof wear, the hooves must be correctively rasped regularly, perhaps weekly in severe cases. Even in mild cases, rasping should be done at intervals of no greater than two weeks.

Not all crooked knees respond to PE. It may be necessary to repeat the procedure six to eight weeks later, and it may also be necessary to staple some cases in conjunction with the second PE. But nothing is foolproof. Some won't straighten no matter what we do. And, conversely, I suspect that some we operate on, even severe cases, would have straightened in spite of what we did. Someday maybe we'll be able to predict both of these.

Transphyseal bridging. Transphyseal bridging, or "stapling," is also effective but is more invasive and more apt to leave telltale evidence or scarring than PE is. In this procedure, metal staples are placed in the radius across the lower growth plate (distal physis) on the long side of the deviation. The theory is that this will prevent growth on that side, while growth continues on the other side. And it usually works.

But the staples must be removed and the timing is critical. If they are left in too long, the joint will end up deviating the other way as the unstapled side continues to grow. Conversely, if the staples are removed too soon, correction will not be complete. It's necessary, then, to remove the staples just before the desired straightening is achieved. And the staples are often bears to get out. All of this has the disadvantage of requiring two general anesthesias and two invasive procedures.

Whichever method you choose, keep in mind that neither stapling nor PE is foolproof. I did both on a foal of my own, and he remained as crooked as ever. And he was the one that was going to pay the bank.

Physeal Dysplasia

Physeal dysplasia occurs in older foals and yearlings, usually being seen between four and five months and sixteen to eighteen months. The involved joints are "big" due to swelling in the growth areas. They are warm and often painful, and lameness will range from negligible to severe. Appearance and joint palpation will give the presumptive diagnosis, but X-rays are needed to verify it.

Treatment

If lameness is present, nonsteroidal anti-inflammatory drugs will ease the pain and reduce inflammation.

This is a mysterious condition, to me anyhow. It is generally accepted that it's a nutritional problem — too much or not enough of something. I think we veterinarians all agree on that. But if it *is* a nutritional problem, why are not all foals (at least all foals of the same approximate age) on a farm affected? A few years ago, a farm of forty-two foals had one four-month-old foal with physitis (physeal dysplasia). There were seven or eight other foals within a week (one way or the other) of this one's age and none of them was affected.

In any event, to properly evaluate the complete ration (hay, grain, pasture) you need an equine nutritionist. I don't feel that your average horse doctor is qualified to do this. (I may well receive hate mail for saying that.)

An older treatment once advocated by many and still used by some is to reduce both the amount of feed and the level of protein in the feed, usually accomplished by placing the affected animal in a dry lot. I don't recommend this approach because Mom is the main source of nutrition at this age, but it's based on the fact that a young foal may overeat on grass.

Osteochondrosis

Osteochondrosis results from a defect in the process of ossification of articular cartilage into bone. The cartilage thickens to a point where synovial fluid cannot supply proper nutrition to it and so it converts unevenly and poorly to bone, and the joint surface becomes uneven. Pieces of cartilage or bone then break off, causing pain and swelling.

Any joint may be involved but the usual culprits are the stifles, hocks, fetlocks, and shoulders. There may or may not be lameness but there is synovial effusion, or excess synovial fluid. Radiographs reveal most cases but not all. In those, arthroscopy is diagnostic.

Treatment

If loose bodies (cartilage or bone) are present, they must be surgically removed. If surgery is declined, stall rest until lameness and effusion stop is effective in some cases. The old treatment of injecting the affected joint(s) with corticosteroids is not recommended. Although they will provide transient relief, steroids actually speed up the degenerative process. In some cases, intra-articular hyaluronic acid is beneficial in affected joints that do not involve loose bodies.

It has been suggested that osteochondrosis, too, may result from nutritional deficiencies. This is supported by the fact that several young horses on one farm may be affected, but it isn't known (at least, I don't know) whether nutrition actually does enter into it.

Prognosis

This varies widely, depending on the articular damage, the joint(s) involved, the size and number of lesions or fragments, and how long the condition has existed. In general, osteochondrosis of the hock has a good prognosis, of the stifle fair to good, and of the shoulder fair to poor. These prognoses depend on successful surgery.

Splints

I don't know whether this next situation falls under the heading of DOD, but I think it must. I have seen nothing in the literature about it (which may only mean that I'm reading the wrong literature), but I have seen two cases and am unable to explain them fully.

I am talking about the occurrence of multiple splints in a young horse when there is no apparent reason for multiple (or even single) splints. The first case I saw began when a correctly conformed colt was about three months old. Three or four splints appeared on the medial aspect of both front cannon bones. By the time he was twelve months old, he had at least ten on both legs. Even his splints seemed to have splints.

The other one began with one splint at about six months. By the time he was a year old, he had four huge, definable splints on each front leg. By *huge,* I mean almost fist-sized. His conformation was good, also. In both cases there was heat but no or minimal lameness or pain on palpation. X-rays revealed typical splint lesions in both horses.

I assume these are nutritional in origin but in neither case were other foals on the farms affected. (See page 150 for more on splint bones.)

Racing or Training?

A question I'm frequently asked is, can a DOD horse ever race or train? Yes. I have seen horses with ankles that looked like a bunch of grapes, knees at right angles, and hocks that not only touched but actually rubbed each other race successfully (if not for long). I have also seen perfectly made horses without a pimple on them that had less than illustrious track careers.

Angular limb deformities, if corrected, seem to have no effect on whether a horse successfully races or trains. The same goes for non-racing animals: most are perfectly usable, but a few are not. And the same goes for physeal dysplasia. I am referring here to the majority of cases; someone can always point to affected horses that couldn't race or train.

Osteochondrosis is much more likely to prevent a horse from running or being a useful riding horse, especially since the problem is often undiagnosed until the horse is two or three years old. Both horses mentioned with multiple splints raced: one moderately well and one like most that I bet on.

Knee Fractures

BACK AROUND 1980, a three-year-old Thoroughbred colt blossomed in midyear. He didn't run in the Triple Crown races, but he ran in all the big races afterward and won most of them.

A major farm, one that already had about thirty-five top stallions, asked me to X-ray this colt's joints. The farm wanted to buy him, syndicate him, race him at four, and then retire him to stud. But first he had to pass my X-rays,

Well, I did X-ray him: his knees, his ankles, his hocks, his stifles. The hocks, hind ankles, and stifles were clean, except for normal wear and tear.

The fore ankles had evidence of old osselets (arthritis) and ringbone. There was a little bit of exostosis (extra bone growth) on one sesamoid bone. None of this was good, but it wasn't horrible, either.

But the knees! Oh, my goodness! Both knees had multiple chip fractures. Both had bone spurs on the carpal bones. The third carpal bone of the right knee had an old, apparently healed slab fracture, a fracture in which a large piece of bone is removed from the rest of the bone. There was no swelling anywhere on either knee.

The trainer said the horse had never taken a bad step. I found that hard to believe; in fact, I didn't believe it. I reported my findings to the farm that wanted to buy the colt, and I was asked my opinion. I said,

"There's no way this horse will stay sound for another year of racing." But I suggested that they get another opinion and left the X-rays. The other opinion was the same as mine. The horse wasn't bought.

The colt went on to race at four, won five more stakes races and another half-million dollars, and never took a bad step. Whenever I've seen the farm owner since then, he just shakes his head.

The books tell us that knee (carpal) fractures occur mostly in racing Thoroughbreds and I'm sure that's true. But I've seen them in a couple of Quarter Horses, a Tennessee Walking Horse, an American Saddlebred, an Appaloosa, three or four hunter/jumpers, and a couple of plain old pleasure horses, in addition to many Thoroughbreds, so I guess no horse is immune. And all of these others had the decency to be lame or have swelling or both, usually both.

Incidence and Causes

Most fractures of the carpal bones are small chips, sometimes no larger than a pencil point. Slab fractures, where a bone is broken into two pieces, are less common. Either knee may have fractures, but in racehorses in the United States, where racing is counterclockwise, it's the right knee that is most often affected. In countries where they race clockwise, it's usually the left knee.

The main cause of carpal fractures seems to be overextension of the joint during exercise. Horses that are back at the knee (from the side, the knee joint appears bent backward) — the worst of all conformational defects, in my opinion — are most susceptible to carpal fractures, as well as to all other carpal problems.

Clinical Signs and Treatment

The onset of lameness is acute, beginning at the time that the fracture occurs, and the severity of the lameness depends on the extent of the fracture(s). Swelling follows within a few hours. In the case of a slab fracture, the horse may not put weight on the leg.

If a chip is not displaced, stall rest may allow it to heal. If the chip is free, or if there are multiple chips, arthroscopic surgery is necessary to remove it/them. After surgery, stall confinement is needed for two to four weeks, followed by being turned out for three to six months. If there is no cartilage damage or arthritic changes, the prognosis for return to previous use is good.

In the case of a slab fracture, the two pieces must be screwed together, followed by six months out of use. The prognosis is the same as with chips.

But that three-year-old Thoroughbred colt was a decided exception to the rules I know about knee injury. Not only should he have been lame before I X-rayed him, he should have been forced to retire shortly thereafter. I guess he just didn't know it.

Carpal Canal Syndrome

I DON'T SEE MANY JUMPERS IN MY PRACTICE and, as I learned, most of the other veterinarians around here don't, either.

Many years ago, a young lady had me look at her jumper. She said he was slightly lame in the right fore. After watching him walk and trot I could see very little wrong with him, so I asked her to get on him. This caused him to be noticeably off, but still not much.

"Watch," she said, and she took him over two jumps.

He was off in the right fore — not much, but definitely off.

I was sure it wasn't his foot, so I flexed and extended the ankle but could elicit no abnormal response. I flexed his knee and he showed discomfort and I noticed a very slight swelling I had not noticed before. It was a little above the knee on the rear of the leg. This was the source of his lameness but I didn't know what the problem was. I told the client that I would have to check with another veterinarian because, even though I now knew where his problem was, I didn't know *what* it was.

This is when I learned that a whole lot of my local colleagues also didn't see many jumpers. I described the horse to several of them and none of them had any ideas. Finally, one said, "I think I can tell you," and he took me into his office where he got a book and looked through it. "Here it is," he said. "Carpal canal syndrome. I've never seen it."

Not only had I never seen it (before), I had never even heard of it. I didn't even know that horses had carpal canals. Maybe they told us in school, but if they did I missed it.

What Is Carpal Canal Syndrome?

Carpal canal syndrome (CCS) occurs mainly in jumpers as a result of trauma from landing repeatedly on a limb after a jump. It is uncommon in horses used for other purposes, but the occasional running horse will come up with it. It results from inflammation and pressure on the contents of the carpal canal, a complex anatomic structure bounded by the ligaments at the back of the carpus (knee), the protruding surface of the accessory carpal bone (the small bone at the back

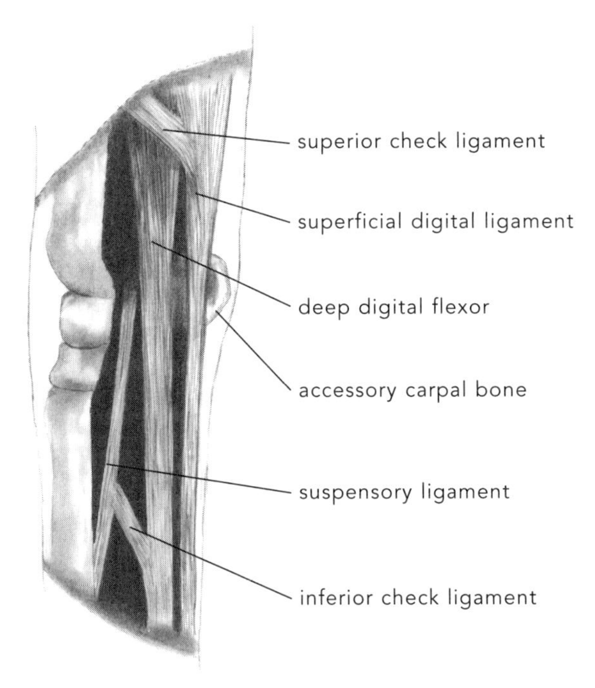

The carpal canal is a complex structure bounded by the ligaments at the back of the carpus (knee), the protruding surface of the accessory carpal bone (the small bone at the back of the knee), and the thick fascia where the ligaments and tendons attach to the back of the knee.

of the knee), and the thick fascia where the ligaments and tendons attach to the back of the knee.

Lameness occurs when trauma to any of these structures results in compression of the soft tissue structures lying within the canal. CCS is occasionally secondary to fracture of the accessory carpal bone. Another cause worth mentioning, although uncommon, is improper bandaging of the knee that puts pressure on the accessory carpal bone.

Clinical Signs

The lameness can range from acute and severe to progressive, insidious, and chronic. Diagnosis is based on clinical signs, which include pain on flexion and swelling at the back of the leg just above the knee. Ultrasound and X-ray help to determine where the problem is.

Treatment

The pressure on the contents of the carpal canal can be relieved in some cases by cutting and removing an elliptical strip of the annular ligament on the inside of the knee. Whether this will be sufficient to allow the horse to resume jumping (or whatever) can only be learned by doing it. Nonsteroidal anti-inflammatory drugs such as phenylbutazone may also be helpful.

The client couldn't afford surgery, so her horse was put on phenylbutazone. It helped for a while, but the lameness eventually worsened and he was turned into a pet. He was okay, but not fully sound when not being ridden.

Since then I have seen two more cases of CCS. Surgery was performed on one (it's surprisingly easy to do) and the horse responded well. The other had been allowed to go too long before the owner had him examined and he had to be retired from usage.

All three have involved the right knee. I don't know if that has significance or is just coincidental. Perhaps they were all right-legged jumpers?

Bone Spavin

Quite often in Western movies, someone will refer to a horse as "spavined." Whenever I hear that I try to get a look at the horse's hocks, camera-angle permitting. On those rare occasions when I do get a good look at the hocks, the horse isn't spavined. It's very disillusioning and enough to cause a guy to disbelieve the entire plot line.

In my experience, back pain in horses is uncommon. Several times owners or trainers have told me that their horses were "back sore," and I have never really known what that meant. And in all but a few I could never demonstrate any problems with the horses' backs.

One is memorable. There was definitely a pain response to simple manual pressure in the lumbar region. Moreover, he also responded to pressure on the gluteal muscles on both sides, but the response was much more pronounced on the left.

He was an eight-year-old gelding of mixed ancestry and was used for trail riding. He was one of four horses owned by a family of trail riders, and all of their horses were fit and well conditioned.

I asked about the possibility of an injury. Had he been *cast,* that is, trapped against a wall in his stall while rolling and unable to get up without help? Had he fallen? Had something fallen on him? The answers were all no.

The principal rider of the horse was the mother of the family. When I admitted my ignorance of the possible cause of his back soreness, she said, "His back hurts him so much he's actually lame in his rear."

Aha! Why didn't she say so before?

I had her trot him on their driveway, both away from me and then in a circle. As he trotted away, his left foot pulled a little inward as it went up and then he slapped it down quickly and it went slightly outward on its downward path. In the circle trot, the arc of the left foot was a bit shorter than the arc of the right foot, but neither arc appeared to be as high as it should have been. On closer examination, the toes of both feet were worn, slightly more on the left.

I was pretty sure it was bone spavin.

What Is Bone Spavin?

Bone spavin, technically osteoarthrosis of the distal tarsal joints (cartilage covering the jointed surfaces of bones breaks down and underlying bone becomes thickened and distorted), is probably the most common source of hind limb lameness in horses. The actual cause is uncertain, but it's usually seen in sickle-hocked or cow-hocked individuals. This horse was slightly sickle-hocked.

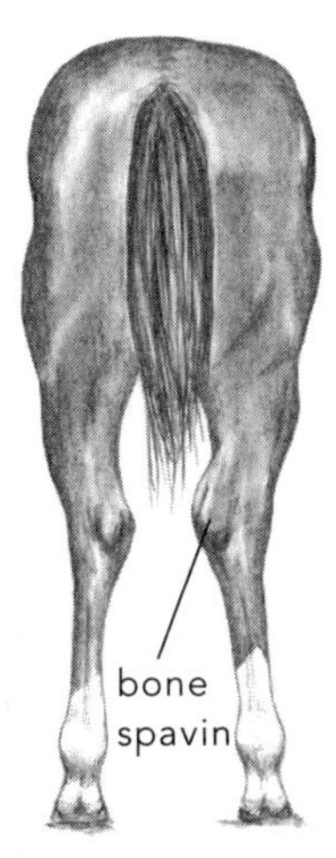

Bone spavin shown in cow-hocked individual

Diagnosis

I performed a spavin test, which involves hyperflexion of the hock. The foot is lifted, pulled straight forward, and held for ninety seconds. This seems more like ninety minutes, as the horse usually complies by giving the holder his full weight.

When the leg is released, the horse is again trotted off. If it is bone spavin, the lameness is increased. It was in this case. The spavin test, regardless of its name, isn't specific for spavin (the pain could be in the hip or stifle), but when added to the other signs, I was convinced that this horse had bone spavin, at least of the left hock and probably of both. (This is a challenging topic to write about; my stupid computer keeps telling me that *spavin* isn't a word. It just did it again.)

Bone spavin is usually present in both hind legs, so the next step was to X-ray both hocks. The X-rays of the left hock showed moderate new bone growth around the distal tarsal joints. There was also new bone growth in the right hock, but it was only a small amount. This is often a visible enlargement and it is what the cowboys see when they call a horse "spavined." I doubt if the scriptwriters know that.

The final step (the next day) was to inject the hocks with a small amount of local anesthetic. If he became more sound (but perhaps not completely so) afterward, it proved bone spavin. He went perfectly sound in fifteen minutes.

Other Clinical Signs

In addition to the signs mentioned previously, many horses are presented for examination with a history of performance alteration: refusing jumps, inappropriate lead changes, wide turns, among other things. The back pain apparent in this case is not a constant finding.

Also, the lameness may be very mild or severe. X-rays may show no bony changes or they may show joint narrowing, irregular joint widening, subchondral cysts just below the surface, or several other abnormalities. The prognosis for bone spavin is good once the joints have fused. This will usually occur naturally eventually, but it is a long and painful process.

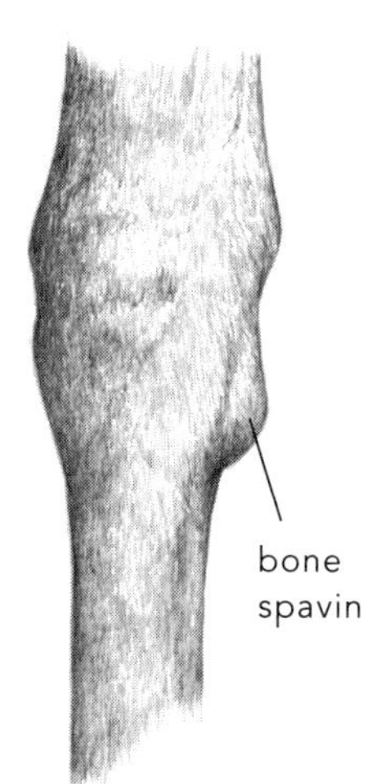

Frontal view of bone spavin on inside of right hock

Treatment

Now it was time to treat him, which turned out to be a fiasco. I started him on nonsteroidal anti-inflammatory drugs and they helped a little, but only a little. We tried this approach for about ten days before it was apparent that the drugs were not going to do the job.

So then I injected the hocks with hyaluronic acid. In retrospect, with the changes seen on the X-rays, I shouldn't have used it and it didn't do a bit of good.

Next I injected both hocks with a long-acting corticosteroid and this worked — for about two weeks. I had been hoping for six months.

I had been working on this horse for more than a month now and my ineffectual treatments had cost the owner a bunch of money. It was time to hit the books or talk with another veterinarian, so I did both. Both the books and the vet said performing a cunean tenectomy (severing the cunean tendon) was a possibility, but both also said that its effectiveness is questionable.

Both also said that fusion of the distal tarsal joints would do the job. It's a surgical procedure that I had never done, but I talked it over with the owner and she wanted it performed, so I referred the horse to the other veterinarian and he did it. I watched the procedure and if I ever encounter another case, I will refer it, too. It's a toughie.

In about six weeks the horse was being ridden with no pain and in six months he was out on the trails again.

Many horses with mild bone spavin respond favorably to non-steroidal anti-inflammatory drugs, hyaluronic acid, and other treatments. Intra-articular, long-acting corticosteroids usually give four to six months of relief, but subsequent injections don't last as long. The steroids may hasten natural joint fusion, however. Chemical joint fusion has been reported as being successful, but I have no experience with it.

Stress Fractures

Most of the horses I work on are Thoroughbreds and they are, or were, racehorses. But I have and do work on other breeds, and while stress fractures are commonly associated with young racing animals, the first case I ever saw was in a Quarter Horse barrel racer.

What Is a Stress Fracture?

A stress fracture is damage to a bone as a result of repetitive activity. It most commonly occurs in horses that are in intense levels of exercise, usually racehorses. A stress fracture can occur in the long bones, pelvis, scapula, or vertebrae.

Stress fractures occur largely because of what humans ask horses to do. In nature, stress fractures are probably pretty rare because horses do what they want to do when they want to, with no extra weight on their backs. True, they occasionally must exert a short burst of speed to escape from a hungry carnivore, but once they escape (or don't, as the case may be), the running ceases and they return to the basics of life: eating, drinking, reproducing, standing majestically on the horizon, and other such activities.

Similarly, pleasure or show horses are less likely to suffer stress fractures because they are not asked to maintain excessive speed for prolonged periods while carrying weight that Mother Nature never intended. But they do happen.

So, as in the case of so many problems that horses endure, we who characterize ourselves as horse lovers create stress fractures.

Equine bone was designed to perform its services for horses in the wild: to carry them from here to there, to let them romp and play for short periods, to run rapidly for a short distance to elude a hungry lion. It was never designed to carry 100 to 150 pounds over distances ranging from a quarter mile to several miles at a sustained speed and often over obstacles. Bone is very adaptive and given time will change, or remodel, to accept these demands. But the key word here is *time.*

With proper and patient training, bone will remodel to the use placed on it, but if the remodeling is not allowed to occur, the result is a stress fracture.

An important consideration that is all too often overlooked or ignored (or just plain not known) is that bone, once remodeled, can "demodel" when a horse is removed from training for a period of time. Thus, a horse that is laid up or one that is turned out for a refresher must be treated as a raw beginner when returned to training.

Clinical Signs

Stress fractures are generally thought of as occurring in young horses early in training, but they may occur at any age, and older horses turned out for the winter (or whatever) are especially susceptible to them.

But there is relatively good news if your horse comes up with a stress fracture: the prognosis in most cases, if caught early and handled properly, is good to excellent for a full return to training.

Which bones are most likely to be affected by stress fractures? That's a good question. None of the veterinary books in my library lists the affected bones in order of occurrence of stress fractures, so I will simply discuss them from the ground up.

- **Cannon bone.** A horse with a stress fracture of the third metacarpus (front cannon bone) or third metatarsus (hind cannon bone) has mild to severe lameness on one side. Palpation will help to determine the area of involvement, but X-rays are essential. Scintigraphy and ultrasonography can also help to diagnose and monitor stress fractures here and elsewhere.

Surgery is occasionally necessary in these cases, but in most cases all that is needed is six to twelve weeks of stall rest, with the progress of healing monitored by periodic X-rays.

- **Radius.** Stress fractures of the radius, the leg bone above the knee, are difficult to diagnose. The horse can't bear weight on the limb, and the lameness may appear to resolve itself with two or three days of stall rest. An incorrect diagnosis of a muscle pull or strain is often made. These stress fractures can be diagnosed by X-ray, but often the problem is not apparent early. Thus, follow-up X-rays at two- or three-week intervals are essential.

Stall rest for four to six weeks, monitored by X-rays, is usually sufficient to allow healing, and the horse may be hand walked after the first two or three weeks.

- **Tibia.** Stress fractures of the tibia, the heavy bone above the hock in the horse's hind leg, are a common cause of acute lameness, especially in young horses in training. As with the radius, these are hard to diagnose. There is a weight-bearing lameness shortly after exercise but by the next day the lameness is apparently gone. Within a few days, the horse is again sound at a trot, but the lameness returns when he is asked for a quicker gait.

There is a tibial torsion test that is supposed to aid in diagnosis, but it involves simultaneously pushing and pulling various joints in the affected limb and many perfectly sound horses care little for this. It has been of little use in my experience, but it must work for someone because it continues to be described in the literature. In my experience, X-rays are much more helpful in making a diagnosis.

Again, rest is the treatment: four to sixteen weeks, depending on the site of the fracture and any complications. Recurrence is uncommon in young animals but does occur in some older horses.

- **Ilium.** Injury to the ilium, which forms the point of the hip in the

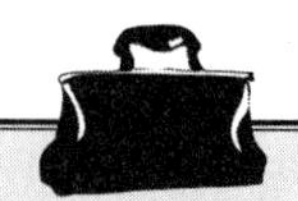

Bone Remodeling

For a long, long time, maybe hundreds of years, we have understood the advantages of proper training in preparing the cardiovascular, respiratory, and muscular systems for extreme physical exercise. Only within the last twenty years or so, however, have we become aware of the fact that bone adapts, too, and that proper training is as important for bone as it is for the other body systems.

On postmortem exams researchers noticed that the bones of horses not being trained for athletic undertakings differed from those of horses of the same ages that were being trained. Further investigation re-vealed that the bones actually changed, or remodeled, with exercise, becoming thicker and stronger in the areas of greater stress. This is a slow process, of course, and the speed of change varies, not much, but some, between horses.

Fractures are the main cause of fatalities in racehorses and other horses in athletic competition, being responsible for perhaps as many as two-thirds of all deaths in horses in hard physical competition. Some of these are the result of direct trauma, but many more are stress fractures, the result of high-speed exercise on bones not ready for high-speed exercise. And on top of outright fractures, many, many more horses lose training time due to conditions such as bucked shins, which are also the result of high-speed exercise on young bones not yet remodeled or ready for such strenuous activity.

While a horse — or a basketball player or a ballerina or any athlete — is being trained, its bones are being damaged by microfractures, but at the same time they are being remodeled. In many horses, it's a race between the two processes.

All of this doesn't take into consideration the horse's conformation and disposition, the fatigue factor, a bad step, and other factors. These things are going to happen but they can be minimized. To reduce the risk of fractures, train gradually, progressively, and consistently to maintain bone health. As with so many things in life, time, patience, and luck are the keys.

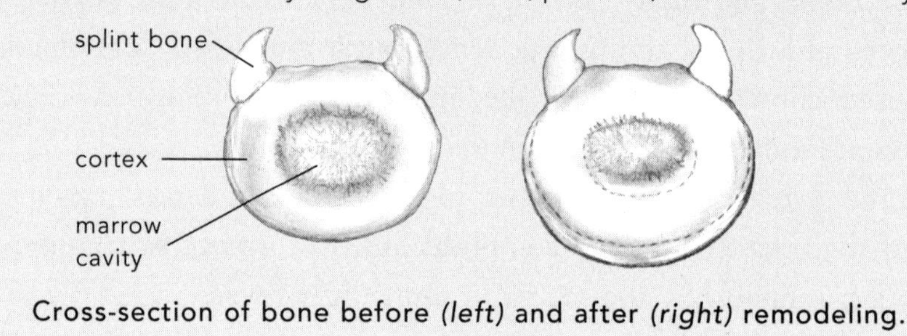

Cross-section of bone before *(left)* and after *(right)* remodeling.

hind leg, is a gradually occurring fracture seen most commonly in young horses. A horse appears to be off in his rear and then suddenly develops an acute lameness. It may be on one side or both, and the pelvic area is moderately to severely painful when palpated. X-rays are of little use, but ultrasound is very helpful.

Stall rest for a minimum of three months and up to six months is necessary, and progress should be monitored by ultrasound.

- **Humerus.** A stress fracture to the humerus, at the shoulder in the front leg, results in weight-bearing lameness characterized by shortened stride and toe dragging. Lameness disappears with two or three days of rest but returns when exercise resumes. X-rays aid in diagnosis.

Stall rest for six to eight weeks should allow healing to occur, and radiographic monitoring is necessary.

Prevention

One way to prevent stress fractures, or at least make them less common, is good management. The bones must be conditioned over a period of gradual training. This allows remodeling in response to the slowly increasing levels of work. It is recommended that bone be given time to adapt to a gait before progressing to the next, more demanding gait. Those who have studied stress fractures and bone suggest thirty days at one gait before moving on to the next.

Horses are not all the same, however, and any lameness or gait alteration must be thoroughly checked out, because a minor stress fracture can develop into a complete fracture if ignored.

The Quarter Horse mentioned earlier with the first stress fracture I ever saw was not the usual case. He was a six- or seven-year-old gelding, a little old for a stress fracture, and he had a fracture of the humerus. He was kept in a stall (which he did not like) for twelve weeks, but he healed just fine and eventually returned to barrel racing as if nothing had ever happened. Since that time I have seen more than a dozen cases, and only one needed surgery.

Splint Bones

The splint bones are the vestigial second and fourth metacarpal (front) and metatarsal (rear) bones. The splint bones add support and stabilization to the bones of the knee and hock (the carpus and the tarsus, respectively). Most horses never have a problem with them, but if you must have a leg issue, this is the one of choice because the prognosis is generally good.

Clinical Signs

Splint problems occur primarily in the front legs. Usually it's the medial splint bone that's involved. Splint problems occur in all types of conformation, but a horse with offset knees is the most likely candidate. A horse will show varying degrees of acute lameness, depending on whether it's a fractured splint or merely a "popped" splint. In either case, there is heat over the area and swelling that is tender to the touch.

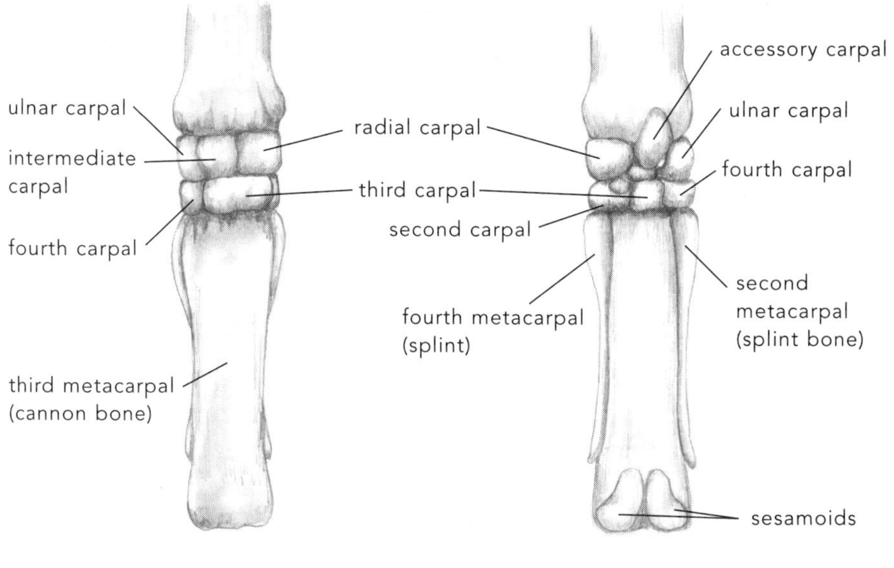

SPLINT BONES

The first thing to do when swelling appears over a splint bone, assuming that your veterinarian isn't there at the time, is to ice it and apply a pressure bandage over it. This will reduce inflammation and prevent any further enlargement and possibly even reduce it (but not cure it). Be sure to call your veterinarian so X-rays can be taken to determine whether it's a fracture or a popped splint.

A popped splint is the result of stress exerted on the bone from exercise; the splint bone tears loose from the cannon (third metacarpal) bone. It usually occurs in the lower third of the bone, but it may happen anywhere in its length. Nutritional causes have been proposed; a mineral imbalance or deficiency may also be possible. A fractured splint occurs in the same way, but it can result from trauma (a kick, for instance). A fracture is also possible when a cast horse struggles to get up.

Treatment

If it's a fracture, removal of the portion of the splint bone below the fracture site must be done surgically. If it's a low fracture, it's a simple procedure that can be done under tranquilization and local anesthesia and no hospitalization is necessary. If the fracture occurs high on the splint, the procedure becomes more difficult and requires general anesthesia. In some cases it is elected to allow the bone to heal, which takes several weeks, during which time exercise must be stopped. A cast will help protect the area.

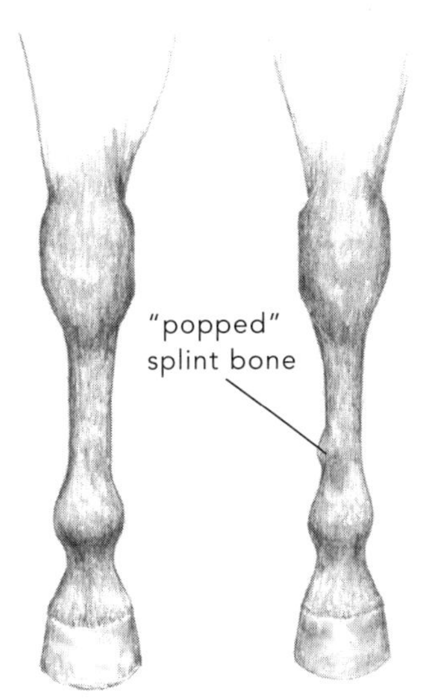

When a splint bone is popped or fractured, the area is warm, swollen, and tender.

If it's not a fracture, ice, pressure bandages, nonsteroidal anti-inflammatory drugs, and rest will combine to resolve the popped splint. An enlargement will probably remain, but it will no longer be tender and there will be no lameness.

The prognosis is good to excellent for return to full use in either case.

Capped Elbow

A TRAINER I KNEW ONLY SLIGHTLY CAME UP TO ME at the track one morning. "Doc Kelley, I got a horse with hygroma of the elbow. Can you come see her?" he said.

Hygroma of the elbow? What the heck is that? I thought.

"Sure, Johnny, I'll be over as soon as I finish here," I responded. I was worming twelve horses for another trainer.

When Johnny left, I asked the trainer whose horses I was worming, "Buck, what's hygroma of the elbow?"

"Never heard of it, Doc. I was fixin' to ask you."

I finished worming and went to my car, not sure what I needed to get to treat a condition that I had never heard of before. Parked next to mine was another veterinarian's car. He was just returning to it so I asked him, "Jim, what's hygroma of the elbow?"

"What's what?"

I repeated the name of the condition.

"I never heard of it," Jim said. "Let me see if I can find it in here," and he pulled a book from his backseat.

There it was: "Hygroma of the elbow, also known by the lay terms 'shoe boil' and 'capped elbow.'" All my life I had called the condition *capped elbow,* although I knew that some people referred to it as *shoe boil.* I guess I knew it had a "real" name, but I had never thought about it. We both learned something that day.

I went to Johnny's barn. "Let's see that hygroma," I said.

He brought out a two-year-old filly with a swelling the size of a softball on her left elbow. I lanced it, installed a Penrose drain, and told him I'd see the horse again tomorrow.

What Is Capped Elbow?

A capped elbow is a fluid-filled subcutaneous swelling at the point of the elbow seen almost exclusively in stabled horses. It's a result of trauma, usually believed to be caused by a shoe hitting it (hence "shoe boil") when the horse is lying down.

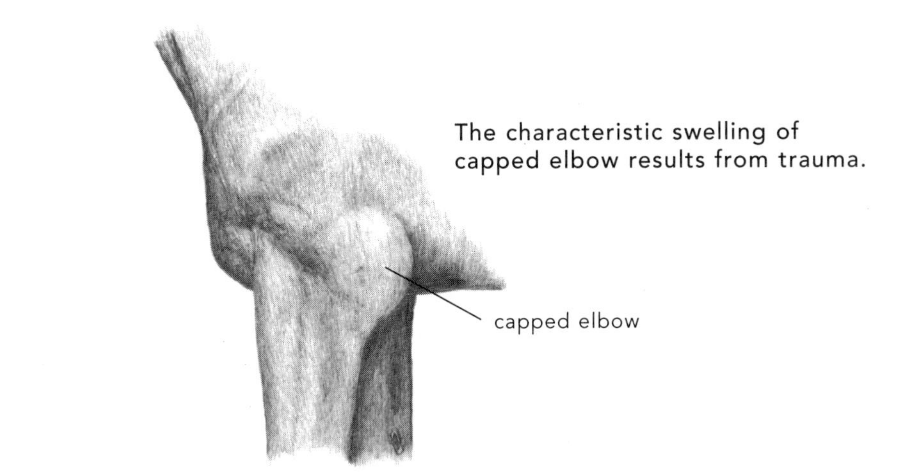

The characteristic swelling of capped elbow results from trauma.

Clinical Signs and Treatment

Capped elbow is very common. I imagine that I've seen dozens over the years. In my experience, it's usually in a young (yearling to three-year-old) horse, though I've seen it in all ages. There is no lameness involved; in fact, it isn't even sore to the touch. If allowed to become chronic, however, fibrous tissue will form within it and then it becomes a problem to treat. Opening the sac and installing a drain for five to seven days usually takes care of it.

If treated early, the prognosis is good. If allowed to become chronic, the fibrous mass must be surgically excised and healing is hard to achieve. There is no way to predict which horses will develop capped elbow, so prevention is difficult, unless you don't let the horse lie down. If a horse develops capped elbow, call your veterinarian.

Locked Stifle

In a period of about two weeks shortly after I got out of school, I was called to see five animals, three ponies and two horses, that dragged one hind foot when first coming out of their stalls in the morning. In a short time, I became proficient at diagnosing and treating what has turned out to be a pretty common affliction. I would estimate that I have seen, over the years, fifty horses of various sizes and uses suffer from locked stifle, or upward fixation of the patella.

It is commonly known that horses can sleep standing on their feet. (I never mastered that but I became quite skilled at sleeping with my eyes open, especially in history and political science classes.) The way they accomplish this is very interesting, albeit highly improbable, and involves the mechanisms of the stifles.

When a horse wishes to rest its hind limbs, it extends those limbs. The patella then elevates to the top of the femoral trochlea and the medial patellar ligament hooks over the medial ridge of the trochlea, thereby locking the joint and allowing the horse to rest the limbs and sleep without falling. (Personally, I think a horse that sleeps lying down is better rested, and horses do tend to sleep lying down during deep sleep.) To reverse this procedure and regain the ability to flex the stifle, the quadriceps femoris muscle contracts, lifting the medial patellar ligament free of the medial trochlear ridge. Then the muscle relaxes and allows the patella to return to its working position.

Sometimes, however, circumstances prevent or hinder the horse's ability to release the stifle. The severity of locked stifle ranges from mild or intermittent cases, which are readily released by a little manipulation or even go unnoticed, to a total lock of the joint that cannot be released.

Incidence and Predisposing Factors

In the literature, it's said that locked stifle generally affects both sides, with one side possibly being more involved than the other, but I have seen it mostly unilaterally. Young horses in poor condition and ponies seem to be the most frequent candidates, but it occurs in both sexes of all breeds. Horses that have been in training and then are forced to undergo prolonged stall rest are susceptible; the resulting loss of condition and muscle tone can lead to upward fixation of the patella.

There are four known causes of upward fixation of the patella: excessively straight hind legs; poor body condition leading to loss in size of the retropatellar fat pad, which keeps the patella away from the underlying end of the femur; poor coordination involving the flexor and extensor muscles of the stifle; and heredity. I think it can also result

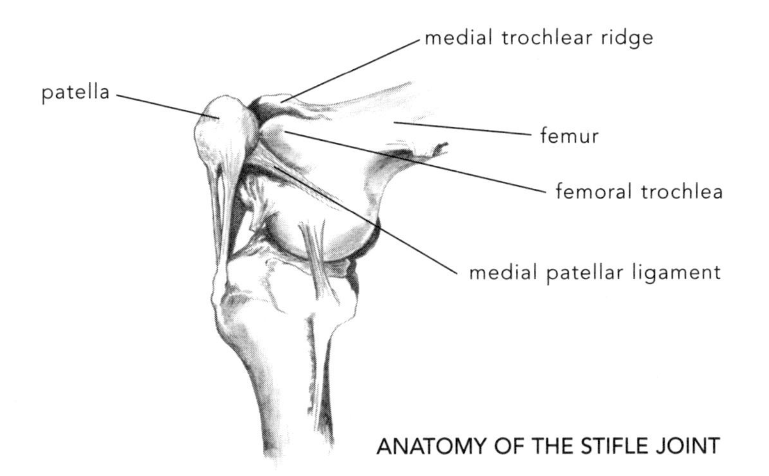

ANATOMY OF THE STIFLE JOINT

when a standing, sleeping horse is startled. This, in my opinion, can cause stretching of the medial patellar ligament as the horse tries to free the patella more quickly than it would normally. This stretching makes it more difficult to release in the future because elasticity is diminished.

Clinical Signs

The signs can vary significantly. In many cases, the actual locking may never be observed. Excessive wear on a rear toe is a clue that it may be occurring because whenever a step is taken with the stifle locked, the toe will be dragged for a step or two. In others, it may occur transiently when the horse first takes a step, then spontaneously resolve. In other cases, the duration of the lock may be a minute or two to a few hours to forever.

The main sign is the affected limb extending backward and not flexing. There is only one condition that can be mistaken for locked stifles: luxation of the coxofemoral joint. In luxation, however, the limb is stiff, *not* extended backward, which is diagnostic for locked stifle.

Treatment

Treatment, regardless of severity, is relatively simple. In young, out-of-condition horses, feed and exercise will take care of it in most cases, unless the horse is genetically or conformationally predisposed to the condition.

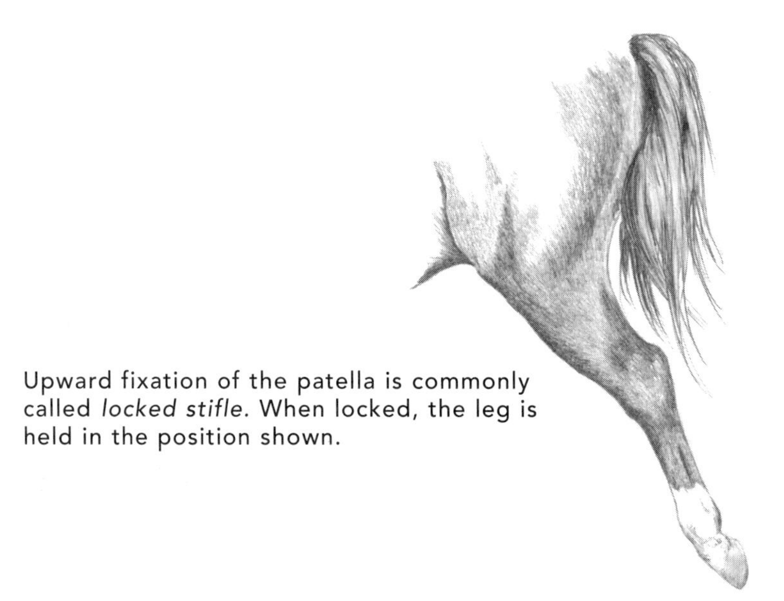

Upward fixation of the patella is commonly called *locked stifle.* When locked, the leg is held in the position shown.

In a horse that must be stalled for a prolonged period, deep bedding and/or shoeing with raised heels reduces the likelihood of upward fixation of the patella.

In those horses in which ready release does not come, backing the animal will usually bring about release. In more stubborn cases, it has been suggested that release can be attained by manually pushing the patella upward. The guy who can do this can also leap tall buildings in a single bound; it has never worked for me.

Another suggested treatment is the injection of both the medial and the middle patellar ligaments with a counterirritant. This is difficult as the dickens to do, does not always work, and is rarely a permanent cure in the ones in which it does work.

The cure — the one that works, and works forever — is surgery. It's a very simple surgery: the medial patellar ligament is sectioned (i.e., cut). It is performed on the standing, tranquilized horse with a local anesthetic. After surgery, the horse needs four to six weeks of stall rest and then a gradual increase of exercise. In those cases where the locking becomes chronic and is severe, surgery is mandatory because in time damage to the stifle joint is inevitable.

Prognosis

The prognosis varies with the severity of the condition and the method of treatment. Joint damage may reduce the use of the horse. In mild, transient cases that spontaneously resolve, the prognosis is good. In the cases that recur frequently or require outside help to unlock the stifle, the prognosis is not as good for continued performance at a normal level. In permanent upward fixation of the patella, the prognosis is poor without surgery. With surgery it is good, as are all other cases with surgery.

The only disadvantage — and I do not consider it to be one — to surgery is the horse can no longer sleep on its feet. I wish there had been a simple procedure to keep me from sleeping with my eyes open in my poli-sci and history classes.

No, I don't. I needed the rest.

Sacroiliac Lameness

My older brother showed American Saddlebreds from the time he was twelve years old or so until he got out of college about ten years

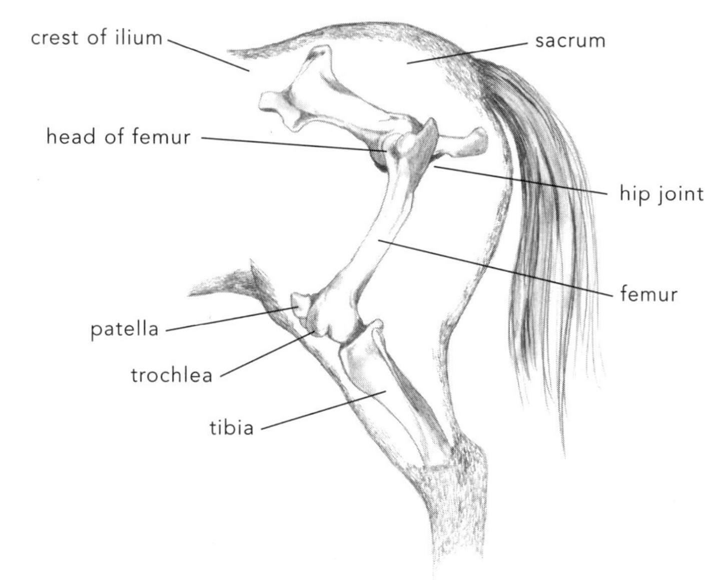

ANATOMY OF THE SACROILIAC AREA OF THE HORSE'S HIND LEG

later. For several years, he had a five-gaited gelding named Cap'n in Command. I was just a little kid, maybe eight or nine, when he got him. I liked Cap; he was sweet and gentle and loved sugar cubes.

I remember that Cap was made to stay in his stall for about three months one year and then he wasn't ridden for another three months. The veterinarian had told my brother that he had a sacroiliac injury. I had no idea what that was, but it sounded bad. After the six months, Cap went back to being shown and he was as good as ever.

There are those who say that sacroiliac problems don't occur. It's a strong joint and essentially immovable. Others, however, insist that the sacroiliac area can be a source of lameness. Since I've been a vet, several people have told me that they have horses with sacroiliac problems. I suppose veterinarians diagnosed them.

Clinical Signs

Lameness that is identified as sacroiliac in origin usually involves only one hind leg and is usually mild but unremitting. Pain cannot be elicited in any conventional manner of testing, and pain relievers do little to improve the situation. How injury occurs, if indeed it does, is uncertain. Torsion is suggested, perhaps from being cast in the stall or from having one hind leg pulled in a way that creates uneven stress on the area. Links to trauma are difficult if not impossible to prove.

Arthritis can also contribute to sacroiliac lameness. Arthritis of the sacroiliac joint is manifested as a sore back, a shortened stride in the rear, and a reluctance to move, depending on the extent of the arthritis.

Diagnosis and Treatment

Diagnosis is by the Sherlock Holmes approach: eliminate everything else and whatever is left must be it. Treatment is basically what was done for Cap: time and rest. Six months is recommended. Because the horse gets better, however, does in no way mean that the problem was in the sacroiliac area. Time and rest do wonders for many things.

Once the horse has recovered, it can be used as it was before. But I'm not saying that sacroiliac lameness actually happens. I know that

I've never diagnosed it, although I freely admit that there have been lamenesses that I was unable to pinpoint and my recommended course of therapy was time and rest.

Nuclear Scintigraphy

It's a good thing that there are a lot of folks out there who are smarter than I am, because otherwise we wouldn't have a whole lot of things that we now take for granted: television, airplanes, computers, frozen peas — the list is long. Heck, we probably wouldn't even have indoor plumbing.

We sure wouldn't have nuclear scintigraphy, which is a diagnostic technique based on the detection of a radiolabeled phosphate compound in bone and soft tissue. The compound is injected intravenously; after passing through the vascular and extravascular fluids, it's taken up by the mineral matrix of bone. The radiation emitted by the compound as it appears in the bone is then detected by a gamma camera. Your run-of-the-mill veterinarian, such as I am, will not have this machine. Some universities and racetracks do.

There are five accepted musculoskeletal indications for the diagnostic use of scintigraphy.

1. To evaluate areas of lameness when X-rays don't reveal the cause.
2. To evaluate multiple sites when the site of lameness can't be determined.
3. To examine the axial skeleton and upper limbs.
4. To determine developing orthopedic problems.
5. To follow the healing process after injury, surgical repair, or both, as an aid in determining prognosis.

In any kind of horse training, both bone damage and bone remodeling occur (see page 148 for box on bone remodeling). The normal result is adaptation of bone density and bone architecture to exercise. An imbalance between the two processes can result in bone damage and, therefore, lameness. Using nuclear scintigraphy, the radiolabeled compound is detected in higher levels in damaged areas.

Scintigraphic examination can reveal areas where problems may develop before there is actual lameness. Usually a period of reduced exercise is all that is indicated, and further scintigraphic exams will reveal when a return to normal limits may be reached.

Right now, scintigraphy isn't available in the field; the cost of the necessary equipment is more than most veterinarians can even dream about. But it is available, even though you have to take your horse to it. It's not for everyone yet, but someday it will be more widely available.

Part III
Breeding and Foaling

The hows and whys of producing new horses
(so veterinarians have plenty to do)

6

Breeding Issues

Fertilization and Fetal Development

That foal you have out there in the paddock began in a most incredible manner: fertilization. (For that matter, so did the grass it's eating and you and everything else organic.) Fertilization is the combination of two cells (a sperm and an ovum) to form the first cell of a new individual. This part seems pretty simple when you compare it to what ensues over the rest of gestation.

None of it is simple, though. Timing is extremely important in getting the sperm and the egg together. Ideally, in horses (we'll ignore you and the grass for the rest of this discussion), the sperm is placed in the uterus within twenty-four hours of the time ovulation occurs, but there is a wide range here. It's generally agreed that stallion sperm is viable for forty-eight hours in the uterus (hence the refusal to allow your problem mare a second breeding the next day), and there are cases of pregnancy occurring when the mare didn't ovulate for up to six days post-breeding.

Though many argue to the contrary, the sperm can be introduced post-ovulation, although the later that breeding takes place after ovulation, the lower the chance that fertilization will occur. Breeding within four to six hours after ovulation is generally successful.

Once the sperm is placed in the uterus, it must travel the length of the uterine horn and enter the oviduct, down which the egg travels. Here the sperm and egg meet, in the upper third of the oviduct, where fertilization occurs.

The fact that the egg is there to meet sperm is pretty miraculous. In fact, ovulation doesn't seem to be a particularly well-thought-out process. The egg is released from the follicle on the ovary into the mare's body cavity. From here, it's up to the oviduct to find it and pick it up, which it generally does. It's a chemical/hormonal thing, but personally I don't see how it ever happens.

Anyhow, the egg going down the oviduct meets a sperm coming up the oviduct, and fertilization takes place. Now there is only one cell, the fertilized egg. At twenty to twenty-four hours, the first cell division occurs, and subsequent divisions follow at about twelve-hour intervals. All this is occurring in the oviduct, but as it divides and increases, the growing structure is traveling downward toward the uterus, which it normally reaches six days after ovulation. Your future champion is called a *blastocyst* at this point. Once within the uterus, movement doesn't stop. The blastocyst continues to migrate. Somewhere along the way it can safely be called an *embryo*. Eventually, this embryo comes to rest in one of the uterine horns, usually near the body of the uterus, and attachment takes place. But a whole lot occurs before that.

For one thing, the little guy is sort of on his own. The mare has supplied a place for him (or, actually, "it"; sex hasn't yet been determined), but she isn't nourishing him, nor will she fully for several weeks. The yolk sac develops around the tenth day post-ovulation and this nourishes the early embryo, but it's gone by about day forty. At that point, early implantation begins and endometrial glandular secretions, which are directly absorbed by the chorionic surface of the early placenta, supply nutrition. The fetus, in fact, isn't fully supported by the uterus until completion of the formation of the microcotyledons (fingerlike interlockings of embryonic membranes and uterine endometrium) at about 150 days. There are thousands of these formed between the uterine endometrium and the chorion, and they make large molecule transfer to the fetus possible.

Landmarks in fetal development are shown in the accompanying chart. At what point the developing foal ceases being an "embryo" and becomes a "fetus" is something about which not all agree. Some sources state that it's a fetus at day twenty-three because internal organs are recognizable; others say day thirty, because evidence of gonad differentiation is found; still others say it's a gradual transition roughly from day forty to day sixty, because during this time the embryo becomes recognizable as a future horse and not, say, a musk ox or a hyena. Take your pick; I'll go with day forty.

The parts of the placenta are, from outside to inside: the chorion, the thick, heavy "bag" that is the first thing presented at foaling; the allantoic space, where urinary waste is deposited; the amnion, the thin

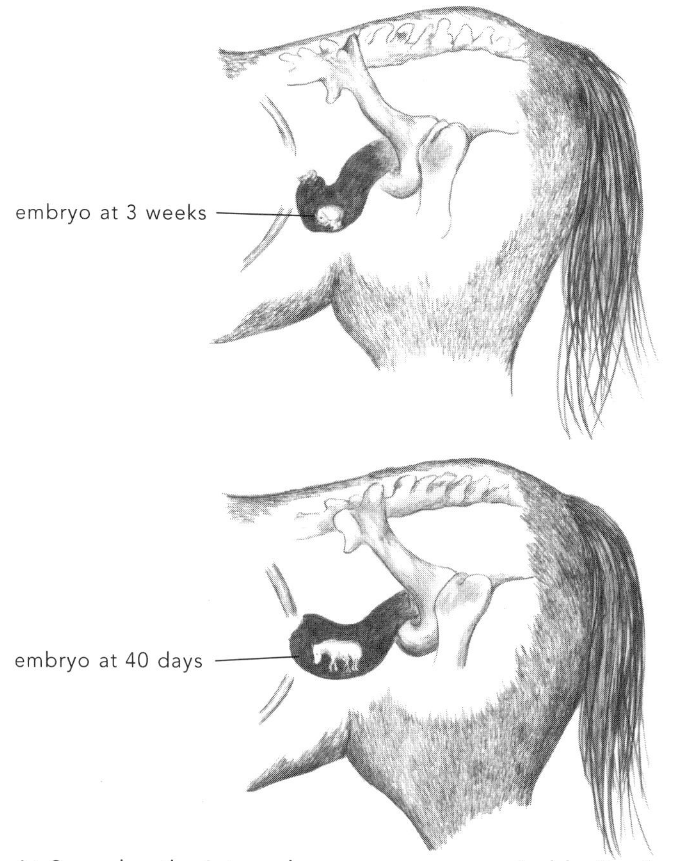

At 3 weeks, the internal organs are recognizable *(top)*, and at roughly day 40 the embryo begins to resemble a horse *(bottom)*.

FETAL DEVELOPMENT	
DAY	OUTWARD CHARACTERISTICS OF FETUS
40	Rudimentary ears, eyelids, and external nares (nostrils), elbows, and stifles; begins to resemble a horse
45	Sex differentiation
55	Eyelids nearly closed; hocks and fetlocks; vulva or penis
60	Eyelids closed; nares become slits; soles and frogs; looks like a horse
80	Points of shoulders and hips; mammary papillae or scrotum
100	Eyes bulge; ears 1 cm long; hooves; hair on lips
120	Hair on chin, muzzle, and eyelids
150	Eyelashes, ergots
180	Early mane and tail
210	Mane hair fills out
240	Hair on ears, poll, tail; vibrissae on chin and muzzle
270	Fine body hair
300	Pad covering soles; full coat

white membrane surrounding the fetus; and the amniotic space, in which is found the developing foal. (See page 166 for more on the placenta.)

During all this time various and sundry hormonal activities are taking place. These several hormones are produced, at one time or another, by assorted parts of the mare and the developing foal and are responsible for everything from ovulation to maintenance of pregnancy to milk production. Their study is interesting but complicated, so we will touch on only one here.

Progesterone is the hormone responsible for the maintenance of pregnancy. Initially, it's produced by the primary corpus luteum (CL), which forms on the mare's ovary after ovulation. This source lasts roughly 180 to 190 days, declining the whole time. A secondary CL forms and produces progesterone from day 45 to 50 and this also lasts through day 180 to 190.

In the meantime, beginning about day fifty, a fetoplacental source of progesterone is produced and takes over as the source of the hormone when the CL sources end. Pregnancy is maintained by this source until foaling. (See page 169 for more on progesterone.)

How you, the horse owner, can apply this to your breeding program is uncertain. Perhaps, though, you can better appreciate what's going on with your mare and future foal and be amazed that reproduction occurs at all.

The Placenta

If you're planning to bring a foal into the world, you should know something about how the placenta develops and what to do with it after birth. Besides, it's interesting, so we'll talk about placentation and a little about twinning.

Different mammal species have various types of placentae and, depending on whom you consider an authority, these are divided into two or four types. The equine placenta is of the *epitheliochorial type* and is the simplest form of placentation. This form consists of six intervening layers: blood vessel endothelium, connective tissue, uterine epithelium, chorion, more connective tissue, and more blood vessel endothelium. The first three are contributed by maternal tissue; the latter three are the responsibility of the fetus. This epitheliochorial type is further subdivided into two types: diffuse and cotyledonary, or multiplex. The horse has the diffuse type. (The pig is the only other domestic animal with this type of placentation, and this distant relationship may help to explain certain aspects of equine behavior, namely, why the mare that must head for the breeding shed at 7 A.M. has wallowed in a mud hole all night.)

The term *diffuse* is pretty much self-explanatory; the entire surface of the allantochorion is covered with microvilli that project into pockets in the endometrium. The only portion of the equine placenta that lacks villi is the region of the cervical star, which is that part of the placenta that lies in the region of the internal os, an opening in the cervix. (If you need to break the placenta at foaling time, the cervical star is the easiest place to do it; frequently it will rupture here with just finger pressure. It is easily identified as a whitish, star-shaped area.)

After parturition (birth, that is), it is extremely important to account for the entire placenta. Various and sundry complications can result if a portion is retained within the uterus, ranging from endometritis (infection resulting from the decomposition of the retained portion of the placenta) to sterility, founder, and even death of the mare.

As soon as you are sure that you have a foal with no problems that need immediate attention, the placenta should be examined. If you have the wherewithal and mare quality to justify the expense of having a veterinarian in attendance at each foaling, let her check the placenta. If, however, your finances and mares are more like those of most of us, learn how to do it yourself or teach an employee how. It isn't difficult. To illustrate just how "not difficult" this is, my daughter was totally competent at placental examination when she was six years old.

Examining the Placenta

To examine the placenta, simply spread it out. This will necessitate touching it and some are reluctant to do this, but don't worry about it; it all washes off. Separate the dark red allantochorion from the translucent amnion and examine each for completeness. Examine all of it. Turn it over; turn it inside out. Missing sections are usually pretty apparent. If any portion is missing or if you doubt its completeness, call your veterinarian and let her look at it.

Also, examine the appearance of the placenta. Look for discoloration, blotches, abnormal character of fluids, and so on; any of these may indicate an infection of the uterus and newborn, and your veterinarian should be informed.

If you are foaling several mares a year, the purchase of a scale of some sort is money well spent. It can be a meat scale or one of those scales hardware stores use to weigh nails; it need only have a twenty-pound capacity. Use this to weigh the placenta. Oft-repeated research has shown that the typical ("normal") equine placenta weighs from ten to fourteen pounds; more than that indicates something is amiss. Once again, call your veterinarian, even if it is fourteen and a half pounds, and submit the placenta to your friendly local pathology lab for an in-depth examination.

Twinning

Now, why don't mares have litters? It has to do with the type of placentation combined with the size of the term fetus, with the latter being the more important factor.

Among domestic animals, the neonate foal's body weight is the highest percentage of its dam's body weight, roughly 10 percent (with a range of 8 to 12 percent). This, coupled with the diffuse epitheliochorial type of placentation, means that the entire uterine inner surface is required to maintain a single viable fetus. In the case of twin fetuses, there is competition between them for adequate placental space within the uterus and usually one or both dies or mummifies due to lack of nutrition. (With the same type of placentation, a 300-pound sow may produce a litter of ten or twelve piglets, but each one weighs only a couple of pounds and there is ample uterine space for all.)

Equine twins are usually terminated at some point without outside influence. One report suggests that as high as 15 to 20 percent of conceptions are twins, but that the vast majority resolves to one or none before we can determine that twins were there in the first place. This particular researcher undoubtedly based his conclusions, in part, on the fact that in mares, double ovulations typically occur 16 to 25 percent of the time.

The fact is, however, that 0.5 to 2.5 percent of equine pregnancies remain twin pregnancies when we are able to determine them, and that figure may be climbing, as many breeders no longer hesitate to breed on multiple follicles as determined by rectal palpation or ultrasonagraphy. And the reason we breed on double follicles is generally related to the desire to get an early foal. (It remains a mystery to me why anyone would want to bring a newborn into a world of five-degree temperatures and snow and ice, when a mere sixty days later that same little guy could enter a world of sunshine, grass, and sixty-five degrees.)

It has been observed by many people in the horse breeding industry, and documented by researchers in ruminants, that multiple follicles occur during the transitional period between the anovulatory and ovulatory seasons of the reproductive cycle. This transitional period occurs, unfortunately, just when we are trying to breed these critters for an early foal next year. In mares housed under lights to encourage early ovulation, this period is January, February, and March (see page 178 for more on the influence of lights); on Nature's schedule, it's usually March and April. If Mother Nature was allowed to have her way and mares were bred in July and August, I doubt if we would see many multiple ovulations and, as a result, the twinning incidence would probably drop to such a low level that it would no longer be a concern.

This will not happen, though, as the horse industry, especially the Thoroughbred breeders, is one of the most tradition-bound endeavors in the world. But maybe, if mares were put under lights earlier, say October 1, we could be beyond the transitional period by mid-February. This would probably create other difficulties, though. Mares are seasonally polyestrous, which means that they come in heat several times a season. By beginning their season artificially with lights, they may have run their course of heat cycles as early as May or June.

Progesterone

I ONCE HAD A HYPER CLIENT. Everything excited him, whether that reaction was justified or not. His blood pressure must have been astronomical.

One year a mare of his that was pregnant at forty-two days was not pregnant at sixty days. This is not unheard of; in fact, it happens a lot. When he heard the news, he went through the roof.

He called me. "Brent, that's my best mare." (I imagine that whatever mare it was he would have called her his "best.") "I can't have any more mares slip. I want to put them all on progesterone for the rest of their pregnancies, to 300 days."

That was a stupid idea and, being close to devoid of tact, I said, “Ben, that’s a stupid idea.”

It’s funny how some people resent being called stupid (actually, I didn’t call him stupid; I called his idea stupid). He out-hypered even himself when he heard that. “Kelley, they’re my mares and I’ll do what I want with them! And you’re my vet and I pay my bills! You’ll damn well do what I say or I’ll get a vet who will!”

He was right. He could very easily find a veterinarian to sell him however much progesterone he wanted, or anything else for that matter. And he did pay his bills, promptly and fully. Everyone should pay as well. I shouldn’t have done it and I still feel ashamed, but I got him all the progesterone that he needed to carry sixteen mares through 300 days of pregnancy. None of his other mares lost her pregnancy and I’m sure he “knew” his progesterone therapy did the trick.

Use and Abuse

Progesterone may be the most improperly used of all the drugs that we give to horses, and that’s saying something in an industry known for overmedicating and incorrectly medicating.

There are hundreds, possibly thousands of mares out there that receive progesterone throughout each and every pregnancy, even though it has never been determined that they need it.

Among the misuses of progesterone are overmedicating (“If 1 mL keeps her pregnant, then 3 mL oughtta *really* keep her pregnant”) and occasional use (“I give her a little swig once a week or so just in case”). I can’t say for certain that these approaches are harmful, but they’re surely not beneficial and they definitely waste money.

I know veterinarians who start all mares on progesterone the day after they ovulate without determining the need, then ultrasound at fourteen or fifteen days. If the mare is not found to be in foal at that time, they withdraw the progesterone and give them prostaglandin so they will recycle, be bred, and go back on progesterone. I guess it’s a great practice builder (in other words, an income generator), but it’s hardly sound veterinary practice.

Now that I've riled some of my colleagues, let's look at progesterone: where it comes from, what it does, and how we can best use the information.

What Does Progesterone Do?

There is no question that progesterone is necessary for the maintenance of pregnancy. Under normal conditions, the hormone is produced at one time or another by the mare, the foal, and the placenta. This is termed *endogenous progesterone.*

During roughly the first 120 days of pregnancy, the production of progesterone is the mare's responsibility. Progesterone is produced by the corpus luteum ("yellow body," or CL), which forms at the site of the corpus hemorrhagicum ("bloody body"), which develops at the site of ovulation on the ovary. There is a primary CL, which produces progesterone for the first 40 days, at which point additional progesterone is produced by secondary CLs. This production continues for the first 150 to 200 days of pregnancy.

Somewhere around day 55 to 60, the placenta begins its production of progesterone and by day 150 to 200, CL progesterone has ceased and the second half of pregnancy is maintained by the fetoplacental source. The accepted serum progesterone concentration necessary to maintain pregnancy is variably quoted as either two or four nanograms per milliliter. Conventional methods of measuring progesterone levels in a pregnant mare are useless from roughly mid-pregnancy to term, because the placental progesterone is not in the mare's bloodstream, and there are no convenient methods to measure the placental source.

Several possible mechanisms have been proposed to explain a mare's failure to maintain a satisfactory progesterone level, including these:

- Primary insufficient production by the CL
- A bacterial infection of the mucous lining of the uterus, which causes release of prostaglandin and the resulting luteolysis (dissolution of the CL)

- Failure of the embryo to prevent luteolysis
- Endotoxins causing luteolysis
- Stress, our old friend

The real problem here is our inability to determine which of these mechanisms causes pregnancy loss. Also, only bacterial infections and endotoxins have actually ever been documented as causes of reduced progesterone production.

Supplementation

Even if the serum progesterone is normal early in the pregnancy, some mares will still slip (abort), but when provided with exogenous progesterone, they will go through a normal pregnancy. I have no explanation for this, but I am aware of at least two mares with normal serum progesterone levels that abort when not on exogenous progesterone; when on exogenous progesterone, they carry their pregnancies to term.

There are several products termed *exogenous progesterone* available for supplementing progesterone. Only two of those currently available have been tested for efficacy in mares, however. Neither has been approved by the FDA for pregnancy maintenance, but both have been used enough to show that they are effective.

These two are the injectable hydroxyprogesterone in oil and the oral altrenogest. The injectable product's effects may be measured in serum progesterone samples, while the oral product will not show a change in serum levels.

The advantage of the injectable is that you know it's in the animal; the disadvantage is that you have to poke holes in your horse. The oral is just the opposite: no holes are necessary but it's possible that part or all of the product may not go to its intended destination, especially if it's given when feed is in the mouth. Horses will spit it out with a wad of hay or grain.

When to begin giving progesterone is uncertain. Many feel that it should be started on the fourteenth day after breeding or after a positive ultrasound finding. In a case of luteal insufficiency or luteolysis due to bacterial infection (endometritis), this is probably too late. Day four (or five) is chosen by some because by this time the egg and the sperm have made contact, while others choose day one. And some prefer to wait until day thirty-two or forty-two or some other arbitrary date, which makes no sense at all to me.

Generally, once begun, exogenous progesterone is continued throughout most of pregnancy, stopping at 300 or 320 days. However, continuing beyond day 120 is probably unnecessary because by that time there is adequate placental progesterone production to maintain pregnancy.

Also, giving it too far into pregnancy may cause problems, such as these.

- Foaling may be delayed or pregnancy lengthened, during which time the fetus continues to grow.
- The exogenous progesterone may prevent the fetus from being expelled if it dies and results in a mummified fetus.
- If the fetus is somehow aborted, the mare may not return to estrus.
- Residual debris in the uterus is not passed and may result in a serious infection.

Some veterinarians believe that when exogenous progesterone is stopped, the dosage should be cut in half for a week or two, but there is no research to substantiate this (which doesn't mean they're wrong).

There is much that we don't know about both endogenous and exogenous progesterone and the use of the latter to maintain pregnancy. What we do know is that a whole lot of mares are receiving it that probably don't need it. And we know that a lot of mares come up empty each year even when receiving it. We also know that there are a lot of foals in the world that most likely wouldn't be here had they not received it.

The Caslick Procedure

The biggest breakthrough in equine reproduction — the single most important thing ever found to increase conception rate and live foal production — was Dr. Ed Caslick's realization that suturing to partially close the vulva prevents vaginal, cervical, and uterine contamination and infection, all causes of infertility. Some may disagree as to the magnitude of this discovery, but they're wrong.

Unfortunately, however, as in the case of so many worthwhile things, the procedure is sometimes abused, mishandled, or just plain botched.

There is the thought, nay insistence, by some that all fillies in training must be sutured. This is as ridiculous as saying that all horses in training must have arthroscopic knee surgery. Of course, the ones that need arthroscopic knee surgery should receive it and those that don't, shouldn't. And the same is true for the suturing of mares.

Indications

In the breeding emphasis on speed and other performance traits in horses, several other aspects of genetics have been ignored. One of these is anal-vulvar conformation. Many fillies now have a deep-set anal sphincter and below it a slanted vulva; it isn't uncommon to see the anal orifice recessed two or three inches deeper than the lower tip of the vulva. Each time a filly such as this defecates, fecal matter runs down the tipped vulva, and some may enter the vaginal vault, especially if the filly is in season. Feces, of course, are full of bacteria, and in the warm, moist environment of the vagina these bacteria thrive and may eventually move to the cervix or uterus. Preventing such contamination is the prime reason for suturing.

Other fillies, while having what appears to be normal or near normal anal-vulvar conformation, lack normal tone in the vulva. The closure is not tight and may even gap open when they are in season. These are usually "wind suckers," and this inrush of air can frequently be heard as these fillies are exercised.

Both types of fillies need to be sutured. By reducing irritation, the procedure may make them better racehorses and performers, and it will definitely make them more successful broodmares. By "more successful," I mean easier to get in foal.

Indications for suturing older fillies and mares once they enter the broodmare ranks are the same. With age, a decrease of tone or an increase in vulvar slant may develop. Additionally, vulvas traumatized in foaling or those of chronically infected mares may benefit from suturing.

Common Problems

There are two basic ways to suture a filly or mare: right and wrong. "Wrong" has many subheadings, and a Caslick's procedure done incorrectly can make matters worse than if the mare was never sutured in the first place.

For reasons that escape me, fillies in training are frequently sutured too low. The completed job looks as if someone inserted a pencil in the bottom of the vulva and sutured down to it. When the sutures are taken so far down, the normal flow of urine is drastically impeded and there is a back flush into the vagina. This is a problem in itself, but if the filly is in season this urine can flow through the open cervix on into the uterus. The uterus was not intended as a reservoir for urine. Because cystitis (bladder infection) is not uncommon in fillies and mares, such bacteria can and will be introduced into the reproductive tract. Likewise, not suturing low enough is useless. Frequently I see mares sutured down only an inch or less. Why? This leaves three to five inches open and vulnerable to contamination.

Another serious problem in suturing is gaps in the suture line. The preferable pattern in performing this procedure is the Ford interlocking stitch, which effectively pulls the two sides of the vulva together. For various reasons, though — interrupted stitches, poor trimming of the edges of the vulva, too wide spacing of the suture material, and so on — gaps can form as the suture line heals. These may be pinpoint-sized or as large as a dime, but size doesn't matter. They allow entry to fecal matter and other contaminants and, because there is vulvar closing below the gaps, this stuff has nowhere to go but inward and upward. A gapped suture line is worse than none.

Breeding and Foaling

Most sutured broodmares cannot be bred without tearing, so the use of a breeding stitch is indicated. A *breeding stitch* is a cross-stitch of soft, heavy suture material called *umbilical tape* that is placed slightly above the lower end of the suture line. It allows for expansion as the stallion enters but prevents, in most cases, tearing out of the suture line.

Some stallions, however, won't breed a sutured mare or one with a breeding stitch. In these cases, the mare must be opened. Some breeding sheds routinely open all sutured mares presented, but this is unnecessary and ridiculous. (They do it anyway.) If a mare must be opened for whatever reason, she should be closed again as soon as possible.

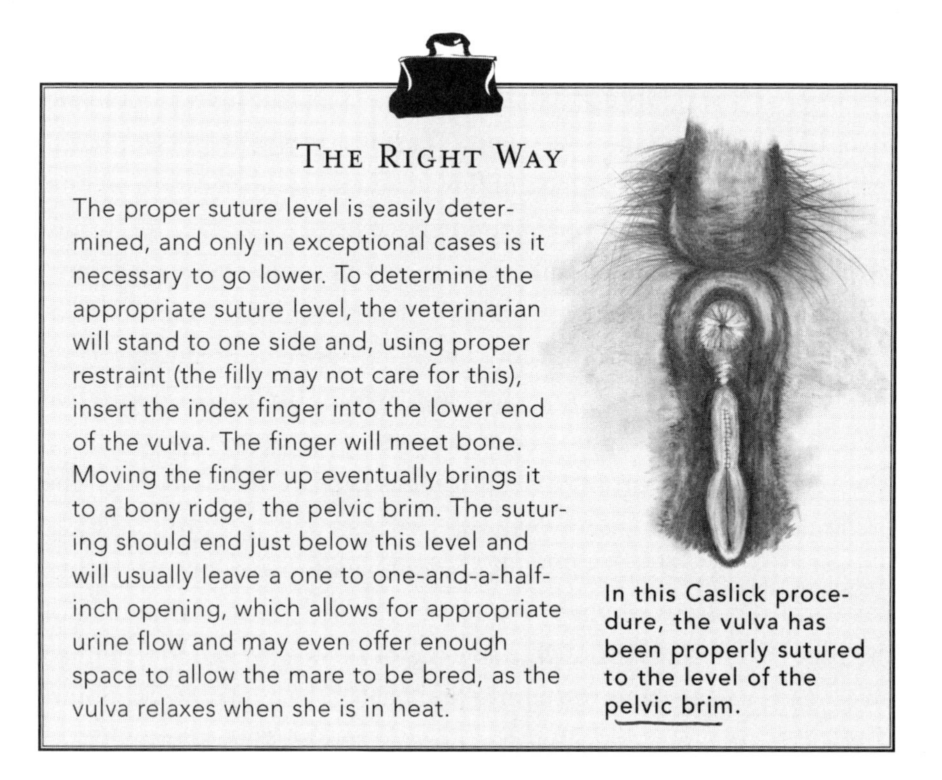

The Right Way

The proper suture level is easily determined, and only in exceptional cases is it necessary to go lower. To determine the appropriate suture level, the veterinarian will stand to one side and, using proper restraint (the filly may not care for this), insert the index finger into the lower end of the vulva. The finger will meet bone. Moving the finger up eventually brings it to a bony ridge, the pelvic brim. The suturing should end just below this level and will usually leave a one to one-and-a-half-inch opening, which allows for appropriate urine flow and may even offer enough space to allow the mare to be bred, as the vulva relaxes when she is in heat.

In this Caslick procedure, the vulva has been properly sutured to the level of the pelvic brim.

Many of the sheds that open mares close them with metal clips or staples after they are covered by the stallion. These are quickly and easily applied, but brutal. If anyone wants to staple a mare, he should first apply some staples to some tender, delicate part of his own anatomy and see if he still thinks it's a good idea.

Another serious problem often encountered is in the trimming of the vulvar lips. Only the barest minimum of tissue should be trimmed off to allow fresh edges that can heal together, but occasionally much too much is removed. Remember, a five-year-old mare carrying her first foal may have to be opened and reclosed every year for ten, twelve, even fifteen or more years. If too much is removed each time, you will eventually run out of vulva.

Eventually, we hope, the sutured broodmare gets in foal. Obviously, the suture line won't allow normal foaling to occur, so she must be opened beforehand or the foal will do so as it enters the world (this usually results in a mess that you will want to avoid). Ideally, the mare should be opened as she goes down to foal and closed again as she gets back up, but both are impractical in most settings.

Opening, then, should be done as close to foaling as possible. Most mares are decent enough to give reasonable warning before giving birth, so when you feel she's sitting on go, have her opened. Your veterinarian can help to determine the proper time.

Closing again should be done within a few hours (six to eight) after foaling, sooner if possible. After that the vulva will have swollen and suturing will become impractical for a matter of maybe several days, during which time bad bacterial bugs may come and go at will (although they rarely choose to go). The uterus is very vulnerable at this time and infections can readily set in.

Proper suturing can mean the difference between a useful performance horse and just another critter, but more important it can mean the difference between a conceiving, producing broodmare and one that produces only feed and vet bills. It's not the only answer and doesn't solve all reproductive problems, but it can help when done properly.

Lights

The mare foaled on Christmas Day. She was due about January 10, so this baby wasn't technically "premature," but he sure was early.

We don't usually have a white Christmas around here, but we did that year. White and *cold.* The foal was weak and should have been sent to one of the neonatal care units we have here in the Lexington area, but his value wasn't enough to justify the expense that would be involved. The farm elected to care for him there, so I made three trips a day to check on him and be sure that the farm personnel were feeding him correctly.

But, as I said, it was *cold;* the highs most days approached twenty degrees. Even though they put heat lamps in his stall, his body temperature could not be maintained. He died on New Year's Eve.

If he had been born two weeks or so early in April or May when it was warm, I think we would have saved him, but Thoroughbreds and other breeds have January 1 as the universal birthday, and everyone wants foals born as close to the first of the year as possible. That way, on the following January 1, when they officially become yearlings, they are pretty close to being a year old. But I think breeding for early foals is stupid. For one thing, mares were not meant to foal in the winter. Their natural breeding season runs from about May roughly through September. When a foal arrives then, there is grass and warmth.

Many, perhaps most, mares are seasonally anestrus, which means that they don't cycle throughout the year. Mares in the Northern Hemisphere cycle from May through September and those in the Southern Hemisphere from November through March, give or take. Because we here in the north want them to cycle from February through June or July, we have come up with a method to convince them that it's time for them to do so: lights. The pituitary gland decides when a mare begins cycling, and it is very sensitive to day length. As the natural day length increases, the reproductive organs become active via signals from the pituitary.

So we fool the pituitary by artificially increasing the amount of light. There are various programs by which to do this, but the easiest is just to create sixteen-hour "days." The mare can stay out during daylight hours, but when she is put in her stall the light is left on until sixteen hours are reached. There is no question that this hastens the onset of cycling. The lights should be kept on for sixteen hours until the natural day length reaches that, usually in late April or early May.

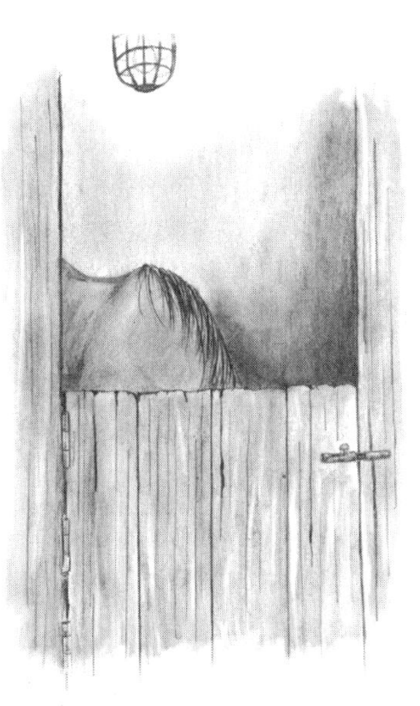

A mare can be artificially induced to cycle with increased light exposure.

The conventional date for beginning the light program is Decem-ber 1. That will cause most mares to begin cycling by early February so, in theory, they can be bred by mid-February and will therefore foal in mid- to late January.

When a mare begins to cycle each year, however, whether it's natural or artificially induced, she often produces multiple follicles, which greatly increases the possibility of multiple fetuses (i.e., twins). This is a bad scenario (see page 166 on the placenta to learn why).

My suggestion for a light program, therefore, is to begin the lights earlier, perhaps on October 1. That way a mare will begin cycling in December. When it comes time to breed her in February, she will have had a couple of cycles, and the likelihood of multiple follicles is greatly reduced. This program increases the need for stall cleaning, but nothing is 100 percent good.

What I don't understand is why on earth anyone would want a January or February foal. In most areas, the weather is atrocious and grazing is nonexistent. I just don't believe it's reasonable to place a newborn foal and its dam out in an environment such as this. And it's a disservice to both to keep them in a stall until the weather is decent. Perhaps in Florida or southern California the conditions are better, but most of us don't live in those places.

Another point, and this is fact, not opinion (as some of the above is): many mares have a certain number of cycles per year, and the sooner they start, the sooner they end. I have seen mares that, because of lights, began cycling in January or early February, didn't conceive on a few breedings, and then stopped cycling in May, just when Mother Nature would make them their most fertile. If they conceived then, they would foal at a time of year conducive to health, well-being, and proper exercise.

To sum this up, a lighting program will enable you to breed your mares earlier in the year, but this approach, in my estimation, is a double-edged sword. When I first wrote about this issue in the *Thoroughbred Times,* one of my colleagues wrote a scathing rebuttal that, in effect, said I was all wet and praised lights and winter foals. He's entitled to his opinion.

I remember one January when the high temperatures were in the teens and the lows in the single digits or lower. A mare was trying to deliver a foal that wouldn't come and I had to help it out. Everyone, including the mare, was shivering so hard that teeth were rattling. When the foal was three days old, the temperature warmed up to the upper twenties and then a blizzard came. This baby, which had not been put outside because of the extreme cold, was then in the barn but now snowed in. She was about ten days old before she could be turned out so that she and her mom could get much needed exercise. It's just not fair.

Teasing

Sometimes it's okay to tease, no matter what your mother told you. And next to mares and stallions, a good teaser is the most important part of a breeding operation. Attempts have been made to circumvent the need for a teaser, but his role is essential.

What Is Teasing?

Teasing is the usual process for finding out if a mare is in season and ready to breed. In chapter 11, on gelding (see page 316), I recommend that most stallions be gelded, with the exception of a valuable one that is needed for breeding. Well, here's another exception.

A *teaser* is a stallion, preferably a very gentle one. He is used to approach the mares to gauge their response to a male horse. If a mare is in heat, she will squat and urinate and usually back up to the teaser, which is known as *showing*. There are exceptions; some mares never "show" while others always do. More than 90 percent, however, will show if they're in season.

SEVERAL YEARS AGO, SOMEONE PATENTED a rod designed to be vaginally inserted in a mare that would supposedly determine in some mysterious way whether the mare was in or out of heat. Several were sold to smaller operations and out-of-the-way farms located far from veterinarians. At least two were sold to a large, foreign breeding farm.

"Kelley," the voice on the phone said, "get the farm one of those rods."

"They're an expensive piece of junk," I said.

"Kelley," the voice continued, "do I pay my bills?"

"Yes, and very well."

"Then get me a rod! Make it two."

Two rods were winging their way overseas two days later. The next time I spoke with the gentleman, he said, "Kelley, those rods are useless." (He didn't exactly say "useless" but this is a book intended for a variety of readers so I choose to paraphrase him.)

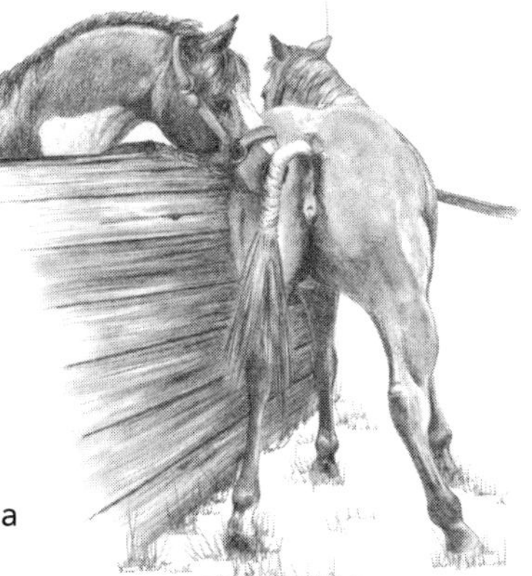

A teaser *(left)* approaching a mare over a teasing board

I agreed that the rods were what he said.

Some small breeding operations, and at least one that is not so small, either have no room for a teaser or don't want to be bothered with one. These operations rely on the counting abilities of the veterinarian and the farm owner to determine when a mare is in heat.

"We bred her sixteen days ago," the owner says. "She ought to be coming back in if she's going to. Spec her." A vaginal speculum is used to visualize the cervix. The speculum exam shows whether the cervix is opening; if it isn't, she may well be in foal. If it is, she's not in foal and will need to be bred again in a few days.

How to Tease

A question generally asked by people new to horse breeding is how to tease. The best way I've found is to lead the teaser up to each mare's stall and let them talk for a minute. If she's in, she'll show. If she's not, she won't. This method makes teasing a one-person operation because nobody has to hold the mare.

This method works a lot of the time, but it also doesn't work a lot of the time because mares don't function precisely on schedule. I certainly don't recommend operating a breeding operation without a teaser, although one client breeds anywhere from twelve to twenty mares a year without one and for years he has maintained a 90 percent conception rate. His place is a definite exception.

One client who has twelve to fifteen mares each breeding season has a very gentle teaser. This guy must have had a draft horse pass through his pedigree because his feet and bones are huge and coarse, though he stands barely 15 hands.

His favorite thing is sleeping. When teasing, he is a little interested in the first couple of mares, but by the fifth or sixth he's ready for a nap. Fortunately, his mere presence causes a few mares to show, but the difficult ones don't. And he doesn't care.

My client loves him, though. He has a home for life.

Some farms with one or two stallions and only a few mares use one or both stallions to tease. Some folks are critical of this, but I can't see anything wrong with it.

Another very good teaser was a gelding that never acknowledged that he had been gelded. Because there was no danger of pregnancy, he was kept with the mares without foals. No one was ever hurt, but usually this is not a good idea, as mares will often pick on geldings.

I DON'T KNOW IF THE FOLLOWING STORY IS TRUE, but I believe it. Before we talk of the teaser, though, I'll relate a couple of stories about the owner to set the stage.

This guy — we'll call him Jorge — was from Latin America. He had some money and owned a farm in the Lexington area where he kept some quality mares. He also acted as agent for horsemen in his native land.

One of his clients from home had a really super filly that was beating everything on the racetrack there, and he wanted to try her in the United States. He called Jorge and asked for advice. Jorge arranged for importation, and he told his friend that he could use his trainer in Florida. Jorge advised his countryman to run the filly in a claiming race first so she could get an easy purse for him. (A claiming race is one in which the horses may be bought [claimed] by anyone who is racing at that meet. It is a selling race.)

Jorge had the filly claimed (for $10,000) by someone else and then transferred to him. He told his countryman that he didn't know what happened. He was very sorry. Jorge later sold her in foal to a popular stallion for $150,000.

Jorge had a good man who broke and trained his young horses. I knew and liked this fellow and had done a little vet work for him, though never on any of Jorge's horses.

One day, however, a colt owned by Jorge received a small laceration and needed a few sutures. Jorge's regular veterinarian wasn't around so I did the repair work.

"Just give me the bill," the trainer told me. "I'll pay you."

Assuming that he would then collect from Jorge, I did.

A short time later, I accompanied a client to Jorge's farm to look at a mare that was for sale. I met Jorge for the first time. The next day

Jorge called me and asked if I would do his vet work. "Boy," I thought, "I really impressed him."

Jorge had about seventy-five horses of all ages, either on the farm or in training. Doggone right I'd do his work.

Jorge told me to stop by and see the man doing his breaking. This was the fellow I knew. When I got there he told me not to do Jorge's work because "Jorge doesn't pay. His last vet just quit because he owes him several thousand dollars," he told me. "The vets always have to sue to collect, and then he offers only a partial payment." And, he told me, he paid me for suturing earlier because he knew Jorge wouldn't.

I called Jorge and told him I was just too busy to take on his horses.

Now about the teaser. While I was on Jorge's farm that one day, I saw his teaser: a solid bay, 16 hands or slightly taller. Later I was told that he was an unraced Thoroughbred, and that every mare sent from the farm to be bred was bred to the teaser the next day if she would still stand. (This was before blood typing was required to register foals.) Amazingly, Jorge never doubled a mare back to the booked stallion. And he had a great conception rate each year. Jorge eventually left the horse business when the horses he bred didn't run well and his clients began to figure out that they were being cheated.

No Signs of Heat

IT HAPPENS EVERY FEW YEARS. Someone has a mare that just won't show to the teaser. Most farms give these mares a little time and wait for the warm weather of spring. ("Spring turns a young man's fancy to thoughts of love." Well, it often works on mares, too.) Eventually, though, the person in charge will turn to the veterinarian for help. Over the years I have found the reason for many of these mares not showing was pretty basic: they were pregnant.

Almost without fail, such mares are seasonal boarders that arrive from out of state to be bred here in Kentucky, and for some reason they had been pronounced not pregnant the previous year.

They aren't all so easy, however. Some mares just don't show any signs of being in season. Ever. Fortunately, though, they're pretty uncommon.

But every year a few people come to me and say, "I have a mare that *never* shows." Most mares, however, *will* show. It just requires a little more effort.

I have come across a farm where the teasing was done improperly. The teaser wasn't allowed to tease the mares for enough time. That was an easy one to correct.

Others are a little more challenging, but here are some methods that may help.

- Place the teaser in an adjacent stall and wait. Constant exposure brings many mares around.
- Twitch the mare when teasing her.
- Tranquilize the mare.
- If the non-showing mare has a foal, remove the foal when teasing.
- Watch the mare before and after she is teased. She may show before the teaser gets there or she may show only after he leaves.

If these approaches fail, check the mare's vulva. Even if she's not outwardly showing her receptivity to the idea of breeding by backing up to the teaser, her vulva will relax and lengthen when she's in heat. There is at least one mare I know that doesn't show, so the farm manager measures the length of her vulva. When she's in heat, the vulva is about a half-inch longer than it is when she's not. In most mares, the length difference is greater than that and it's easily seen.

The mare that truly won't show still cycles. Your veterinarian can do periodic speculum exams, and this way it can be learned when she's in heat; her cervix will be open. These are called "spec mares."

There *are* mares that don't come in, though. One year in the middle of the breeding season dozens of mares around this area refused to cycle. I'm sure there was a reason but if anyone knew it I wasn't told.

Prostaglandin is a hormonelike drug that is used to bring mares

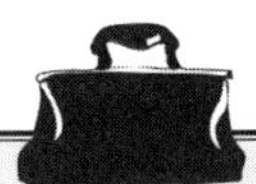

Not Too Shabby

For many years I owned a red-and-white-spotted Welsh pony–sized teaser named Patches. Patches was given to me by a client who was afraid of him, and that client in turn had gotten him from a friend for the same reason. It seems that Patches had repeatedly kicked everyone who ever handled him.

In the twelve years that I had him, Patches never kicked me. Other things and other people, however, were different stories. I guess he and I understood each other.

Patches was the greatest teaser that ever lived. He was worth his weight in gold. A mare could not fool him. If she was rearing and kicking and destroying the whole farm and Patches liked her, she was in season. If he really liked her, even if she wasn't showing, she was ready to be bred. On the other hand, if a mare was falling down in love and showing all the signs of a mare absolutely ready and he didn't like her, she was lying.

There was one time I doubted him. I was teasing a mare that I had boarded for a long time. I knew her to be extremely honest. If she showed, she was in heat, and she never showed when she wasn't. This particular time she showed weakly. Patches didn't like her, so I was a little confused.

"Go on, Patches," I urged. "Work on her. She can show better than that." I poked him gently in the ribs.

He took a step back and turned toward the next stall.

"Oh, no, son," I said. "You're not through here."

There were Dutch doors on the stalls in this barn, and the mare was backed right up to the closed lower half of the door, winking her vulva.

"Come on, Patches, touch her," I ordered, and pulled him closer to the door. He tried to refuse, but I tugged his nose over the door until it touched her on the rear.

Ka-blam! She exploded! She reduced the stall door to splinters with a vicious double-barreled kick. Then she kicked through the wall. Patches squealed and retreated. So did I.

He had been right all along. I apologized to him and never doubted him again.

Most teasers are not as good as Patches was, and it's too bad. He made life easier.

into heat. It causes lysis (dissolution) of the corpus luteum. Prostaglandin didn't work on these mares, even when repeated doses were given. Eventually they came around, but I don't know if it was because of us or in spite of us.

Most mares are seasonally anestrus. What that means is a mare will cycle part of the year and not cycle the other part (although some will cycle year-round). If a mare is in anestrus, you can pump drugs into her twenty-four hours a day and get nowhere.

A mare not under lights may not begin cycling until April, so until then nothing can be done. And a mare under lights (see page 178) may begin cycling in late January, cycle five or six times, and return to anestrus by mid-June.

All of these possibilities must be considered when trying to figure out why a mare won't show to a teaser. When in doubt, consult a veterinarian. (See page 180 for more on teasing.)

Foal Heat

Opinions differ radically on whether to breed on foal heat, a mare's first heat after foaling. Some breeders insist on it, some refuse to even consider it, some insist that it only can be done on the ninth day after foaling, and some say that if the foal doesn't scour the mare will not conceive. Others, fortunately, feel that each mare is an individual and should be treated as such.

What Is Foal Heat?

Foal heat is the first heat cycle after a mare foals, usually around the ninth day. One of the classic signs associated with foal heat is diarrhea ("scours") in the foal. There is a wide variance in timing, however. As you'll see, some may come in at day three or four (but these are rare), and some may not come in until day eighteen or twenty. Some mares apparently don't always have a foal heat, not coming in until perhaps day twenty-five or thirty.

Many years ago, I had a one-mare client who bought his mare at a breeding stock sale. It was his first experience with horses but he had read volumes and thought he was ready when foaling time came.

When the time arrived, though, the mare went down and strained but nothing came out. He called, and I came to find one leg of the foal bent backward at the knee. With a moderate amount of difficulty, I straightened the leg and out came a scrawny, weak, sickly foal that had to be helped to stand for the first twenty-four hours. Also, the mare retained the placenta and it was twelve or fourteen hours before we could get it to pass.

"Doc, I wanna breed her on foal heat," my client told me as I was picking up an extremely dark and heavy (it must have weighed twenty pounds) placenta.

"Oh, man," I said, "there's no way." And I went on to enumerate the reasons: a difficult delivery, uterine contamination (from my arm), a sickly foal, a retained placenta, and an abnormal placenta.

"But," he protested, "I've read that a mare gets in foal easiest on foal heat."

By the time the foal was two days old, the mare had developed a nasty discharge. The normal discharge following birth may vary from clear and thin to dark, even blood-tinged, and thick, but this was particularly unpleasant and odorous.

Again my client voiced his intention to breed on foal heat and again I told him not to, adding the obviously abnormal discharge to the previous list.

On day three, believe it or not, the mare began teasing in. My client called. "When can I breed her?" he asked.

"You can't," I replied.

He booked her for the next day (four days after foaling). She conceived and carried a normal, healthy foal to term.

Another client, a veteran horseman who owned or boarded between twenty and thirty mares each year, attempted the morning after foaling to book each mare for nine days later. Fortunately, few stallion managers would book that far in advance, so my client would wait until seven days after foaling and book for two days later. This led to some very exciting breeding-shed scenes, as many mares had no interest in mating when confronted by the stallion.

This client's mares had about a 20 percent conception rate on foal-heat breedings. One day he said to me, "I don't even know why I bother. Mares just don't get in foal on foal heat."

In another case, we sent a client's mare to be bred on her foal heat, which happened to be twelve days after foaling. While at the shed, the stallion manager asked my client when she had foaled.

"Twelve days ago," he answered.

The farm owner happened to be there and heard this. He became very angry and told my client that he was never again to bring a foal-heat mare beyond the ninth day to his farm. "I won't allow my stallions to be wasted on mares that can't get in foal!" my client was told.

One more. A client had a mare that had earned more than $100,000 on the track. When he retired her, she conceived on her first stallion cover. When she foaled the following year he elected to skip her foal heat and she wound up barren and remained that way for three years before finally deciding to have another foal, on a June cover.

She foaled in late May and this time, in an attempt to gain a better foaling date, he bred her on her foal heat, around the first of June. She conceived.

The next year he again bred her on her foal heat, had an early May foal, and repeated the procedure for the next several years; eventually one foal was born in late January.

When her foal heat came around that time, the breeding shed was not yet open, so she had to be passed. She never got in foal again. Of course, since she was then fourteen or fifteen, it may just have been Mother Nature deciding she was through, but my client firmly believes to this day that she would have conceived had he been able to breed her on that last foal heat.

Breeding during foal heat is useful when a mare is properly evaluated (see page 190), but many people don't understand this and misuse it. It should *never* be done routinely or skipped routinely.

Opinions Differ

If you read books and journals, you find statistics that tell you several things, among them:

- Mares bred on foal heat have a higher conception rate than those bred on subsequent heat periods.
- There is a much higher percentage of fetal loss in mares bred on foal heat.
- Mares bred on foal heat are more apt to develop a uterine infection than mares bred on later heats.

I don't know the criteria used that resulted in those conclusions, but I agree with the first one. Using a few simple guidelines, foal-heat breeding can be successful, with no abnormal rate of fetal loss and no greater chance of infecting a mare's uterus than with breeding on any other heat.

When to Breed on Foal Heat

The first and most important factor when considering whether to breed on foal heat is the quality of foaling. Other important questions concern whether foal and mare are normal and healthy.

1. Was the foaling normal (easy delivery, no retained placenta, delivery relatively on time, and other factors as expected)?
2. Is the foal normal (strong and vigorous, not weak and sickly)?
3. Is the placenta normal (complete, with good color and feel, not black or brown or leathery or heavy or missing a portion)? Weigh it. More than fourteen pounds indicates that there may be a problem.
4. Does the mare have an abnormal discharge, in either appearance or odor?
5. Is the foal heat "on time," that is to say eight or more days after foaling (the later the better)? Before eight days, it is unlikely (but not impossible) that the uterus will have shrunk (involuted) sufficiently. Your veterinarian can determine this by rectal palpation. Even if the foal heat doesn't come until

two weeks or later, if the uterus is still large enough to put the foal back in it, the foal heat should be skipped.

6. What is the condition of the vagina and cervix? Again, this is best determined by your veterinarian by a speculum examination at seven to ten days after foaling, or when the mare starts to show. Bruising or discoloration, and especially tears, are a "stop" sign for foal-heat breeding.

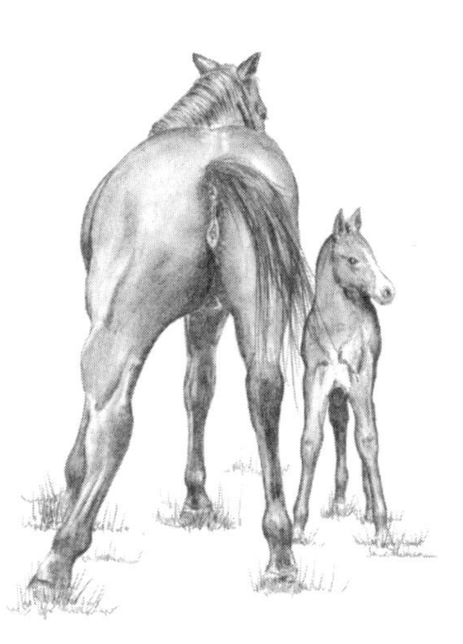

Opinions differ radically on whether or not to breed on foal heat.

By answering these questions satisfactorily, foal-heat breeding can be very helpful to a breeding operation. One unsatisfactory answer, however, means that the foal heat should be passed, and it is a good idea to culture the mare on her next heat period. (A culture taken on a foal heat will almost always yield bacterial growth, and it doesn't mean the mare is infected.)

And about our first case history, the mare that was bred four days after giving birth to a sickly foal: don't try it. Not everyone is as lucky as that guy.

A Year Off?

"I think I'll give her a year off."

I've heard that many times. For one reason or another, a mare foals late — the end of May, June, even July — and her owner wants to try to get her back to an earlier foaling date. He figures if he doesn't breed her, he can get her in foal again next February. (See page 178 on lights for information on breeding schedules.) Well, maybe he can. Or maybe he can't.

First, although I haven't seen statistics lately, the month when most Thoroughbred foals arrive is April. Number two is March. And three is May. Even with a year off, a mare probably won't get in foal until late spring, if she gets in foal at all.

Second, research several years ago in Germany concluded that a mare not in foal for any reason has only a 50 percent chance of conceiving the next year. Two empty years, 25 percent; three, 12.5 percent. (This study included all empty mares, whether they just missed a breeding year or had their ovaries removed; the odds are real bad on the latter.) Modern technology and veterinary knowledge may have altered these figures slightly, but a mare is still a mare.

Most people who give a broodmare a year off assume that they're doing her a favor. We all tend to anthropomorphize, but I really don't believe that mares think that way. And if you're a commercial breeder, you're certainly not doing yourself a favor. Remember that the mare "benefiting" from your compassion is eating all the time.

Okay, so why not let a mare that has produced six foals in a row, for example, have a year off? As the German study indicated, the statistics are against you.

And she'll eventually take off a year on her own. How many mares do you know that have a foal every year? I knew a mare that had eleven

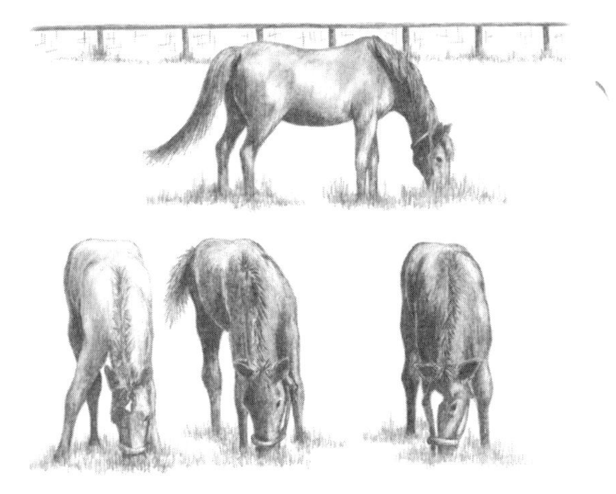

A mare "baby-sitting" weaned foals reassures them.

foals in a row. I read of one in California that had fifteen in a row. But even they eventually took a year off without being given one.

A client had a mare that had produced, I think, seven foals in a row. He gave her a year. She spent that year staring at and longing for the foals of the other mares. She didn't have a foal again for three years and that was her last.

There are reasons to give a mare a year off, but none of them involves a healthy mare that foaled on time and produced a normal, thriving foal without complications.

When Not to Breed

Here are some reasons not to breed your mare. There may be other reasons that I have missed, but these are the usual ones. (Note that the months given are especially critical for market and commercial breeders, as most breeding sheds close around the first of July.)

- A dead foal in mid-June or later
- A sick or unthrifty foal born in mid-June or later
- An older mare (over seventeen) that carries more than two weeks past her due date and foals in June or later
- A mare of any age that goes more than two weeks past her due date for two years in a row (it may become a habit)
- A bruised cervix or vaginal wall after a June or later delivery
- A dirty, or infected, mare
- A torn vulva or cervix after the end of May (or earlier, depending on severity)
- A difficult pregnancy in a mare foaling after mid-June
- Dystocia, retained placenta, or any other abnormality at or during delivery in June or later (or earlier, again depending on severity)
- A late foal heat in a mare that foaled in mid-June or later
- A sick mare
- The stallion is unavailable in June or July for any number of reasons: injured, ill, breeding shed closed, and so on.

At least one farm I know of stops breeding on May 15 each year. I have no idea what the annual conception rate on this farm is, but I'm sure that it's not exemplary. The farm is a market breeder and wants only early foals.

I have also known farms that only breed their mares every other year. That's unwise if conception rates matter. As I've said before (causing the ire of at least one colleague), I can see no rational justification for breeding early for a January or February foal, but that's just me. If you want a blizzard baby, go for it. But don't do it at the cost of a nice, warm May or June foal.

You can always try for a frosty foal after your mare takes her own year off (or is given one by a subfertile stallion, but that's another story).

Selecting a Sire

An overseas client called and asked me to examine a young horse that he was considering buying to use as a breeding stallion in his country. The horse was in New York and I was in Kentucky, so it wasn't a simple matter. I couldn't just pop over some afternoon.

So I called the farm in New York, and they agreed to give prostaglandin (a hormone that will cause a mare to come in season) to three mares on a Monday, and I planned to arrive on the following Saturday. At least one of the three would be in season by then, and that way I could perform a thorough reproductive exam on the stallion.

The farm was about 30 miles from New York City, so I flew to LaGuardia and rented a car. Have you ever driven in or around New York City? I'd rather have my teeth pulled with pliers.

Eventually I got to the farm, and one of the mares was ready to breed. First, though, I looked the stallion over to see whether there were any conformational defects. A stallion with poor conformation is a poor prospective sire because of the danger of his passing on faults to the foal. This horse wasn't perfect, but he wasn't bad. My only complaint was that his shoulders were a little too straight.

Next I had them show the stallion the mare, so he would drop his penis so I could examine it. Grabbing a horse's penis may prompt an unfavorable reaction, but this young fellow took it in stride. The penis was normal.

I placed an equine condom on him and let him mount the mare, which he did eagerly. That's a good sign; not all stallions have a decent libido.

I examined the semen collected in the condom under a microscope. There was both a sufficient quantity and quality of sperm and good motility of the sperm.

Next I examined the stallion's testicles. Studies have shown the average width of the scrotum across the widest point in successfully fertile stallions is 90 to 112 millimeters, and this horse was exactly 100 millimeters (I measure with calipers). Also, the testicles should have good tone and be of approximately the same size. His were fine.

But even though everything checked out as normal, the real proof of a stallion's fertility lies in his ability to get mares in foal. Stud farms arrange for test mares to be bred to stallion prospects, and this horse had not yet had any test mares. (Many years ago, a top racehorse checked out perfectly normal on all examinations and tests, but fewer than 10 percent of the mares bred to him actually produced foals.)

I explained everything to my client, and he asked if I had any reservations about the horse. I didn't, he was purchased and exported, and he proved to be very fertile.

Key Points in Choosing a Sire

The important points to remember when considering a sire are these:

- Good conformation
- Satisfactory libido
- Good performer
- Ability to impregnate mares

It's nice to have a potential sire examined thoroughly, but unless you're dealing with million-dollar horses and insurance companies, it really isn't necessary.

Libido

Libido in stallions varies. One super racehorse had to stand around and watch other stallions breed before he got the idea.

Every time. But when he did breed a mare, he usually got her in foal.

Another very fine horse, when presented with a mare, would put his head on her rump and practically go to sleep. But he, too, was normally fertile when awake.

Then some have libido problems of a different sort. They want to breed so badly that they're dangerous and can be handled only by experienced stud grooms.

Artificial Insemination

Artificial insemination (AI) can be considered, but stallion semen doesn't lend itself well to AI, and AI is not allowed in Thoroughbreds. I do have considerable experience with AI in Trakheners, however.

There are Trakhener mares around here but apparently no top Trakhener stallions, so the cycling of the mare and the acquisition of the semen must be carefully orchestrated. We check the mare to determine the time of ovulation, then the out-of-state stallion farm is called. They collect the horse and ship the semen by air. The semen is picked up at the airport, and we get it into the mare as soon as possible. Several quality foals have been produced in this manner.

Penile Trauma

SEVERAL YEARS AGO A JAMAICAN CLIENT called from Jamaica. One of the stallions on his farm was not impregnating his mares.

The horse was in his early twenties, and for nearly twenty years he had been doing well, but this particular year all of his mares were coming back in heat. It was the first of April and he was 0-for-9. He approached his task with his same ardor and enthusiasm but to no avail. My client wanted me to come down and see what was wrong.

But, as I said, it was the first of April and both the breeding season and the Little League season here in Kentucky were in full bloom. Getting away would be tough, but coming up was a weekend with no ball games scheduled; I was able to arrange things with my Kentucky clients so I could be gone for two days.

I arrived in Kingston on the south coast of Jamaica late Saturday morning and was driven across the island to the farm in the mountains on the north coast. By 2 P.M. I was looking at the stallion. I had seen the old boy before on earlier trips to the island but, as he had never had any problems, I had never had reason to do more than say hello to him.

They brought out an in-season mare and the old guy immediately grasped the idea. Then I saw the darnedest thing: his erect penis started out normal but about halfway down it took an abrupt left turn at roughly a 75-degree angle.

The farm owner told me the story. When the horse was five or six, more than fifteen years earlier, he was breeding a mare that did not care for the idea. She was bouncing around, wiggling, and trying to sit down. All of a sudden the stallion squealed, dismounted, and immediately pulled his flaccid penis back into its sheath. And there it stayed. He refused to attempt to breed the mare again and, indeed, would not breed any mare for more than a week.

This all happened more than thirty years ago, and at the time equine veterinary science in Jamaica was not very well developed, so nothing was done for the horse. When he bred again, his penis was at the above-described angle. He needed help to enter mares, but nothing else was affected. He had apparently been the victim of pretty serious penile trauma.

Interestingly, it turned out that when I was asked to look at him, he was not stopping his mares because he had a very low sperm count and a high percentage of abnormal sperm, a bad combination, especially at his age. It had nothing to do with his old injury. So he was retired from breeding. I have seen mares act badly in several ways — sitting down, turning, bucking, and so on — without damage to the stallion's penis, so apparently it takes some effort to damage a penis. I've also seen damage occur for no apparent reason.

Penile trauma can range from a mild inconvenience, wherein a stallion may miss a couple of days of breeding, to a more serious state causing him to miss a month to an entire season. And if worse comes to worst, his breeding career can be ended.

Predisposing Factors

I have read and have been told that the most common cause of penile trauma is a kick from a mare, either before or after breeding, but I have never seen an injury to a penis caused by a kick. Of course, that does not mean that forty-two stallions a day are not kicked in the penis; all it means is that I have never seen it.

In my experience, the most common cause is difficult to pinpoint. A stallion mounts and enters a mare with no problem and dismounts with a swollen penis. A mare jumps or sits or shifts during copulation, and once in a while there is an injury to a penis, but 99.99 percent of the time, of course, there is no problem. Likewise, a mare stands perfectly, and occasionally a penis is injured for no apparent reason. There are other documented causes.

Stallion rings are sometimes used to prevent a stallion from getting an erection and masturbating. A too-small stallion ring can cause severe damage to a penis, and if left on too long can eventually cause loss of the penis. If stallion rings are used, they must be checked regularly and often.

Breeding stitches can also cause penile damage. A properly done breeding stitch will not adversely affect a stallion, but unfortunately not all are done properly. It is the custom now of many breeding sheds to routinely remove a breeding stitch when a mare with one is presented, apparently without concern for whether she tears when bred. She is then stapled when she does tear. As I've said before, apply staples to some tender part of your own anatomy, then if you still think it's a good idea you can do it to horses. A better idea would be to apply a proper breeding stitch in the first place and leave it alone.

Clinical Signs

Penile trauma usually causes internal hemorrhage and edema. The penis may be discolored (bruised) and swell to twice (or more) normal size. There may also be lacerations, which must be sutured.

Urethral obstruction, either from swelling or laceration and indicated by difficult urination, may result from trauma to the penis. I am happy to say that I have never seen this, but drainage of the bladder must be maintained in this situation. A catheter may have to be sutured in place to accomplish this.

Treatment

To treat edema, elevate the penis by bandaging or otherwise holding it up against the lower abdominal wall. If the penis cannot be fully retracted, ointments must be applied to prevent it from drying out. Cold-water hosing two or three times a day, twenty to thirty minutes at a time, is necessary for both edema and hemorrhage; once the danger of further swelling has passed, warm-water massage will help to disperse the swelling.

Sexual rest is important until healing is complete. An erection increases penile blood pressure, which will cause further swelling, and the act of breeding itself may aggravate the initial injury. Once healed, and time is the main consideration, an injured penis is as good as ever.

A FARM OWNER CALLED. "There's something wrong with my stallion's 'thing,'" he reported.

I was pretty sure what the "thing" was, but I had to ask to be sure. When I got to the farm, I saw that the "thing" indeed had something wrong with it. It was swollen to more than twice normal size, which was noticed right after a breeding.

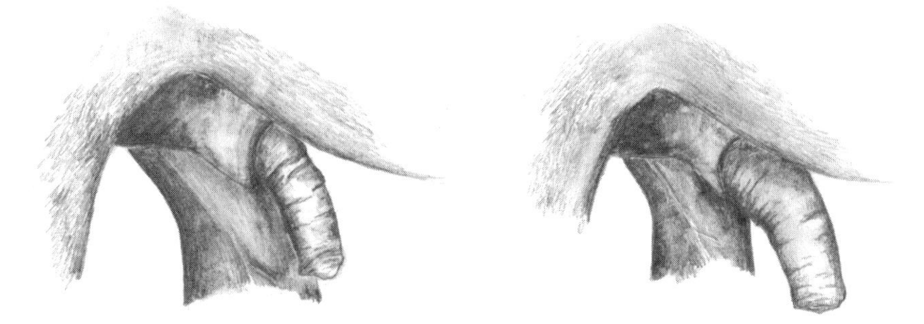

A normal penis *(left)* and a penis swollen from trauma *(right)*. Trauma to the penis usually causes internal hemorrhage, edema, or both. If the penis cannot be fully retracted, ointment must be applied to keep it from drying out.

It was hemorrhage, and I outlined the treatment procedure to the client and his stallion manager. I told them that they had to pretty much play it by ear as to when he could be bred again. It could be a few days to a few weeks and during that time "he *must* have sexual rest!" I emphasized that point.

This was not an outstanding horse but he had a $10,000 stud fee and his book was full. I realize that turning away a potential $20,000 a day for a possible prolonged period is tough to do. The owner realized this, too, and in two or three days he called me into his office.

"Close the door," he said. I did.

In a lowered voice, he said, "Dr. Kelley, I *need* for this horse to breed. I'll pay you well for this."

He paused. I waited, suspecting what was to come.

"Look," he continued with the same reduced volume, "I want you to artificially inseminate his mares. No one will know." Artificial insemination is not allowed with Thoroughbreds.

I was not sure how no one would know because I felt certain the van driver or the employee from the mare's farm would realize that, as robust and as vigorous as I was in those days, I was not a stallion. I explained again about erections.

"Oh," he said, "I thought you said he couldn't be bred."

7

The Pregnant Mare

Slipped Mares

There are those who say that animals don't mourn. Maybe *mourn* isn't the right word for it, but I've seen dogs search a house tirelessly for a departed master and then lie sadly near where that master used to sit. And whimper. If that isn't mourning, I don't know what it is.

I've seen mares that aborted in late pregnancy, presented a stillborn foal, or had a foal die search for the lost baby. They look longingly at foals alongside other mares. They call out to them. If they're turned out with mares with foals (a bad idea but it's done by some), they'll often try to take another mare's foal. Many times a mare will not cycle normally after her loss. Maybe *mourning* isn't the word, but it sure sounds and looks like it to me.

I don't know how or when *slip* came to mean "abort," but when a mare aborts it's said that she "slipped." It's a heartbreaking event, and not only for the mare. Anticipation of a foal is one of the great joys of breeding horses. That next foal could be *the* one: the stakes winner, the great jumper, the top barrel racer, the champion.

Why Does It Happen?

Mares can abort at any point in pregnancy. Slipping in the first two trimesters often goes unnoticed. For this reason, a pregnant mare should be checked periodically to make sure that she's still in foal. I usually check a mare at 18 days after she's bred, then at 32, 42 or 45, 60, 100 to 120, and 180 days. If a mare is found to have lost the fetus, she should be teased and cultured when she comes in season. One of the main causes of abortion is endometritis (uterine infection), and that must be cleared up if rebreeding is planned and even if it isn't planned.

If the aborted fetus is found, or if the foal is stillborn or dies, a post-mortem examination needs to be done. Knowing the reason for the abortion or death is necessary so it can possibly be avoided in the future. Also, the mare should be cultured.

In the case of a stillborn foal or one that dies, leave it with the mare for a while (at least eight to twelve hours). This enables the mare to understand that her baby has died and greatly reduces the "mourning."

Aftercare

Cut the mare's feed back. She's no longer eating for two. If she has produced milk, pay close attention to her bag. Mastitis (inflammation of the mammary glands) can be very serious in a mare. If her bag doesn't dry up in a few days, apply camphorated oil to it for several days. If it still doesn't dry up, consult your vet.

And take it easy on the mare. It's a tough time for her.

Nutrition of the Pregnant Mare

With everyone trying to have January and February foals, those little guys need to be especially strong, vigorous, and healthy when they arrive to contend with winter conditions. Even if they don't arrive until May or June, they still need to get here in good shape.

Unfortunately, the occasional foal arrives in the world neither strong, vigorous, nor healthy. And some mares consistently produce foals that are not strong, vigorous, or healthy. These are always problems, but a little diagnostic work, some decent veterinary care, a little tender loving care, and some quality management usually sees them through.

I ONCE HAD AS A CLIENT an entire farm that consistently produced foals that didn't thrive. I did the farm's work for three years and it wasn't until the last year that I found out what the problem was.

This farm had, if I remember correctly, sixteen mares. They had decent, middle-of-the-road pedigrees and ran the gamut of sizes that you would expect to find in a group of that number. None of them carried any excess weight, though. They weren't skinny but they could all use a pound or two.

I began to do the work there around Halloween. The first foal was due in late January and it arrived on time, more or less. But it was small, weak, and spindly. I suggested that we do some blood tests to see if there was something we could correct, but the owner said he didn't want any done. The foal was nearly two weeks old before I considered it to be out of the woods.

The next two foals were not due until early March and they, too, arrived within a week or so of their calculated dates. Both of these were small and one was very weak.

And so it went. If memory serves me correctly (and more and more it doesn't), the farm had ten foals that year, and every one of them was smaller than average and about half were weak. One — surprisingly the only one that arrived in decent weather (June; it had been a cold, wet spring) — died. And one mare didn't produce milk.

At times I'm a little naive. I chalked it up to bad luck, although the farm owner didn't seem to be concerned in the least.

My first complete breeding season there was not spectacular. Thirteen mares conceived but three came up empty in late pregnancy. Again, the foals ranged from small to small and weak. One died within an hour of birth and another died at about a week of age. The owner didn't want postmortem exams. And, again, he didn't seem to mind. And another mare, a different one, had no milk.

I suggested that we test his pasture, hay, and feed to see what his horses were either missing or getting too much of. He didn't see any reason to do any of that.

I also suggested that we take blood samples from the mares and foals in an effort to determine why all the foals were scrawny. No, he said, that was an expense that he didn't need. Besides, "They all grow out of it," he said. Those that live, I thought.

That year, I think twelve mares got in foal, but only nine produced foals. Again, the foals were small or small and weak. And, once more, one died. And a mare didn't produce milk.

When one especially weak foal arrived (it survived, but I was sure it wouldn't), I said to myself but in the presence of the old man who worked on the farm, "Why the devil is this happening?"

"What?" asked the old guy.

"Why are all these foals so small and weak?"

"Oh," he answered matter-of-factly. "It's because he don't feed the mares."

And he explained it to me. It seems that the owner had had a couple of severe dystocias (difficult deliveries) several years before, accompanied by large veterinary bills. The foals involved were pretty good sized and he blamed the dystocias (and the vet bills) on their sizes; he also had lost both a mare and a foal. Ever since then, the old man told me, he had reduced the mares' feed so their foals would be small and therefore easily delivered.

Here is what he did. He stopped giving the mares grain in mid-pregnancy and fed them only enough cheap hay to maintain a little body condition. Stress "little."

He succeeded. There were no dystocias after the feed adjustment was made. He also averaged only about a 70 percent conception rate and a 60 percent live-foal rate. And some mares didn't produce milk as a result of their poor nutrition.

I tried to explain the facts of nutrition to him, but he wouldn't listen. I told him that I could no longer do his veterinary work under those conditions. "There's plenty of vets around," he replied.

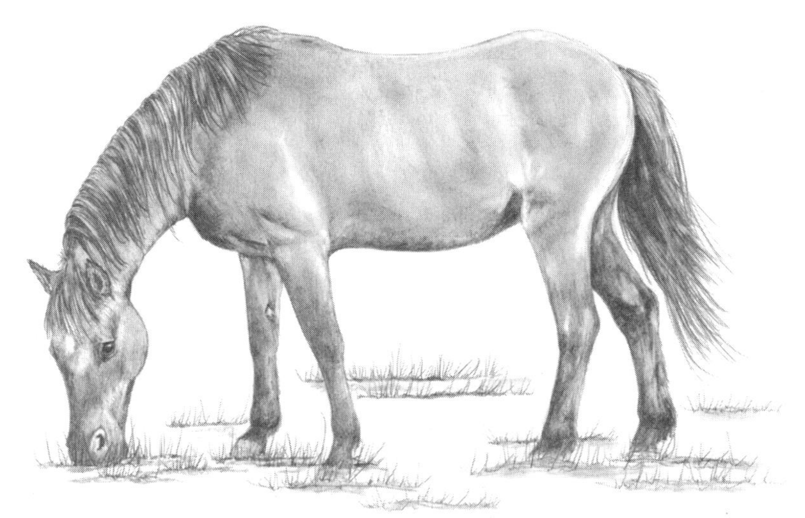

Good grazing is important to the nutrition of the pregnant mare.

Okay, for those out there who don't know: a mare's peak nutritional needs are in the last third of her pregnancy and the first ten to twelve weeks of lactation. This allows her to grow a strong, vigorous, healthy foal and have enough to feed it when it gets here, even if it is in the middle of winter.

Nutritional Needs of Mares During the Last Trimester of Pregnancy and the First Twelve Weeks of Lactation

Nutrition	Last Trimester	Early Lactation
Total feed, percentage of body weight	2.25–2.50	3
Total feed, pounds	22–30	30–36
Concentrates with grass hay, pounds*	3.5–10	5–10
Concentrates with alfalfa hay, pounds*	1.5–8	3.5–8
Percent crude protein, total diet	12–14	16

*Concentrates shouldn't exceed 30 percent of total ration by weight. Mares are different, and slight adjustments may need to be made in some cases to maintain correct weight.

But be careful. "Peak nutritional needs" doesn't mean fat. And remember: cheap feed or hay can be very expensive in the end.

The chart on page 205 shows the basic requirements for 1,000- to 1,200-pound mares.

Tall Fescue

I THOUGHT I COULD MANAGE AROUND THE PROBLEMS of tall fescue, but I was wrong. I had been doing it for years with no apparent difficulty. But it caught up with me all at once.

A very expensive and talented mare belonging to a client was way overdue, with no signs she was even remotely thinking about foaling. Another mare, one belonging to me and of considerably less value, was right at her foaling date and it appeared that she was going to be on time.

The person who normally watches the mares at night was sick and could not come to work one night. I was alone and had no one to help when my mare started to foal about 10:30 P.M. (Fortunately, it was late April and warm; had it been cold when everything went wrong that evening I probably would have left the horse business.)

The foal from my mare was presented upside down with premature placental separation. When it finally got into the world (with much help from me), it was dead. Delivery had taken more than an hour, even assisted, and the little guy just couldn't last that long.

It was nearly midnight when I finished with my mare, and as I was leaving the barn I looked in on the first mare, which was at least three weeks overdue. She was down and straining and trying to deliver a foal about the size of downtown Duluth. With much straining on her part and much pulling on mine (although I am never sure how much good I actually do when pulling), a half-grown behemoth filly was born, alive and hungry.

The next problem was feeding her. The mare had no milk, not even a hint of mammary development. Luckily, right across the aisle was my mare, with milk and without a foal. She was an older mare (twenty-one) with a kind disposition and had been wondering why her foal was not on its feet and nursing. (I think it's a good idea to leave a dead foal with a mare for several hours, so she will come to understand that it isn't going to get up.)

I took her placenta and rubbed it on the live filly and presented the foal to her. She readily accepted her, although I don't promise that this approach is a good idea. A mare may not accept another foal and may hurt or even kill it. Next, I took the dead foal over to my client's mare, which had not gotten up after an hour-plus, being exhausted from trying to push a 170-pound object through a 100-pound opening. I laid the dead foal by her and put her placenta over it. When she was able to rise, she accepted it as hers.

The problems with both mares and foals were due to tall fescue *(Festuca elatior;* formerly *F. arundinaceae),* which grew abundantly on my farm and on all those around it.

What's Wrong with Tall Fescue?

For ages, horsemen have suspected that tall fescue causes problems, but only in the last twenty-five years or so have their suspicions been proved correct. It has been shown that grazing tall fescue during late gestation can cause agalactia (no milk), hypogalactia (reduced milk production), dystocia, premature placental separation, thickened placentas, retained placentas, and delayed parturition (delivery) — all problems that you don't need when trying to foal a mare.

The fescue itself doesn't cause the problem; rather, the culprit is an infection within the plant. A specific fungus that produces alkaloids

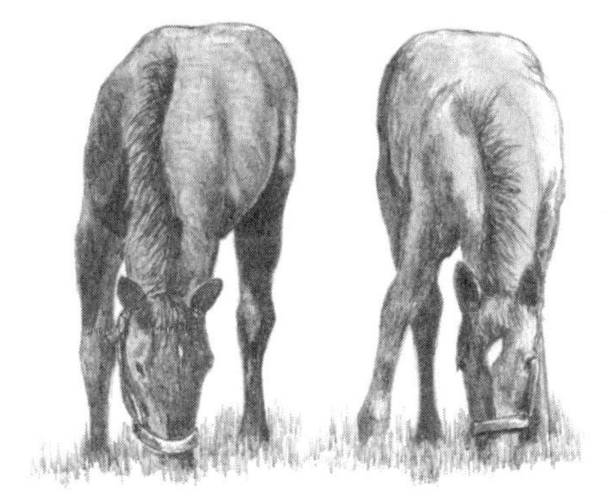

Allowing horses to graze on tall fescue can lead to many problems.

spends its entire life cycle within the fescue stems and leaves. These alkaloids are the real bad guys. The fungus is also in the seed, so it's actually there from the beginning.

The alkaloids inhibit prolactin secretion by the anterior pituitary gland, and prolactin is important in mammary gland development and milk production. This explains how agalactia or hypogalactia can be caused. Unless something has been learned very recently, it isn't clear how the other problems come about, but they do. The box lists all the things we currently blame on tall fescue.

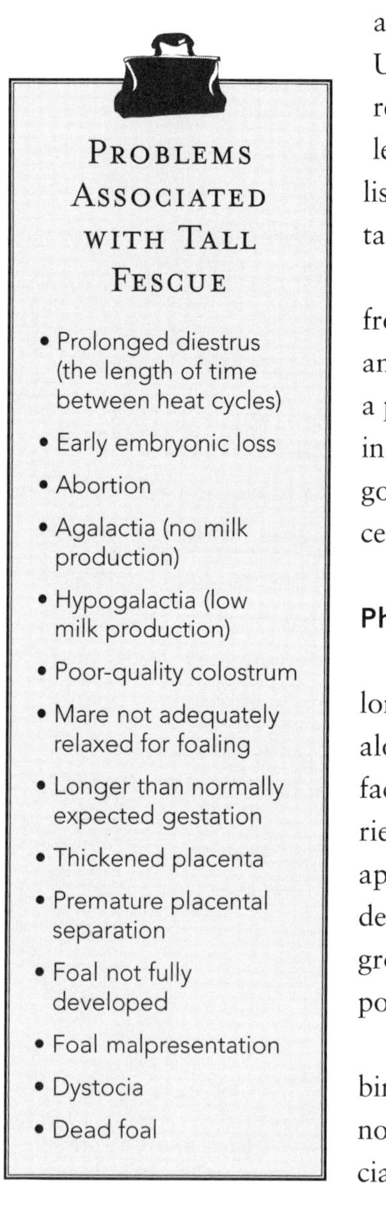

Problems Associated with Tall Fescue

- Prolonged diestrus (the length of time between heat cycles)
- Early embryonic loss
- Abortion
- Agalactia (no milk production)
- Hypogalactia (low milk production)
- Poor-quality colostrum
- Mare not adequately relaxed for foaling
- Longer than normally expected gestation
- Thickened placenta
- Premature placental separation
- Foal not fully developed
- Foal malpresentation
- Dystocia
- Dead foal

Infected fescue can't be differentiated from uninfected fescue without laboratory analysis. A 5 to 10 percent infection rate in a pasture may be enough to cause problems in some mares; 50 percent infection is a good bet to cause difficulties; and 75 percent and above is a sure thing.

Physical Effects

One reason foals die at birth after a prolonged pregnancy is their size, and that alone can cause dystocia, but there are other factors as well. The foals, even though carried longer than expected, frequently appear to be immature with poor muscle development, abnormal teeth, and overgrown hooves. Also, the foals often fail to position themselves properly.

And the mare seems unready to give birth. The pelvic ligaments and muscles are not fully relaxed and, in addition to dystocia, there can be damage to the tissue of the uterus, cervix, vagina, and vulva. The placenta is thick and may not rupture, resulting in premature separation.

In addition, there may be alterations in the estrous cycle of mares that graze tall fescue and an increased occurrence of slipping (early embryonic loss).

Prevention and Management

The best way to prevent these problems, of course, is not to allow your mares to graze tall fescue. Unfortunately, the plant is everywhere and will take over a field if given a chance. Complete pasture renovation works, but it's expensive and time-consuming, and if an adjacent field has fescue it will be back.

Other management methods work but nothing is 100 percent. See the box for recommendations.

Endophyte-free fescue is less hardy and more difficult to establish than regular fescue, but be aware that if infected tall fescue is present, it will win out eventually, because the fungus actually seems to help the fescue thrive.

The main problem in mares grazing tall fescue is lack of milk production or a reduced milk output, with associated reduced colostrum quality. Although there are three products helpful in overcoming milk production problems, only one is recommended for use in mares. Domperidone, given orally for the last two to four weeks before the expected foaling date, reportedly prevents these problems.

Even with domperidone, foaling should be attended, and you should be

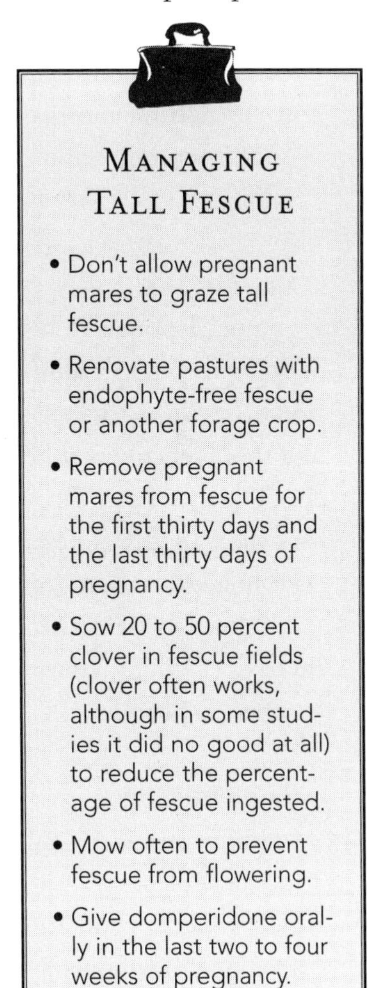

Managing Tall Fescue

- Don't allow pregnant mares to graze tall fescue.
- Renovate pastures with endophyte-free fescue or another forage crop.
- Remove pregnant mares from fescue for the first thirty days and the last thirty days of pregnancy.
- Sow 20 to 50 percent clover in fescue fields (clover often works, although in some studies it did no good at all) to reduce the percentage of fescue ingested.
- Mow often to prevent fescue from flowering.
- Give domperidone orally in the last two to four weeks of pregnancy.

ready for any problems. A source of colostrum must be on hand as well as a milk replacer, and a nurse mare should be available if she should be needed. This is a real problem in most areas. If at all possible, your veterinarian should be present at the time of foaling. It's a cheap precaution when compared to the potential loss of a foal.

Back to the three horses with which we began this tale. My client's mare did not get in foal that year but did the following year. My mare, aged to begin with, never had another foal, and three years later became a pet for an elderly couple who loved horses. The foal out of my client's mare grew up with her adopted mother's kind disposition and her natural mother's considerable ability, which proved to be a profitable combination.

Iodine

Dr. James Rooney, in his marvelous book, *The Lame Horse* (Neenah, Wisc.: Russell Meerdink Co., 1998), states that proper bone maturation in horses is affected by excessive iodine in the pregnant mare's diet, and the chief culprit is kelp fed as a feed additive. It seems everyone has that book or has borrowed it, and although Dr. Rooney clearly says that the bad guy is kelp, many people have asked me about allowing their horses access to iodized salt.

Iodine is essential for the thyroid gland to produce the hormone thyroxine, which controls the body's metabolic rate. Roughly three fourths of the iodine in a horse's body is in the thyroid gland.

Iodine Deficiency

Goiter, primarily in young animals, is the result of iodine deficiency, which leads to decreased production of thyroxine, the lack of which in turn stimulates the pituitary gland to produce an excess of thyrotropic hormone. This leads to enlargement of the thyroid gland. Iodine deficiency is not a problem in much of the United States, but it can be a problem in the so-called goiter belt, which extends from the Great Lakes region west to the Pacific Coast.

Foals born to mares deficient in iodine usually are born dead or die soon after birth. If alive, they are born with goiter and are weak, unable to stand and nurse. Contracted tendons are also seen.

Although iodine deficiency is the primary cause of goiter, it may also be caused by high levels of calcium, and there are also goitrogenic substances in some feeds (carrots, cabbage, soybeans, linseed). These substances slow the thyroxine-secreting ability of the thyroid gland, so, although iodine deficiency causes goiter, goiter doesn't necessarily mean iodine deficiency.

In adult mares, reproductive efficiency is affected by iodine deficiency. Abortions, prolonged gestation, and irregular estrus are the primary manifestations.

Excessive Iodine

So far this discussion has been about iodine deficiency, but my clients' concerns were about excessive iodine. This can occur, but you really have to work at it. The recommended daily level of iodine is one milligram (1 ppm). Iodine is evidently easily transported across the placenta and mammary glands, so any excess will go directly to the fetus/foal. For a problem to develop, however, the level of iodine per day must be 40 to 50 mg, or forty to fifty times normal.

The foal resulting from a mare fed iodine at these levels looks and acts as would a foal from an iodine-deficient mare: goiter, weak, dying or dead. The excessive iodine may prevent thyroxine synthesis or release. Any diet that includes excessive iodine should be avoided.

To the best of my knowledge, kelp has been an ingredient in the rations of all mares that have borne foals with excessive iodine-induced goiter. It would, therefore, seem to be a good idea not to use feeds containing kelp.

Even in iodine-deficient areas, the iodine requirement is usually met by simply allowing free access to iodized salt. Supplementation beyond that is both foolish and asking for trouble.

Surprise Foaling

THE PHONE RANG AT 4 A.M. It was the breeding season, so a middle-of-the-night call was not unusual.

The voice on the other end said, "Doc, come quick! I got a foal."

I didn't recognize the voice. "Who is this?"

"Whitey Tremble." Whitey was a trainer. I didn't know he had any mares, so I said, "I didn't know you had any mares, Whitey."

"I don't. I'm at my barn at the track."

It happens every few years. A filly or mare that was not supposed to have been bred delivers a foal. I went straight to the track, and Whitey was waiting for me. A two-year-old filly had a nice, vigorous little filly by her side. Stress "little."

"She hadn't been training well the past two or three weeks," he explained. "Now I think I know why."

I've seen a few fillies or mares unexpectedly foal (actually, one aborted) over the years, and all of them were surprises to the people responsible for their care, or so they claimed. These female horses ranged in age from two to five (although most of them were two-year-olds), and there was "no way" that they could have been impregnated. Not all were racehorses; two were pleasure horses. I have primarily a breeding farm practice, so if I've seen several, then I must believe that this phenomenon is not all that rare.

How Does It Happen?

I also believe that someone knows who the sire is in some cases. It wouldn't surprise me if some of these fillies and mares were used as "test mares" at 3 A.M. for a retiring stallion, to determine whether he was fertile and knew how to breed. Also, some horses get out of their stalls. Some in-season fillies or mares will go looking for love if they gain their freedom. Or a colt in a stall three or four down the aisle from a young filly may go to great lengths when no one is looking. He'll know she's in season even if the people involved don't.

As yearlings, colts will try to get into the fillies' field, but the biggest problem is they may be allowed to run together because the management believes they're "too young" to reproduce. Fillies will sometimes reach puberty as early as ten months; the average is fourteen to fifteen months. Colts get there three to four months later on the average, but twelve months is not unheard of.

Clinical Signs

These "unauthorized" foalings are almost always a surprise because external appearances are deceiving. Just as some women look pregnant only a few weeks after conception and others don't look all that pregnant on the way to the hospital to give birth, so it is with horses. Don't expect a big belly, especially in a young filly that is being ridden or trained.

A very observant owner, groom, or trainer (and I really mean *very*) may recognize a difference in a pregnant filly or mare, but bear in mind that the changes seen in pregnancy, whether they are physical, mental, psychological, or physiological, are gradual. Some changes will be noticed, but a whole lot more won't be, especially if they aren't being looked for.

A man bought a three-year-old Quarter Horse filly from a farm in Ohio and loaded her in his two-horse trailer to bring her home, which was in Paris, Kentucky. When he got here, he discovered that it was a good thing that he had a two-horse trailer because he now had two horses. She had foaled on the road. Both mother and child were fine.

But frequently the foal resulting from these liaisons is weak and scrawny because its dam was not fed properly. And a two-year-old filly may not have a suitably sized birth canal, and dystocia may result.

Another problem that I've seen in very young horses (two-year-olds) that foal is a lack of milk production — not enough or none. I don't know whether it's due to their age or the fact that they're not being fed properly for mammary development.

The lesson here is this: Separate the sexes at weaning and keep them separated. Otherwise, you're asking for another mouth to feed.

Gestation Length

DOGS ARE EASY TO PREDICT: sixty-three days. Pigs are *real* easy: three months, three weeks, and three days. Breed a dog and sixty-three days later you will have a litter of puppies 99 percent of the time. Breed a sow and 114 days later she will have piglets 99 percent of the time.

But mares? Eleven months? Not often. Three hundred and forty days? Usually pretty close. Eleven months and eleven days? That's fairly accurate a lot of the time. But the mares don't know this schedule.

Breed a mare and, assuming she conceives (an iffy proposition), 340 or so days later you may have a foal. Or you may have a two-week-old foal. Or you may not have a foal for quite a while yet.

I have seen dozens of mares that carry foals longer than the 340-day gestation period that is considered normal. Of course, there are circumstances responsible for this in many cases. Colts, for instance, are often carried longer than the calculated date (and fillies sometimes shorter).

Mares that have been on progesterone for too long may go over. A mare that has been barren for several years usually goes long (*if* she gets in foal). Older mares (sixteen or seventeen years old and up, especially those older than twenty) often seem to carry forever.

But some have none of these excuses. One young mare carrying her first foal breezed past eleven months, past 340 days, past 350 days. I suggested to the young woman who owned her that she had the wrong breeding date. Absolutely not! Okay, then, that breeding was unsuccessful and she was bred on her next cycle by something on the farm. Impossible! There were no male horses there, not even a teaser. Not even a gelding.

Well, she made it to 361 days and produced a vigorous, healthy, normal, albeit large foal. She went a full year the next time, and her shortest gestation in the five or six years I was her veterinarian was more than 350 days.

One mare went thirteen months to the day. (The Jockey Club required all sorts of affidavits to register that one.) Another, after several normal-term foals, suddenly had two in a row at a year, plus or minus a couple of days, and then reverted to 340 or so days.

Several years ago, a client bought a mare at a breeding stock sale. She was from a dispersal sale, and he paid $300,000 for her. This was back in the days when $100,000 mares still brought oohs and aahs from the spectators. We will refer to her as 300K.

She was ten, her two foals that raced were high-class stakes winners, and she was in foal to a young horse of incredible popularity. Her calculated due date (341 days) was easy to remember: April 15.

She made a small bag in early March — that is, her mammary glands enlarged in preparation for milk production — but even though this is borderline worrisome, it isn't unusual. And her bag did not grow. In the wee small hours of March 19, I received a frantic call from the farm manager. "300K is foaling! Get over here!"

I got there just in time to see 300K give birth to a normal foal. No signs of prematurity or dysmaturity. Vigorous. Hungry. After 316 days of gestation. 300K had not had a foaling bag that afternoon, but she did when she got up after delivering.

Okay, we figured, an error was made on the breeding date reported to the sales company, which is not an unheard-of occurrence. But the next year she did it again: 318 days — a vigorous, healthy, normal foal. The longest she ever carried a foal while my client owned her was 326 days. He was worried that year because she was going so long.

I have never known another mare to do that and produce a normal, healthy foal, but where there is one there is surely another.

Most mares are pretty much on time (within four or five days of expected delivery), though, and some are almost like clockwork. I once owned a mare that produced eleven foals for me (none of which could outrun me, but they were all beautiful and sold well enough to support her). Until her last one at age nineteen, they all arrived at 340 or 342 days. That last one almost made it to a year.

Be aware that long-lived sperm can mess up your calculations.

One year a client's mare was bred on a beautiful follicle, but unfortunately ovulation didn't follow when I expected it. Two days later we tried to double breed her, but the stallion was booked. A couple of days after that the follicle was still there, but the stallion was still busy. Finally, six days after breeding, she ovulated. (Any vet who says this has never happened to him is either fibbing or doesn't work on horses.)

She conceived. Some stallions have very long-lived sperm and this was evidently one of them. The owner figured her expected foaling date from her breeding date. (He always used 340 days.) He became worried when 345 days arrived and she still had no foal. At 350 days, she delivered. That was 344 days after ovulation, right on time as far as I was concerned.

Go Figure

What all this comes down to is this: there is no set period of gestation in mares. I guess 70 percent will foal between 340 and 345 days, and probably 85 percent will foal between 336 and 350 days, but there are some mares that just don't follow the rules.

And most mares will give fair warning; the outward signs (udder development, waxing, vulvar relaxation, for example) will all be there, but there are tremendous variations.

For instance, 300K went down year after year with only a minimal bag, if that, and got up thirty to sixty minutes later with a full milk supply. I once owned a mare whose bag looked like a Holstein cow's for four or five weeks before she was due but always went between 340 and 350 days.

Late-Pregnancy Colic

Colic cases range from very mild, transient discomfort — most of which are probably never noticed or recognized by the people responsible for the care of the horses — to agonizingly painful, fatal conditions, even when caught and treated early. The treatment, of course, depends on the cause, but pain relievers are important in all cases, and the animal's response, or lack of response, is a helpful diagnostic and prognostic tool.

What follows is not a general discussion of the assorted causes and treatments of colic, because they're too numerous and varied to discuss here, and excellent treatises on these topics are available in many books and journals. Rather, this is the story of what may be an obscure cause of colic. I say "obscure" because, as with so many colics, this may go unnoticed and, therefore, it actually may be quite common.

What Is Colic?

Colic is not a disease or condition in itself; it's a group of signs, characterized by pain or discomfort, that may originate from different areas of the body as a result of various causes, any of which can occur in late pregnancy. (See page 70 for more on the causes of colic.)

"SAVE HER, DOC! I don't care about the foal! You've got to save her! Do anything, but save her!" Rodney was pleading.

Rodney was in his late twenties, out of college, and employed in a well-paying position by a large national company with a Lexington office. He wasn't married, apparently didn't date much from what I heard, and lived with his widowed mother, who had been left financially comfortable by her late husband.

Rodney liked horseracing a lot and decided that he wanted to get into the sport. Rather than purchase a yearling or horse in training, however, he decided it would be more fun, satisfying, and rewarding to acquire a broodmare and raise and race her foals.

Rodney did his homework. He studied pedigrees, sire production, sales averages, and other matters and went to the November breeding stock sale at Keeneland racetrack, where he bought a pretty nice, middle-aged broodmare for about $50,000. (We'll henceforth refer to her as Pretty Nice.) She had won several races and enough money to support herself and was a half sister to a couple of stakes winners. She herself had produced a stakes-placed winner of more than $100,000 and two other very useful runners from four foals of racing age. And she was in foal to a young stallion whose stud fee was somewhere between $15,000 and $40,000.

Rodney decided that he personally wanted to give Pretty Nice all the care she needed. He didn't own a farm, so he boarded her at a public boarding farm where I was the veterinarian for several owners who kept their pleasure horses there. He asked the girl whose horse resided in an adjacent stall if she knew a good vet. Not knowing any other vet, she gave him my phone number. That's how I came to work with him.

Rodney tended to Pretty Nice each day at 6 A.M. before going to work and then at 5 P.M. after he left work. In the evenings he'd usually stay for at least two hours, often more, doing things to or for Pretty Nice, who became very important to him. Everyone is partial to his own horses, of course, but Rodney became convinced that Pretty Nice was the best mare in captivity, a Broodmare of the Year in waiting. And he wasn't the least bit bashful about expressing that opinion.

This is a lengthy introduction to what comes next, and I include it so the reader will better understand Rodney's response to what follows.

Pretty Nice was due to foal in mid-May, so Rodney had several months of bonding time. And he used it well. He called me if anything even remotely out of the ordinary occurred with his beloved mare.

On the evening of April 20 he called. Pretty Nice had not eaten, and now she was lying down. Although my first thought was that she was foaling or aborting, this turned out not to be the case. In the half hour it took me to get there, she began to roll. She was in rough shape.

What I think was going on with Pretty Nice is something that I have never read about but that I know occurs because I saw it on a postmortem exam. (Of course, there may be dozens of articles on it that I've somehow missed. Another possibility is that it's so common that no one has bothered to write about it and I have lived a sheltered life.) The fact that I've seen four or five similar cases over the years leads me to believe that it happens more than the lack of reports would indicate, but I'm the first to admit that my diagnosis may be wrong. All of the cases I've seen were during the last month of pregnancy, including the one I saw on postmortem, which adds to my conviction that this condition does indeed occur. With that disclaimer, here is what I think was happening to Pretty Nice.

Pinched Intestine

A section of Pretty Nice's intestine had become trapped between the fetus and something else, probably the pelvis. This would result in the same signs as any severe colic and would produce the same outcome as a twisted intestine. In other cases in which I've suspected this (I don't know how to prove it), the mares attained relief by rolling on their back, enough back-and-forth movement apparently freeing the pinched intestine, and the mares eventually went on to uneventful foalings. (The mare that died had apparently been in bad shape all day and wasn't found until it was time to bring in for her evening meal. At that point she was beyond saving and died within minutes of my arrival.) Pretty Nice's pain didn't abate, however, even with a lot of vigorous rolling. There was minimal response to the usual colic medications, as was the case with the other mares in which I had suspected this condition. Around 11 P.M., she was no better and Rodney was getting frantic. I told him that we were approaching an extremely serious stage, and action had to be taken soon or we'd lose the mare.

"What can be done?" he asked, pacing and wringing his hands.

"Surgery is a definite possibility, but I think if we get the foal out the problem may resolve itself," I said. "The foal will have to be taken if surgery is done anyway, but by inducing labor the compromised intestine may be released."

"Well, then, do it!" he commanded.

"The foal's the problem then. It's not due for at least three weeks," I explained. "If we induce labor, it may be too weak to survive. And it'll need to eat if it's viable. Pretty Nice has no milk yet."

Rodney didn't care. He wanted the mare to be saved. "I don't want my mare to die!" He was shouting.

I manually dilated Pretty Nice's cervix and gave her an injection of oxytocin to induce labor. An hour later she delivered a small, weak colt that was unable to stand.

She, however, was. Within five or ten minutes of delivery she got up. She went down two or three times but within an hour she was essentially acting normal.

Rodney was delighted, but then I called his attention to the pathetic little colt in the corner of the stall.

"We might be able to save him," I told him. "We need to try."

With the mare apparently out of danger, Rodney agreed. I went home and got some frozen colostrum. In the hour of my absence, Rodney sat on the stall floor with the little guy; bonding occurred quickly because when I returned he insisted that he be saved.

As we gave the colostrum by stomach tube, Rodney asked, "Will he make it?"

"I don't know," I answered.

"Save him!" he ordered. "You've got to save him! Do anything you have to, just save him!"

This was before neonatal intensive care units existed in the local equine clinics, so Rodney took time off from his job and we fed the colt by tube for about ten days, at which point the foal began drinking from a bucket. By two weeks he could stand, and from then on he developed as naturally as a bucket-fed foal could. Rodney put him in training, but he never raced and eventually Rodney gave him away as a pleasure horse at the age of four.

Pretty Nice was not bred that year but went on to have four more foals for Rodney. Two were winners but none came close to duplicating the success of her earlier offspring. She was struck by lightning and killed at the age of eighteen, and Rodney was inconsolable. He didn't buy another mare, sold his three horses in training, and apparently ceased to be a racing fan. I never saw or heard from him again.

8

Foaling

Care of the Pregnant Mare and Foaling

After years and years of attending to the needs of pregnant mares and delivering foals, I tend to forget that it isn't second nature to everyone. I have even found longtime horse folk who don't know what to do and what to have on hand for the big day. Unbelievably, the mare has not been properly cared for during late pregnancy, and the few items needed for foaling aren't even available. It's all pretty basic, once you learn it.

General Care

Pregnant mare care begins with good general horse care: worming, vaccinations, and proper nutrition. A pregnant mare has no specific housing requirements. Actually, if the weather is warm and the grass is good, she has no housing requirements at all.

Worming

Worming, of course, is essential to the well-being of all horses. A bimonthly schedule and a rotation of products are best, although some of the new products are effective for three months. Your veterinarian can advise you on which wormers she feels are most effective. If, however, grazing is poor, you have a large population of horses on limited space, or both, worming should be done more often. (See page 288 for more on parasite control.)

It's not a good idea to worm a mare within four to six weeks of foaling, however. With the products now available it may be perfectly safe to do so, but worming may also stress the mare unnecessarily, which could lead to a premature foaling. Do worm her the first or second day after she foals, however.

Vaccinations

Vaccinations depend somewhat on the use of the mare and the environment of the stable. If she is an only horse with no outside contact, routine flu, tetanus, rhinopneumonitis, encephalitis, and rabies vaccines are necessary and should be given on a schedule outlined by your veterinarian.

If, however, she is going to compete or be shown (both of these can easily and safely be done through the first seven months of pregnancy), the vaccination program needs to be a little more strenuous. Training centers, racetracks, show grounds, and other similar facilities are incubators of all diseases known to veterinary science and probably to several that aren't known. Also, if she is stabled where there is a transient horse population or other horses that show or compete, extra precautions need to be taken.

In these cases, flu and rhinopneumonitis vaccines should be given quarterly after the initial doses. Other vaccines, such as those for strangles (a bad idea, as it is not terribly effective and often makes the horse sick), equine viral arteritis, botulism (a good idea), and Potomac horse fever, may be given if your veterinarian recommends them, although depending on the circumstances they may not be necessary. A very important vaccination is a tetanus toxoid booster a month before the mare foals. Don't forget it! This provides protection to both the mare and her foal.

Nutrition

Nutrient requirements of a pregnant mare are the same as those of a nonpregnant mare through the first two thirds (roughly seven and a half months) of pregnancy. At this point, the requirements increase. Each mare is different, but generally a mare at foaling needs 50 to 60 percent more feed than she required in mid-pregnancy. This new level should be reached gradually, beginning with a slight increase as she enters the last trimester. The protein level should not exceed 15 or 16 percent, nor should it be lower than 13 percent.

A very important fact often overlooked or ignored even by veteran horsemen is that a mare has even greater nutrient requirements when she is lactating. Her feed should continue to be increased until the foal is sixty to ninety days old, then the amount gradually lessened until weaning, at which point she should be back down to her regular level.

Good-quality roughage, both hay and pasture, is always important. Try to avoid fescue if at all possible. It isn't particularly nutritious and can cause problems in foaling, with the fetus, or in milk production. If you have fescue in your pasture, see page 206 for more information.

Items for a Foaling Box

There are a few things that you need on hand for use when the mare finally decides to foal, so gather them up beforehand and put them aside in the barn in a foaling box.

- Several rolls of gauze for wrapping the mare's tail
- A few disposable plastic sleeves or gloves
- A bottle of strong (7%) iodine for the foal's navel
- A shot glass or 6 mL disposable syringe case for applying the iodine
- A commercial phosphate enema
- An inexpensive retractable ballpoint pen

In addition to these items, you might want to keep a twitch on hand in case the mare won't allow the foal to nurse.

How You Can Help

Before the big day, check to see whether the mare's vulva has been sutured. Even people who have owned the same mare for years often forget this. If you don't feel confident that you can tell, have your veterinarian do it. If she is sutured, she must be opened before she foals or she'll tear. It's important not to open her too soon, as this may invite contamination.

Ideally, opening should be done as the mare lies down to foal, but realistically it needs to be done by your veterinarian a few days before the calculated due date. It's also important to resuture her the day after she foals. (See page 174 for more information on the Caslick procedure.)

If you are lucky enough to be there when foaling begins, go in the stall with the mare, slowly, carefully, and quietly. Don't alarm her and don't have a crowd with you. I once had a dentist for a client. He had seven kids, and when his mare foaled, he had all seven with him in the stall. If I were the mare, I would have stopped right there.

Foaling

When the mare begins to foal, wrap the tail with a roll of gauze. It keeps it out of the way and prevents it from being covered with placental fluid.

The first thing you'll see protruding from her vulva is a large sac that will rupture, spewing placental fluid everywhere. If it doesn't break within a minute or two, you need to break it for her. There's a place called the cervical star where the placenta will break easily (see page 166 for more information), but if you're inexperienced you need to use an instrument to pierce it. Remember, though, there's a foal in there, so don't use a sharp instrument. A ballpoint pen with the point retracted will do a very good job. I have probably gone through thirty pens doing this, and I'm experienced.

Once the water breaks (or is broken), check the foal's positioning. Using a disposable glove or sleeve, slowly and carefully slip a hand into the vulva. You should feel a foot. Keep going in another few inches, and you should feel another foot. A few more inches should reveal a nose.

If this isn't the case, or if you can't tell, there may be a problem. Call your veterinarian immediately or, preferably, have someone else call because you need to get the mare up and make her walk. As long as she's

When Should You Call a Vet?

As a veterinarian, I believe that when a mare starts to foal, a vet should be called. But Mother Nature does a pretty good job when allowed to. I'd guess that more than 99 percent of all mares foal by themselves with no problems, but if a problem should arise, the foal and perhaps the mare might be lost.

Mares are very inconsiderate. They usually foal between 10 P.M. and 2 A.M. This has been statistically proved, so if you want to see your mare foal, plan to lose some sleep. Monitors that sound an alarm when the mare begins to foal are available, and using one of these sure beats trying to stay awake night after night, watching and waiting.

But when is a veterinarian really needed? Call the vet immediately if a foal is malpositioned and if the delivery is prolonged and takes longer than 30 to 35 minutes. You'll also need to call the veterinarian if any of these statements apply:

- The placenta is abnormal (too heavy, discolored, too thick, etc.).
- The foal is unable to stand after two or three hours.
- The foal can't or won't suck.
- The foal is weak.
- The foal is colicky.
- The foal strains to urinate, produces no urine, or urine comes from the umbilicus.
- The foal is lame or has swollen or warm joints.
- Blood comes from the umbilicus.
- The mucous membranes are abnormally colored.
- Capillary refill time is greater than two or three seconds.
- There is excessive tearing or blepharospasm.
- There is rapid or heavy breathing.
- There is anything abnormal.

Even if everything seems normal, it's a good idea to have the veterinarian examine both mare and foal the morning after delivery. Some people balk at the expense of calling a veterinarian, but it's a cheap precaution when compared with the time and expense already invested in the foal.

walking, straining will be reduced or stopped. If the mare's allowed to stay down and strain, a malpositioned foal can be wedged within her pelvis so tightly that nothing short of surgery will extricate it.

Check the Foal

When the foal is finally out, check its nostrils to see whether placental tissue is covering them; if there is any, pull it away to clear the airway. The absolute next thing you must do is put iodine on its navel. Pour the iodine into the shot glass or syringe case, roll the foal onto its side, and invert the iodine container over the umbilical stump, holding it there for several seconds. This aids in preventing bacteria from entering what amounts to an open wound. Not surprisingly, the foal thinks little of this procedure, and it will usually flail about with its legs, so be careful. Those little feet can hurt. If the umbilical cord has not broken, call your vet. There is an easy way to break it, but it's best done by someone who knows how.

A word of caution here: check the foal's sex. I've seen dozens of colts that have had their sheaths iodined. It's close to the umbilicus and it hangs down, but it definitely doesn't need iodine.

Observe the Mare

The mare may or may not get right up. Either way it's fine. If she does get up, she may continue to have contractions and go back down and roll. Try not to let her roll on you or her foal.

The mare should pass the placenta within twenty or thirty minutes. If she still retains it after three hours, call your veterinarian. A retained placenta can lead to serious problems.

Standing and Nursing

The foal should try to get up within a few minutes to a half hour. If after an hour or so it still can't get up, or won't try, help it. This is one of life's more frustrating things to try to do. Be aware that the foal will do just the opposite of what you want. If you push it right, it will go left.

Eventually, either by itself or with help, standing will be accomplished. Now comes the search for food. This is a *really* frustrating experience for all. The foal will aim its muzzle seemingly everywhere but the right place and continue to miss the mark. If it's the mare's first foal (and in some older mares), the udder may be tender. The foal may make meaningful contact only to have the mare squeal and pull away. In some cases, she may even kick at the foal. If this occurs, a tranquilizer, a twitch, or both may be necessary to make her stand for the foal. Once the initial pressure is relieved by nursing, she'll probably be fine.

After the foal nurses and moves around, it should have a bowel movement. If it hasn't had one by the morning after foaling, give it the enema you packed in your foal kit. A foal is born with hard fecal matter called *meconium* in its rectum, and it must be expelled or colic will result. The meconium is pelleted and black or dark brown in color; you can easily tell when it's been passed. Some people advocate giving an enema at birth or shortly thereafter, but many, if not most, foals will have a bowel movement on their own once they have nursed and put forth a little activity.

Turn Them Out

Get both mare and foal outside for a few hours, at least. They both need the exercise. Be sure to turn them out alone; a newly foaled mare is often very protective and may kick at other horses. The foal instinctively runs behind its dam and can be seriously injured. I have seen two foals killed in this manner. Even if the weather is miserable, get them out for a little while.

Difficult Labor (Dystocia)

It was 3 a.m. on January 18. Snowing. Twenty degrees. I was in a barn, a nice, modern barn, but a barn nonetheless, and barns are cold when it's 20 degrees outside. I hate January foalings.

And this mare was having a terrible time. She was trying to deliver, but her foal's head was turned down, and both of its front legs were bent backward at the knees. It was definitely *dystocia:* slow or difficult labor or birth, usually caused by abnormal positioning of the fetus.

And hard labor is another reason why I hate January foalings. There is no way to reposition a foal in a mare and still remain bundled up. I had placental fluid all over me; it was warm when it first came from the mare, but it chilled all too soon and so did I. I was freezing.

But I got the little guy straightened and we had a live, if somewhat weak, foal. He would live, but every year some foals won't arrive alive, even though they enter the birth canal that way. And some will take their dams with them, victims of dystocia.

Incidence

Fortunately, dystocia is uncommon, although there seems to be a variance among breeds. In Thoroughbreds it is estimated that 3 to 5 percent of all births follow a difficult delivery, but in draft and pony breeds it's higher, with some estimates approaching 8 to even 10 percent. Also, there may be a familial predisposition. Over the years, I have attended three mares with dystocias that were themselves the products of dystocias.

What Happens

Difficult labor is an emergency. Once the membrane surrounding the fetus ruptures, delivery should occur within twenty to thirty minutes, so time is of the essence.

Once foaling has begun, the mare's uterus continues to contract either until the foal is delivered or until the foal cannot be delivered and a combination of fatigue and depletion of the hormone oxytocin causes the uterine contractions to cease. By that point, the foal is usually wedged irretrievably in the birth canal, often resulting in the loss of both mare and foal.

Be Attentive

We all know of foals that have entered the world unattended, with neither mother nor offspring any the worse for wear, but that is no reason to allow a mare to foal without an attendant present or one of the new foaling alert systems in use. Even if the help is inexperienced, an attendant can tell time and call for help if no foal is lying beside the mare within a reasonable period.

If someone is present to help out, making the mare get up and walk can minimize a dystocia by causing the uterine contractions to stop or become less intense. The mare will not want to do this and will have to be forced. One person pulling on the lead shank and another walking beside her swatting her with a broom usually will keep her moving until the veterinarian arrives.

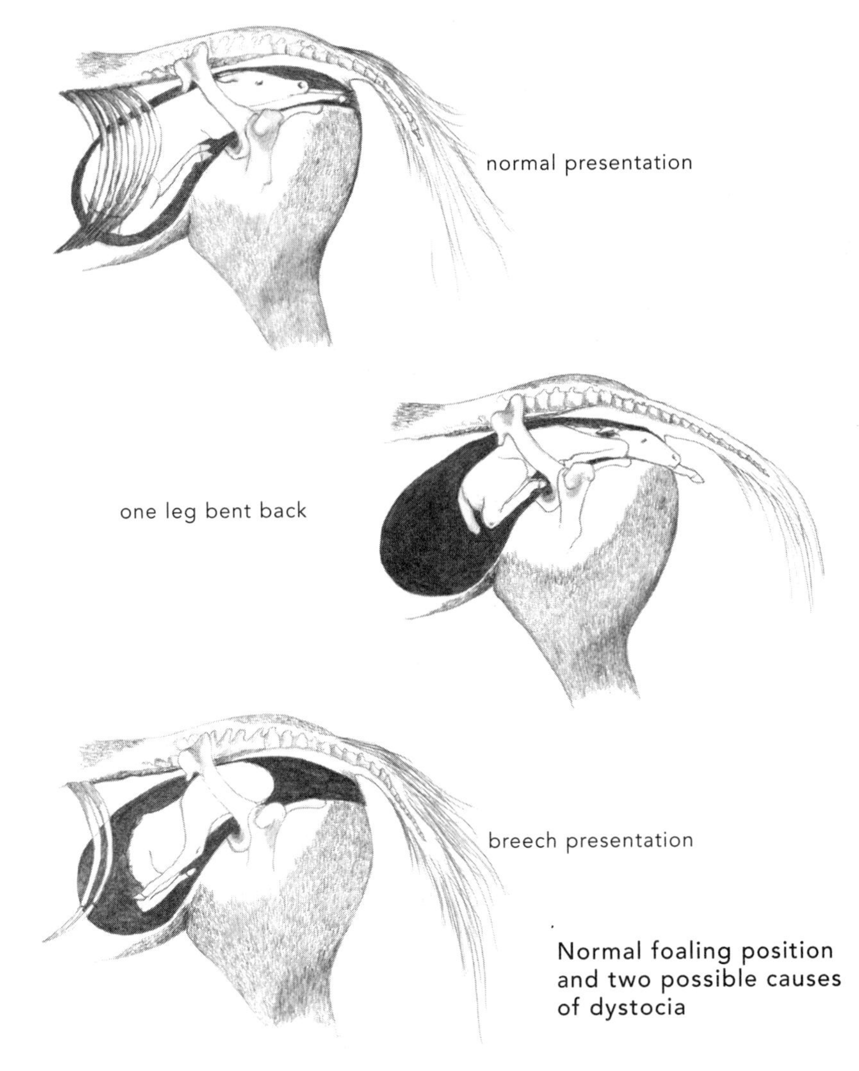

Normal foaling position and two possible causes of dystocia

Possible Causes

When the veterinarian arrives, the reason for the dystocia must be determined. As already noted, it is usually due to fetal malposition, but fetal size can also be a factor. Although the dam is the primary determinant of the size of the foal, a large sire/small dam combination can occasionally create a problem. I have seen fetal size as a cause twice, once in a very small pony mare and once in a very large draft mare, and the grim outcome was the same in both cases, as the owners would not or could not justify a cesarean section. Less common, and a scenario that I have never seen, is previous damage to the pelvis resulting in a birth canal too small to allow even a normal-sized foal to pass. Also, twins coming at the same time will cause dystocia. And, finally, fetal malformation is extremely rare but can result in dystocia.

How to Proceed

Once the cause of the dystocia is determined, there are five options to consider when attempting to deliver a live foal, maintain a live mare, and ensure that the mare's reproductive tract isn't damaged or compromised. These five options, in decreasing order of desirability, are manipulation of the fetus, traction, fetotomy, cesarean section, and euthanasia.

- **Manipulation of the fetus.** Manipulation consists of repositioning the fetus so it can be delivered. If the head is turned, straighten it; if a knee is bent, straighten it; if a hock is flexed, straighten it. It all sounds deceptively simple but repositioning an incorrectly presented foal is the most difficult thing I have yet encountered in veterinary medicine.

Gravity is a great help in manipulation. By anesthetizing the mare, placing her on her back, and elevating her hindquarters, the fetus can more easily be repelled so working space is gained. This is not feasible in most foalings without taking the mare to a clinic, but twice we have put chains on a mare's hind legs, swung the chains over a beam, and attached them to a tractor. The mares were none the worse for wear and delivered healthy foals. Whatever works.

• **Traction.** Traction, which involves pulling the foal, can be resorted to after first lubricating the foal and vagina generously if it is a tight fit or if the positioning has been corrected and the uterine contractions have ceased to propel the foal. Traction can also be applied as a last resort when the foal is wedged too tightly for manipulation or if it is dead. Traction is rough on both the live foal and the mare, and uterine prolapse (inversion of the uterus) is an occasional consequence.
• **Fetotomy.** Fetotomy, or dissection of the foal so it can be removed in pieces, is usually done only when all else fails and the foal is dead. There are occasions in which it must be done on a live foal to save the mare, which should be the primary goal in the first place. Usually it requires removing the head so it can be gotten out of the way in order to manipulate the legs. I'm glad to say that I have had to perform only one fetotomy in my career.
• **Cesarean section.** Cesarean section is the absolute last resort if the mare or foal is to be salvaged. Mares do not tolerate this well, are very slow to recover, and, if they survive, are quite often unable to bear more foals. The only situation I can imagine that would justify a cesarean section is if it's a young, extremely valuable mare, but it isn't my call.
• **Euthanasia.** Euthanasia may be necessary if there is uncorrectable damage or if the owner chooses it for financial or humane reasons.

Complications

In addition to the possible complications following dystocia mentioned above (dead foal, dead mare, dead foal and mare, or a mare that loses her reproductive capability), there are lots of other possibilities. Uterine contamination causing a uterine infection is the main problem. One factor that all complications share is the need for veterinary attention.

I don't think a dystocia can be predicted — I know I can't do it — but difficult labors are going to happen. By being there and being attentive, the odds of a loss can be minimized.

Red Bag Foal (Placenta Previa)

A CLIENT HAD A MARE THAT HAD PRODUCED several foals with no problem. Then she had a red bag foal. Then the next year she had another red bag. This brought questions from him. Will she continue to have red bag deliveries? Is it common to have two in a row? Can red bags be prevented?

What Is Placenta Previa?

In a red bag delivery, properly called *placenta previa,* the placenta doesn't rupture, and the foal is delivered while still enclosed in the membranes. Movements of the foal probably will cause some placentas to rupture. In attended foalings, rupture is easily accomplished by tearing or puncturing the placenta at the cervical star, the whitish area on the otherwise reddish brown placenta. This is where nature intended the placenta to break. If you can't accomplish this with your fingers, a ballpoint pen with the point retracted works well. If all else fails, use scissors, but be careful: there's a foal in there.

Incidence and Predisposing Factors

Placenta previa isn't common. I have seen fewer than a dozen cases. In unattended foalings, it's a potentially serious problem because a foal can easily suffocate if the bag isn't broken.

I've read various accounts about why red bags occur. One theory attributes red bag deliveries to the age of the mare or to the number of pregnancies she has had, or both. Because each pregnancy requires the generation of a new placenta, I'm not sure what these factors have to do with anything.

Another popular theory is that a mild infection occurs that apparently toughens the placenta. Maybe. Several red bag foals are weaker than expected, and this is compatible with a mild infection. But I have seen myriad foals with infections of the placenta, in which the placenta was no tougher than a normal one. If anything, it may even be more fragile.

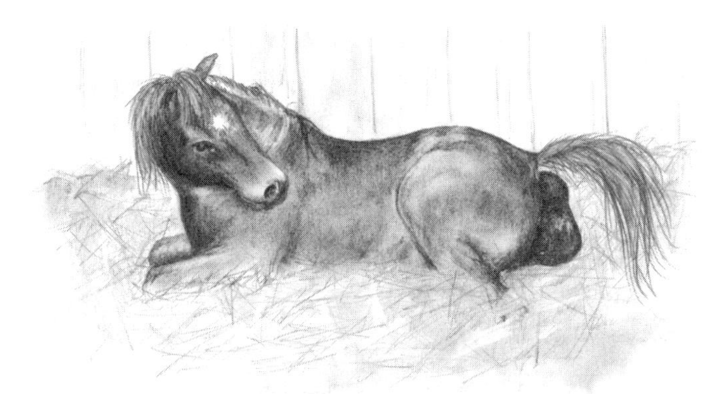

In a red bag delivery, the placenta does not rupture and the foal is delivered while still enclosed in the membranes.

I once heard that red bag is more likely to occur in mares that have been heavily stressed. That's a plausible theory because, directly or indirectly, stress is probably the cause of all things bad in this world, from hangnails to heart attacks.

The theory that I like best is this one: it is linked to any or all of those previously listed factors. In the cases that I've seen, there was no common denominator I could discover.

Now to answer my client's questions. Will the mare continue to have red bag deliveries? I don't know. I've never seen another mare that had two or more in a row, which also answered his second question. Is there anything to do to prevent red bag foalings? I don't know. I wish I did. I wish I could predict when they're going to happen. (At this point I know he was glad he asked. He could have gotten the same answers from the clerk at the grocery store.)

9

Care of the Foal

Problems of the Newborn Foal

Someone once said, "If one tenth of the things that can go wrong with foals did go wrong with them, there would be very few horses." I don't remember who said it (it may have been me), and it may be a slight overstatement, but it's nonetheless true that many things can go wrong with baby horses that can prevent them from developing into useful adults. Indeed, some of these problems can lead to death if not addressed in a timely and proper fashion.

Some of the problems, both the potentially fatal ones and the ones that "only" make a horse undesirable to a possible owner, arrive in the world with the foal. Fortunately, a good many are correctable if caught early. We'll touch briefly on several of the more common problems of newborns, starting at the head of the foal and working back.

Entropion

Entropion is the inversion of one or both lower eyelids. It's most often seen in premature or dehydrated foals. The signs typically associated with entropion are lacrimation (tearing) and blepharospasm (holding the eye closed) and, if uncorrected, it may lead to corneal ulceration, which, in turn, can lead to blindness or partial blindness.

This is easily remedied in many cases by simply rolling the lower lid outward with the thumb at frequent intervals, but most cases require the placement of a few sutures in the lower lid to hold the lid everted. The sutures may be removed in a few days to a week, depending on the severity and duration of the entropion. It's also a good idea to apply a small amount of an appropriate ophthalmic ointment several times a day. Your veterinarian will advise you on this.

Legs

Next are the forelegs. (Much of this information may also apply to the hind legs.) Because the legs are the most important part of a creature designed to run, problems here are common. The biggest problem with potential racehorses, of course, is that the legs don't go fast enough, but lack of speed is not a correctable fault.

The easily corrected leg problems of a foal include angular deformities, contracted tendons, and supernumerary digits.

Angular Deformities

In foals with angular deformities of the legs, time may be the best remedy. Many will correct themselves, although restricted exercise is sometimes beneficial. If self-correction is slow or nonexistent, there comes a time when a decision must be made to do something to correct the problem, specifically periosteal elevation. Your veterinarian can help you decide when intervention is needed. Periosteal elevation is simple and remarkable, although it doesn't always work. It's less successful in severe angular deformities, but it may be useful when combined with other, more invasive techniques (see pages 132–134 for details).

Contracted Tendons

Contracted tendons illustrate well what Dr. Foley told us in veterinary school: "Ten years from now, half of what we tell you now will be wrong. And we don't know which half." Back then (nearly thirty years ago), we learned to exercise foals with contracted tendons, providing, of course, that the foal could stand. The theory was that the animal's weight and eventual fatigue would "stretch" or lengthen the tendons, promoting recovery.

Okay, so now we find that that approach was wrong. Stall rest, with the tendons wrapped in support bandages so they *won't* fatigue, is now a major part of the treatment. The other part is a high dose of intravenous tetracycline (in theory, tetracycline binds to excessive calcium, which is believed to be the cause of contraction). Tetracycline is readily available in 99 percent of the feed stores and tack shops around the country, but *don't* administer this yourself. Consult your veterinarian. Tetracycline can, and will, kill the foal if given incorrectly.

Supernumerary Digits

I have seen two cases of supernumerary digits. As far as I know, they have absolutely no effect on a horse. They occur below the knee or hock and vary in their extent of development, ranging from what appears to be small portions of hoof to a little tiny toe. Simple surgical excision is all that is necessary; and the sooner it's done, the easier it is on everyone concerned.

The first of the two cases I have seen was on a Tennessee Walking Horse farm that had more cats than was reasonable. Probably 80 percent of these cats had six toes on each foot. I don't think extra digits is catching, especially between species, but it sure was a strange coincidence. Also, as a matter of interest, Antonio Alfonseca is a successful major league pitcher who has six fingers and six toes on each extremity, so this "problem" really isn't a problem.

Umbilical Problems

Now we get to the body, or, more precisely, the belly. In this area we find two potentially lethal, yet easily repaired, conditions: umbilical hernia and pervious urachus. They both occur in the same place, but I have never seen a foal having both conditions.

Umbilical Hernia

An umbilical hernia is formed at birth but may not be evident until days or weeks later when a bulge of varying size is noticed on the underside of the belly.

These hernias range in size from about the diameter of a pencil to a couple of inches across. They often repair themselves, even the larger ones, so unless a loop of intestine enters one, they are best observed and left alone. "Left alone" doesn't mean ignored. Just because there is no intestine within a hernia today doesn't mean there won't be some there tomorrow or next week. The hernia itself is not the problem; the danger of a loop of intestine entering it and becoming strangulated is. If you don't feel qualified to evaluate this yourself, have your veterinarian examine it periodically.

If the hernia doesn't reduce on its own, or if the intestine is involved, one of two simple procedures can be performed. If the hernia is small (that is, if you can't insert two fingers into it), it can be clamped. If the intestine isn't involved, delay this procedure until fall or winter when the fly problem no longer exists.

If the opening is two finger-widths or larger, surgery is the treatment of choice. This can be done whenever you choose, but in the case of intestinal involvement it should ideally be performed as soon as possible.

Pervious Urachus

Urachus was *not* one of the conspiratorial senators involved in Caesar's assassination. Those were Cassius, Brutus, Casca, and some other guy whose name escapes me at this sitting. The *urachus* is the structure within the umbilical cord that carries urine from the fetal bladder to the allantois. Usually the urachus closes at birth, but sometimes it remains open or partially open, and it may even reopen (rarely) a day or more after birth. When this occurs, urine leaks from the umbilical stump. It may be only a small, occasional drip or it may be a steady stream, but in either case the umbilicus is moist and infection results. Umbilical infections such as this may lead to an *acquired pervious urachus,* the term for the condition that results from an infection.

Due to a lack of inspection, this condition frequently goes unnoticed. Simply feel the umbilical stump once a day for a few days, beginning on the morning after foaling. (The foal won't like his belly being touched, so be careful.) If it's wet, call the veterinarian. Failure to close the urachus may lead to a fatal infection.

Fortunately, this condition is easily repaired if caught early. Cauterization with silver nitrate sticks two or three times a day for several days resolves this 99 percent of the time.

Inguinal Hernia

The problem of an inguinal hernia occurs a little farther back on male foals. I've seen twice as many foals with supernumerary digits as I have with inguinal hernias, and the one I saw corrected itself, which I understand most do.

The inguinal ring is the hole in the abdominal wall through which the testicle descends and the spermatic cord passes. An inguinal hernia occurs when a small amount of intestine enters the ring. Evidently, most of these reduce themselves within a few weeks, but if this doesn't happen, there are two courses of action.

One is a bandaging technique that I have read about in two different publications. Apparently this external figure-eight bandage holds the intestine within the abdominal cavity while the inguinal ring reduces in size. If you ever choose to have this done to your colt, I hope I'm not your veterinarian because I suspect that this is easier to describe than it is to do.

The other method of treatment is surgery, the approach depending on whether the intestine is strangulated, in which case colic signs are seen. Inguinal hernia presents with something other than testicles in the scrotum and may include signs of colic. (By the way, the testicles are there at birth. They don't descend later, regardless of what you may be told. If they're not there at birth, you have a *cryptorchid,* a male with retained testicles. See page 316 on gelding for more information.)

Ruptured Bladder

Books lead one to believe that a ruptured bladder is more common than my experience would suggest. It can occur in either sex, but it usually affects colts. The foal's bladder is full, and as it is squeezed through the birth canal, rarely the full bladder ruptures. The reason that it happens more frequently in colts is because the urine can be easily expressed in a filly (it's a straight shot), but in colts it has to go around turns through a long tube.

The only sign initially is a foal that doesn't urinate, because the urine is filling the abdominal cavity as it runs from the ruptured bladder. This is bad news and immediate surgery is the only treatment.

Meconium Retention

Finally we reach the end of the foal. By "end," I mean the rear. In chapter 8 on foaling, I discuss meconium (the hard fecal balls a foal is born with) and the need to get it out of the little guy (see page 227). A lot of times — most times — the stimulation of nursing and getting up and moving around takes care of the situation, but many people feel that a prophylactic enema is a good idea anyway. Personally, I wait awhile before resorting to this, but an enema won't hurt (unless the foal kicks you).

Occasionally, though, the meconium is high in the intestinal tract and is loosened neither by nursing, activity, nor enema. A foal exhibits intense abdominal pain, and frequently in the middle of a bout through which no living creature could possibly survive, it will cease its throes of agony, get up, calmly nurse, and then return to its death scene. Call the veterinarian if no meconium is passed after an enema or at the first signs of pain.

Panic by everyone ensues, but a little mineral oil and permeatrate adminstered by the vet via nasogastric tube should move the offending meconium out and everything will be fine.

These are only a few of the problems that can affect a newborn foal and are the most easily recognized and corrected. There are other problems that can enter the world along with the foal that can also be remedied if recognized early. Failure of passive transfer and neonatal isoerythrolysis are relatively common and potentially fatal; they are discussed next.

Failure of Passive Transfer

IN THIS AREA WHERE HORSES ARE BIG BUSINESS, there are people who keep *nurse mares,* mares whose only purpose is to be leased out to Thoroughbred and Standardbred breeders who have orphaned foals. These nurse mares act as surrogate mothers for the orphans.

The nurse mare folks also usually maintain a colostrum bank, which is a freezer full of colostrum for use by foals that were unable to get colostrum from their dams for whatever reason. It's a big business. Some veterinary clinics also maintain a supply of colostrum.

I think it was 1983, in late April or so. No nurse mares were available, and the colostrum supplies were depleted. Some of the large farms maintain a colostrum bank for their own use, but the regular suppliers had none. In a two-week period that year, my clients had five

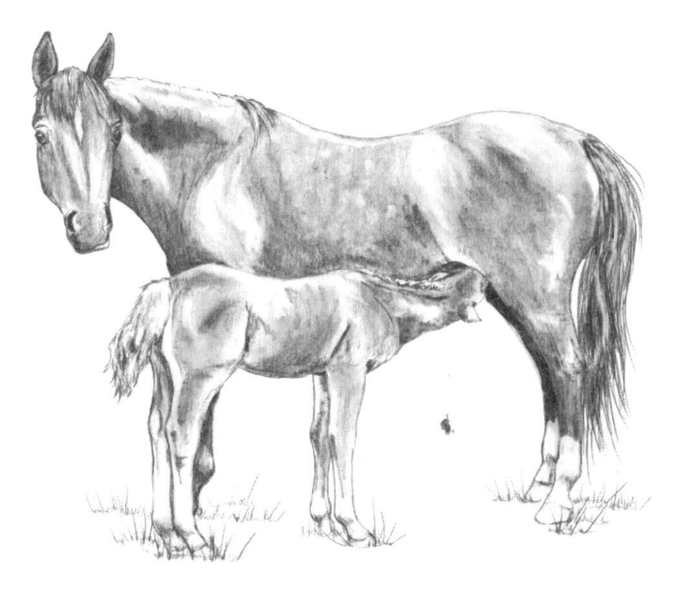

It's essential that a foal receive colostrum (first milk) from its dam.

mares die in foaling or shortly thereafter. All of the foals lived, but the problem of feeding them was significant.

I always kept a small amount of colostrum on hand if I ever had a need for it, and I had enough for the first two of these orphans. A client let me "borrow" some from a mare of his that foaled on the same night that the third orphan arrived, but we were in trouble for the last two. These last two were both nearly twenty-four hours old before we could find a colostrum supply for them, and we got it into them as quickly as we could. The last one had briefly nursed her dam; the mare died about three hours after foaling.

How Are Antibodies Transferred?

The foal gets needed antibodies via colostrum. The antibodies are selectively transferred from the blood of the mare to the colostrum in the last two to four weeks of pregnancy, probably as a result of alterations in estrogen and progesterone levels during this time. These are antibodies for a variety of the common microorganisms to which the mare has been exposed, which is the main reason it's recommended that a mare's vaccinations, especially tetanus, be boosted approximately one month before she's due to foal.

The foal relies on the supply of antibodies (primarily immunoglobulin G, or IgG) in the colostrum for protection against pathogenic and opportunistic microorganisms that it may encounter in its first few weeks of life before it is able to produce its own.

The absorption process of the colostral antibodies is more involved than the level of detail I'm including here. Suffice it to say that the antibodies are absorbed through the small intestine and enter the foal's circulatory system, where they can be measured a few hours after nursing, reaching levels approximating those of the mare at about twenty-four to thirty-six hours after birth. At about twenty-four hours after foaling, the small intestine loses its ability to absorb the antibodies, so the window of opportunity is relatively brief.

These antibodies from the dam are essentially depleted from the foal by 90 to 180 days. Somewhere in this time frame, say 90 to 120 days, a vaccination program for the foal should begin, in response to which it will create its own antibodies.

All five foals were bottle fed, which is a harder to do than to say. (The foals don't want to be handled, don't want the bottle, and resist in every way possible.) The first three foals did okay. One of the last two did okay, too, but the one whose dam lived long enough for her to nurse never thrived and died at one month old. She never developed any antibodies, even though we gave her intravenous plasma from a cross-matched donor. In retrospect, we should have given her oral plasma when she was a few hours old, but because she had nursed a little we thought we might be okay. That's a mistake I've never made again. She was a victim of failure of passive antibody transfer (FPT).

Eventually nurse mares became available, and two of the remaining four foals were put with surrogate moms. The other two were placed on buckets and did very well. One of them grew up to be a stakes winner of nearly a half-million dollars.

What Is Failure of Passive Transfer?

FPT and neonatal isoerythrolysis (NI, or jaundice, discussed on page 245) are both conditions in foals related to the mare's colostrum. In FPT, the foal doesn't get enough colostrum and is therefore deprived of antibodies it needs to combat disease; in NI, the foal gets enough colostrum, but the colostrum has the wrong antigens. FPT, then, makes the foal less able, or unable, to combat pathogens that it may encounter. With FPT, any infection becomes extremely serious, and death is often the outcome.

Contributing Factors

There are three possible causes of FPT.

- **Colostrum low in antibody levels.** This occurs in foals of improperly vaccinated mares. Shame on you if this happens to your foal.
- **Inability of the foal to absorb the antibodies.** This occurs infrequently and unpredictably. Stress on the foal may be a factor, but it may also occur when the foal cannot or will not nurse for a prolonged period after foaling, during which time the gut's ability to absorb the antibodies is diminished.

• **Failure of the foal to receive colostrum or insufficient colostrum.** This is probably responsible for 85 percent of the FPT normally seen in practice. The rare agalactic mare that is unable to produce milk doesn't pass on antibodies or anything else to her foal for obvious reasons. Agalactia need not be dwelled on; just remember that you must quickly round up some colostrum for your foal, in addition to milk replacer (or a mare replacement) if the mare doesn't give milk. If the mare has not produced a bag as foaling nears, it's a good idea to begin the search for an alternative source of colostrum, just in case.

Severe dystocia may cause a mare with a seemingly normal bag prior to hard labor not to have a bag after the foal has been straightened out and delivered or surgically removed. This is undoubtedly stress-related, and though the milk usually returns, by that time her foal may be too old to benefit from the colostrum.

Prematurity (usually defined as foaling before 320 days of gestation) is also a problem. Although the preemie foal's gut has the ability to absorb antibodies, the mare has not yet produced colostrum.

The most common cause of a foal able to nurse not receiving colostrum is lack of colostrum in the mare's milk. A major reason for this is the mare streaming milk prior to foaling, thus losing colostrum. This may occur as a result of several situations, all involving hormonal changes and including prolonged gestation (355 days or more), placentitis, twinning, premature placental separation, and the occasional mare that thinks some other mare's foal should be hers and lets her milk flow when the other baby is seen or heard.

Another reason a foal may not receive colostrum is the death of the dam prior to nursing.

Force-Feed the Foal

One last thought on FPT: if a foal is slow to nurse for whatever reason, and after about four to six hours it still hasn't, milk the mare and have the veterinarian intubate the foal with the colostrum. Then you have a bit more time to hook the little guy up to his dam.

Determining Antibody Level

The levels of passively acquired antibodies in a foal may be measured in a serum sample. An IgG level of 400 mg/dL is accepted as the minimum to satisfactorily prevent most infections. There are lab tests that will give a precise determination and quick field tests that will give an accurate estimation, but the main problem is time. The minimum 400 mg/dL level may not be reached until the foal is twenty-four hours old. By the time it's discovered that a deficiency exists, the foal's small intestine has already lost the ability to absorb antibodies. On the other hand, and I don't know how often this happens, a foal's twenty-four-hour serum sample may contain an extremely high antibody level of 2,000 mg/dL or higher. I don't know why, but these foals frequently become very sick. Watch them. If it's known in advance that there is a good chance a foal may be deprived of colostrum (for example, if the mare has no udder development as the calculated foaling date nears, or if the mare has been streaming milk for two or three weeks), a little preplanning proves beneficial.

Treatment

As already mentioned, in areas where horse breeding is a major industry there is often a source of frozen colostrum; a veterinary clinic or nurse mare operation may well have a supply available. Get some, thaw it when the mare foals, and have your veterinarian give it via stomach tube.

Alternatively, you can build your own colostrum bank. If a mare presents a dead foal or one that dies within a few hours of birth, milk her out several times over the next twelve to eighteen hours and freeze the product. Colostrum may also be borrowed from another mare if you're fortunate enough to have one foal at the same time or know someone who has such a mare. Two to four ounces may be taken from a mare every three or four hours without adversely affecting her foal. Just in case, it's a good idea to plan ahead; borrow from a foaling mare and freeze it, then you'll have it if and when you need it.

If, however, colostrum just isn't available, oral administration of plasma or serum by the veterinarian will solve the problem. Because plasma and serum contain lower antibody levels than does colostrum, a very large amount — a few liters — may be necessary. If you learn at twenty-four hours of age that your foal is antibody-deficient, the remedy becomes a little more challenging but is still manageable. Intravenous plasma should be given by the veterinarian, paying attention to the donor. (See the next section on NI.)

There are now commercial products, both oral and intravenous, that may be given to foals that are denied colostrum. The products contain needed antibodies and are very useful; some people give them prophylactically.

Also, general nursing care, particularly keeping the foal warm, dry, and comfortable, and shielding the FPT foal from stress are necessary until its own immune system kicks in.

Jaundiced Foal (Neonatal Isoerythrolysis)

This condition comes under the heading "Things that can go wrong with my foal no matter how careful I am." And there are several things that fit that description.

Neonatal isoerythrolysis (NI) is also known as *jaundiced foal* and *hemolytic anemia* of the newborn. The usual result is a dead foal if it isn't treated, but early recognition can often save the little guy.

It is widely preached that the colostrum is extremely important for the newborn foal. It should be received within a few hours of birth. In NI, it's important that the foal *not* receive colostrum, at least not his dam's colostrum.

Isoerythrolysis is a two-dollar word that means the foal's red blood cells (erythrocytes) are being destroyed within the foal's circulatory system. (We'll use some other big words here; they will serve to show that I really did pay attention at those continuing education courses that I've had to attend.) The erythrocytes are destroyed by *alloantibodies* (*allo-* means "other") in the colostrum that are absorbed into the foal's circulatory system along with the antibodies necessary for protection from disease. These alloantibodies are produced by the foal's dam in response to alloimmunization by foreign red blood cell alloantigens that the foal inherited from the stallion. More simply put, the blood of the stallion and the blood of the mare are not compatible, and this incompatability is inherited by the foal. Thus, in effect, the foal's immune system turns against it.

Clinical Signs

A foal appears to be normal at birth and nurses normally and acts normally, until enough red blood cells are destroyed to initiate signs of trouble. These signs may appear as early as four to six hours or as late as a week. The earlier the signs, the poorer the prognosis. Foals that don't show signs until three to four days or later frequently recover unassisted; foals that show signs before twelve hours usually die, even with vigorous intervention.

There are three main signs of neonatal isoerythrolysis in the foal:

- **Depression.** This may be the first symptom noticed. The foal appears to be weak and lethargic but will not lie down on its own; if placed in recumbency by a handler, it will get up again and resume its weak, lethargic actions.
- **Icterus (jaundice).** The mucous membranes and sclera (white of the eye) are yellow, sometimes warning-light yellow. This is most easily seen in the conjunctiva, the tissue surrounding the eyeball. Roll back the foal's upper eyelid for a clear view.
- **Hemoglobinuria.** The urine is red, because the hemoglobin released by the destruction of the red blood cells is filtered by the kidneys and excreted.

Diagnosis

None of the three signs is diagnostic for NI, not even all three together, but the suggestion is strong, and further steps must be taken in the presence of any of these symptoms. A blood count is essential. A low red cell count accompanied by a low packed cell volume, in combination with the other signs, zeroes in pretty well on NI. Cross-matching the colostrum with the foal's blood, which results in lysis (breaking) of the foal's red blood cells, is a further aid in diagnosis.

A definitive diagnosis can be made by demonstrating alloantibodies on the foal's erythrocytes, although I'm not sure why anyone would want to waste precious time with a laboratory test that confirms what you already strongly suspect. With all the other signs, treat the foal as if it has NI; submit blood work for analysis to avoid problematic breeding in the future, but do not wait for results before treating. You could easily have a dead foal by the time the results are analyzed.

Treatment

The first and most important step in treatment is to stop the foal from getting any more colostrum from its dam and to locate another source of colostrum, as well as a source of milk replacement. The veterinarian will cross-match donor colostrum. You should leave the foal with its dam; this can safely be done by muzzling it. Milk the mare out and discard the milk. The veterinarian will cross-match the mare's milk with the foal's blood once or twice a day after the foal is twenty-four hours old; many can go back to nursing at this point, but it's not uncommon to still have an unfavorable reaction in a cross-match for many days. Even so, it's generally safe to allow the foal to nurse again after forty-eight hours of age, because its gut should have lost its ability to absorb the alloantibodies by then.

The foal's red blood cells, though, have been and are being destroyed, and something must be done until its bone marrow can produce replacement red cells. Therefore, in most cases, a transfusion is necessary. The blood donor, of course, should not possess the same alloantibodies that are already at work, so the dam is not an option. Blood-typing can readily identify a suitable donor, but that's not practical under field conditions and, besides, you have an emergency. Cross-matching is easy and satisfactory, although not foolproof. A cold-blooded teaser or riding horse makes an excellent donor, as does a pony, but whatever donor you choose, a cross-match is a cheap and wise precaution.

Depending on the severity of the anemia, the amount of blood transfused will vary greatly. A mildly affected three-day-old foal may respond to one liter; a severely affected twelve-hour-old foal may require several liters and still not come around. Each case is individual and must be treated as such.

Prognosis

A foal that does not show signs of NI until it is four or five days old will usually survive, often without a transfusion. One that shows signs in the first few hours of life will probably not make it, even with extensive care. It's safe to say that the prognosis is serious before twelve hours; guarded, at best, from twelve to thirty-six hours; fair from thirty-six to ninety-six hours; and favorable beyond that.

Textbooks tell us that the condition occurs only in mares that have had several foals. Not true; I've seen it in a first foal. Textbooks also tell us that once it occurs with a mare, all of her subsequent foals will also be victims of NI. Also not true; I've seen two mares that have had NI foals (one had two and one had five) and then had a foal with no problems. But for the safety of an NI mare's future foals, assume that it is true. The foaling must be attended. If any mare has had a previous foal with NI, this foal should not be allowed to nurse until proper diagnostic steps have been taken. Showing up a half hour late and finding that the foal has already nursed decreases the odds of a happy outcome.

And, of course, if a mating of mare X to stallion Y has produced an NI foal, obviously don't breed X to Y again.

Foal Diarrhea

Approximately 80 percent of the foals that I see in my practice undergo a bout of diarrhea at some point in their first month or so of life, and generally it's at the time of the mare's foal heat, her first heat cycle after giving birth. I don't know if that's high or low when compared with other practices, but because that's roughly what I've seen for nearly thirty years, I suspect it's fairly typical.

Foals were given a tail for a purpose. When they're grown, tails are useful as fly shooers or face swatters. (Your face, not theirs.) But when they're babies, that little tail is very useful as a handle. It helps immeasurably when handling a youngster because he/she doesn't want to be handled. One hand under the throatlatch or around the neck in front of the shoulders and one hand holding the tail should enable anyone to handle even the most fractious foal.

But sometimes that tail is slippery, especially around eight to twelve days after birth, and no one wants to handle a little guy's tail then.

The vast majority — 90 to 95 percent — of the foal diarrheas I see, and I imagine the foal diarrheas that anyone sees, are the so-called foal-heat scours typical between eight and twelve days after birth. This is rarely more than a mild inconvenience, but it can become more serious.

Although foal-heat diarrhea is by far the most common and the least dangerous diarrhea in young foals, there are many other causes of diarrhea that can be very debilitating and even fatal. There are various causes, some infectious and others not, and each has different (some very subtle) clinical signs, different causes, and different treatments.

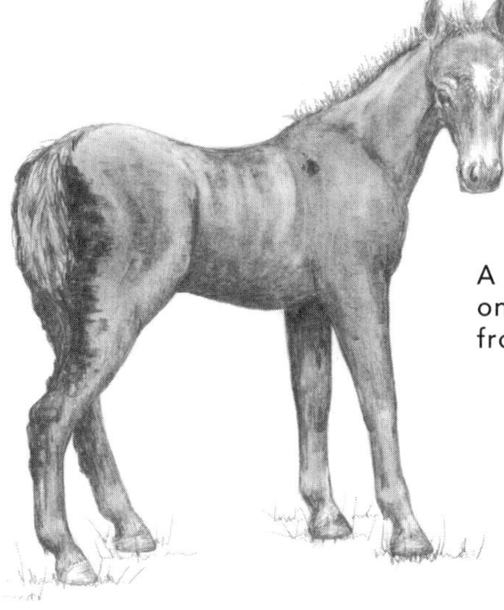

A foal with evidence of diarrhea on its rump should be kept away from other foals.

Foal-Heat Scours

As I've said, the most common foal diarrhea is foal-heat scours. This occurs somewhere between three or four days and fourteen to sixteen days of age and usually coincides with the mare's first heat cycle after foaling. The reason is unknown, although many possible causes have been proposed, including hormonal changes in the mare; alterations in milk composition; excessive milk intake; bacterial or viral agents; physiological changes in the foal's gastrointestinal tract; ingestion of discharges from the mare's vulva; and strongylosis. All are noninfectious. Most of these theories have been discarded, and thinking centers on roughage ingestion or physiological changes in the foal.

Foal-heat scours is an inconsistent condition. I know of one farm that has not had a case in years (about forty foals), and to the best of my knowledge nothing different is done there than at any other farm. Also, I know of at least one mare that has never had a foal with foal-heat scours, even though she routinely has her foal heat at ten or twelve days. The foals in adjacent stalls and in the same paddock scour right "on time" each year.

As interesting as this may be, however, it really doesn't matter much because uncomplicated cases (as most are) will pass in two to five days, and these foals never become debilitated. The only treatment necessary is the application of petroleum jelly to the foal's rump so the diarrhea doesn't scald (remove hair and cause irritation to the skin). Some say the administration of an intestinal inoculant, a preparation of normal intestinal bacteria, will shorten the duration of the diarrhea, but I'm not sure this is true. And how would anyone know whether the duration was shorter, anyhow? An occasional foal appears to cramp with this diarrhea; for these give about two ounces (60 mL) of bismuth salicylate (Pepto-Bismol) daily if necessary, to ease the discomfort and also to slow the gut motility slightly.

If the diarrhea persists or if the foal runs a fever or becomes depressed or dehydrated, diagnostic steps should be taken because it is no longer (or never was) simple foal-heat scours.

Noninfectious Causes

The noninfectious causes of foal diarrhea are usually little more than an inconvenience, especially when trying to hold an affected, rambunctious foal.

- **Overeating** is a noninfectious cause of diarrhea in foals and can occur at any age. A serious potential side effect here is founder, although that condition is rare in foals younger than six months of age. (Some believe that it's impossible for a foal less than six months old to founder, but I don't promise that.)

The diarrhea associated with overeating is rarely watery, frequently accompanied by flatulence, and commonly shows undigested grain in the feces (if the overeating involves grain). Diarrhea occasionally occurs in foals of mares that produce an overabundance of milk; in these cases, milking the mare before the foal nurses will aid in prevention. The overall treatment is to reduce the foal's feed ration and monitor its intake.

- **Parasitism** is another noninfectious cause of foal diarrhea. *Strongyloides* will cause a watery diarrhea in foals two to four weeks of age. *Strongylus* will cause intermittent diarrhea in foals a month old or older and is accompanied by a mild fever, depression, colic, and weight loss. Treatment of both consists of the administration of the proper anthelminthic medicine to kill the parasite once it's been identified through fecal samples.

Infectious Causes

The infectious causes of diarrhea are potentially life-threatening and require prompt action. Viral diarrheas typically occur in the first month; bacterial diarrheas are primarily problems in newborns, but some affect older foals as well.

- **Rotavirus** affects foals in the first month of life. Before the diarrhea appears, the foal is febrile and depressed. Once the greenish gray diarrhea begins, dehydration occurs rapidly. Typically, all foals in a group or barn will be affected. Rotavirus has also been implicated as a cause of gastroduodenal ulcers (see page 71).

Diagnosis may be made by virus identification. Treatment consists of intravenous fluids, oral electrolytes and glucose, and antibiotics if a secondary bacterial infection is suspected.

- **Salmonellosis** can occur at any age but is most severe in the newborn. The diarrhea is watery and may be bloody; its characteristic odor is almost diagnostic in itself. Depression, fever, and dehydration accompany the diarrhea. Fecal cultures are used for diagnosis, but a blood test that shows leukopenia (a reduction of the leukocytes in the blood) is enough to warrant treatment for salmonellosis. This consists of fluids, electrolytes, oral gut protectants, and antibiotics (gentamicin or trimethoprim sulfa).
- ***Escherichia coli (E. coli)*** causes a watery diarrhea in newborns, accompanied by fever, depression, dehydration, and sepsis. This often occurs in foals that don't receive typical immunity from the mare via the colostrum (known as passive transfer). Blood and fecal cultures are necessary for diagnosis, and treatment is the same as for salmo-

FOAL DIARRHEA

TYPE	CAUSES	DESCRIPTION
Noninfectious	Foal-heat scours	Occurs in most foals 3 to 16 days post foaling (typically 8–12 days)
	Overeating	Rarely watery, often containing undigested grain
	Parasitism	Usually watery, with mild fever, depression, and weight loss
Infectious, viral	Rotavirus	Occurs in first month; greenish-gray diarrhea and dehydration
Infectious, bacterial	Salmonellosis	Any age; watery, possibly bloody, odiferous
	Escherichia coli	Newborns; watery, with fever, depression, dehydration
	Actinobacillus equuli	Newborns; septicemia and enteritis
	Clostridium perfringens	Severe, bloody, with dehydration and depression
	Corynebacterium equi	Watery in 3- to 6-week-old foals; fever, weight loss

nellosis. If failure of passive transfer is indicated, a plasma transfusion is required. (See page 240 for more on failure of passive transfer.)

- ***Actinobacillus equuli*** infection also occurs in newborns and it, too, is associated with failure of passive transfer. Septicemia and enteritis will accompany this infection. The organism can be cultured from the blood and joints. The treatment is the same as for *E. coli* infection, accompanied by antibiotic joint flushes.
- ***Clostridium perfringens*** has several variations. Types A, B, and C will cause a severe bloody diarrhea with dehydration and depression. It mainly affects newborns but can occur in older foals as well. Diagnosis is by anaerobic fecal culture. Treatment consists of high levels of penicillin, fluids, and gut protectants.
- ***Corynebacterium equi*** causes a watery (or nearly so) diarrhea in foals three to six weeks old. There is fever, weight loss, nasal discharge, and maybe a cough and peritonitis. Gentamicin or erythromycin and gut protectants are the treatments.

The most important aspect of treatment in all of these cases is fluid and electrolyte replacement. Bismuth salicylate is the gut protectant of choice; it also aids in neutralizing bacterial toxins. The correct antibacterial agent is necessary to control the infection, and proper and timely worming will eliminate some diarrheas and lessen the severity of others. (I once had a client who refused to worm his foals until they were six months old; he didn't want to "stress" them. He had problems with foal diarrhea and unthrifty foals.) Regardless of the cause of the diarrhea, keep the foal's rear clean and protect it with petroleum jelly or some other water-resistant ointment.

Foals with diarrhea should be kept away from other foals, and ideally the handler should have no contact with other horses. Because that's impractical in most situations, the sick foal should be handled last each day, and the handler should clean and disinfect him/herself thoroughly after working with it. Even stall cleaning equipment (rakes, forks, etc.) should be used only for the sick foal's stall or disinfected between stalls. Once vacated, the stall must be disinfected and left idle for at least a few weeks. The soiled bedding should not be mixed with other bedding or spread on the fields.

These are not the only causes of diarrhea in foals, but these are the typical ones, with causes that we can identify.

ONE YEAR ON A FARM, four of seven foals had a diarrhea of three to four days duration during the first week. It began on the third or fourth day; they were depressed but had no fever, backed off but didn't stop nursing, and became very mildly dehydrated. Lab tests revealed nothing. These weren't the first four foals or the middle four or the last four foals; they were four at random. Each was put on antibiotics and given fluids, and all four recovered quickly. Two of the four later had normal foal-heat scours at about eleven or twelve days.

These cases didn't fit any of the descriptions of the identified causes of foal diarrhea, which proves that there is more out there than veterinary science is aware of. But we knew that.

Neonatal Maladjustment Syndrome

Once every year or so, I will have a client call about a foal that acts funny. "He was born yesterday (or the day before) and everything was okay, but this morning he can't seem to find the mare," I am told. "He gets in a corner and can't get out. I think he's gone blind."

I suppose some foals do go blind, but I've never seen one that did so soon after birth. What these little guys have is termed *neonatal maladjustment syndrome* (NMS), and they are commonly called "wanderers" or "barkers" due to the strange barking sound some make.

Of the dozen or so afflicted foals I have seen over the years, the majority had mild cases. The signs described are the only ones seen, and a little tender loving care, mainly ensuring nutritional intake, will carry them through, but some progress to the point of convulsions or coma. I don't know why some are so much worse than others; perhaps in the more serious cases the early signs aren't noticed or are ignored and the condition is allowed to progress.

Clinical Signs

Here is a description of everything that may occur, though not always, in a case of NMS. Birth is apparently normal, and standing and nursing occur uneventfully, but twelve to twenty-four hours later, give or take, the foal appears to become lost and wanders around the stall. Getting caught in a corner is a common occurrence; the foal walks into the corner and cannot seem to make the turn that will get him back out again.

He will stop nursing and appear either to have no interest in his dam or not to recognize her. Even if there is interest in nursing, he may not be able to find the udder or hook onto it, and his sucking reflex is noticeably diminished. These signs plus the wandering make him appear to be blind.

Next, the foal's movements become jerky and he becomes ataxic and stumbles. He may fall suddenly. Within a short time there is a quick onset of convulsions. He falls or flips backward and will lie with either rigid limbs or frantic paddling motions, accompanied by banging his head against the floor. At any point after the foal's gait becomes altered, the "barking" sounds may begin.

Between convulsions, the foal is hyperreactive to sudden noises and these noises may trigger further convulsions. Rarely, the foal will go into a coma and, if not fed, will die.

Short of entering a coma, many of these foals will recover over a period of a few days, with or without treatment, although there may be residual sight or mental deficiencies.

Fortunately, most foals don't go through all of this and most survive with no aftereffects other than a large veterinary bill. Those complicated by other factors — infection, prematurity, congenital defects, dystocia, or other disorders — have much reduced chances of making it, even with proper therapy.

Diagnosis

The cause of NMS is unknown, but is undoubtedly related somehow to a central nervous system disorder. Postmortem findings cannot establish whether the lesions found are the cause or result of the condition.

Premature, weak, or just plain stupid foals will show the same early signs as NMS, but the signs in these conditions are present from birth and do not wait to develop as they do in NMS. Convulsions and coma may result from both hypoglycemia and septic meningitis, but both conditions can be ruled out by additional physical and laboratory findings.

Treatment

In uncomplicated NMS, treatment must be aimed at controlling the convulsive seizures, preventing self-inflicted injury, and maintaining nutritional requirements; concurrent problems, of course, must be treated accordingly. As the course of NMS may be several days, this is not as easy as it sounds.

The foal is unable to nurse, so he may be fed his dam's milk via nasogastric intubation until his suckle reflex returns. NMS foals are usually highly reactive to tactile stimulation, so passing the tube will be a challenge for the veterinarian. To prevent the need for multiple intubations, and to allow the person responsible for the care of the foal to feed it, the veterinarian should tape or suture the tube in place.

The convulsions are controlled with anticonvulsive medication. Because repeated doses may be necessary, and because hitting a cooperative foal's vein is hard enough without having to hit the vein of a hyperreactive, convulsing foal, a catheter should be placed in the foal's jugular vein.

Because of the danger of the foal injuring itself when convulsing, the stall must be bedded extremely well. Also, the walls should be cushioned either with padding or by lining them with hay or straw bales. And a padded helmet can help to protect the foal from head and eye injuries.

Prognosis

Foals with uncomplicated NMS will usually recover, although there may be some lasting neurological signs in some. If the condition persists for a week or more, or if there are concurrent problems, the survival rate is greatly reduced.

The key to NMS, as with most other problems in horses, is early diagnosis, which hinges on careful observation by those responsible for the foal's care. Eventually a cause will be found and that will make prevention and control easier; in the meantime, observe and report any abnormalities to your veterinarian.

Tyzzer's Disease

There's only one good thing about Tyzzer's disease: you'll probably never see it. I thought I'd never see it and the reason I am including it here is because I did see a case. Admittedly, as a veterinarian I am more apt to see unusual diseases than a horse owner is, but I would have told the person that owned the foal involved that he would probably never see it and, unfortunately, he did.

There's one small consolation if you ever do encounter it: you can probably do nothing about it, so there should be no guilt feelings about not catching it soon enough.

What Is Tyzzer's Disease?

Tyzzer's disease occurs in foals from one to six weeks of age. It's an acute bacterial infection caused by *Bacillus piliformes,* which probably enters the foal's body by ingestion. Once in the foal, the bacteria cause liver damage, inflammation of the heart tissues, and colitis.

Clinical Signs

Typically, a previously healthy-appearing foal is found dead, but occasionally a foal is found seriously ill; it is feverish (or hypothermic), recumbent, convulsing, and suffering from diarrhea and possibly jaundice. An examination reveals signs of cardiovascular collapse, septic shock, and liver failure. Typical symptoms also include poor capillary refill, petechial hemorrhages, an exceptionally rapid heart rate, and cold extremities.

Diagnosis and Treatment

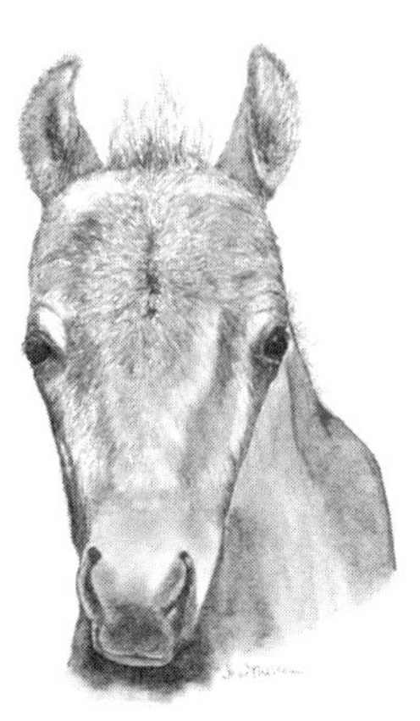

Tyzzer's disease occurs in foals 8 to 42 days after birth.

Diagnosis is based on clinical signs, and treatment is generally considered futile, although there is a report of successful treatment of one tentatively diagnosed case of the disease. If treatment is attempted, it should consist of fluids with added dextrose and bicarbonate, plus high levels of systemic antibiotics (such as potassium penicillin and amikacin) and general therapy for septic shock. Before initiating therapy, however, bear in mind that the prognosis is exceptionally poor.

As previously mentioned, Tyzzer's disease is extremely uncommon and doesn't (or, perhaps more correctly, hasn't been known to) occur in outbreaks, but it may be endemic on some farms, with a foal being affected once every several years. Rarely, more than one foal may be affected in some years, but, basically, Tyzzer's disease seems to be a "luck of the draw" condition. (This information was gleaned from the literature because, as I said, I've only seen one case and it was enough. The foal was down and showing all of the signs described, and it died before I could start fluids. And I hurried.)

Windswept Foal

A CLIENT HAD A MARE THAT HAD THREE windswept foals out of five before he sold her. Two of the three straightened up, but the third didn't, and he had a large stud fee invested in it; that's when he decided that the mare would be better off eating someone else's grain.

What Is a Windswept Foal?

The term *windswept* describes the appearance of the foal's hind legs. One hind leg is forward and held under the body, with outward deviation below the hock. The other leg is held away from the body, behind the first, with inward deviation below the hock. The pelvis is at an angle to accommodate this conformation, or may in fact be the cause of the condition. Scoliosis, contracted tendons, or both often accompany the windswept condition. It's a congenital condition; the foal is born that way. In humans, it's described as bow-legged on one side and knock-kneed on the other.

There are varying degrees of the windswept condition. Some are so mild that the disorder is almost unnoticeable, and others are so severe that the foal can't stand and eventually must be euthanized. Most of the mild cases resolve readily, and so do some that aren't so mild.

Predisposing Factors

There is a reason for windswept foals, but if someone knows the cause, I haven't been told. Many consider it to be just the luck of the draw — simple bad luck — but I don't accept that, and I'm pretty sure there are other veterinarians who share my feeling.

There are several suggested reasons for it. A very popular suggested cause is *in utero* positioning. Genetics is also popular, as is the ever-reliable nutrition. Those last two are "when in doubt" causes: when in doubt about almost anything, blame feed or inheritance.

But I have a few ideas. How about low levels of a toxin, such as poison from a plant that's only eaten accidentally or when grazing is poor? (I guess this falls under nutrition.) How about fescue? Endophyte-laden fescue causes all sorts of wild and crazy things, so why not windswept? (See page 206 for more on fescue.)

I'm sure (although no one else may be) that its origin is neural, so how about anoxia (oxygen deprivation) somewhere during gestation? Why neural? Cerebral palsy is a defect of motor power and coordination resulting from brain damage. Human babies so affected often have a tipped pelvis and they may hold their legs in an almost windswept fashion.

I've provided perinatal care for the one mare I know of that has had multiple windswept foals. I think that rules out bad luck, and I'm pretty sure that it also eliminates *in utero* positioning. I guess we can't eliminate nutrition, but I don't see why one mare out of a group receiving the same ration would produce a windswept foal while none of the others did. I can't think of an argument against genetics other than the fact that I don't like it as a reason: too many things are blamed on inheritance.

Treatment

Although many windswept foals do resolve themselves, others don't and correction is very difficult. Periosteal elevation (PE) has been tried. In PE, the appropriate area of the periosteum (the sheath covering a bone) is cut and an instrument like a chisel with a bent end called, appropriately, a *periosteal elevator* is inserted between the periosteum and the bone as far as can be reached in all directions. Somehow this allows the bone to grow instead of being limited by a restricting periosteum. Straightening of the leg is the result; it works remarkably consistently in cases other than windswept. Though it has been successful in some cases of windswept, it has done absolutely no good in others. My feeling is that the ones that straightened after PE would have straightened on their own without it. (See page 132 for more information on periosteal elevation.)

The prognosis for windswept foals that straighten is good, but for those in which there is also scoliosis, the prognosis for the foal to grow into a useful animal is poor, as it is for those that don't straighten. I have seen two windswept fillies that remained that way and were later bred and neither produced windswept foals, but one had difficulty delivering her two foals and she was not bred again.

Some day we'll learn more about windswept and what causes it. Much of

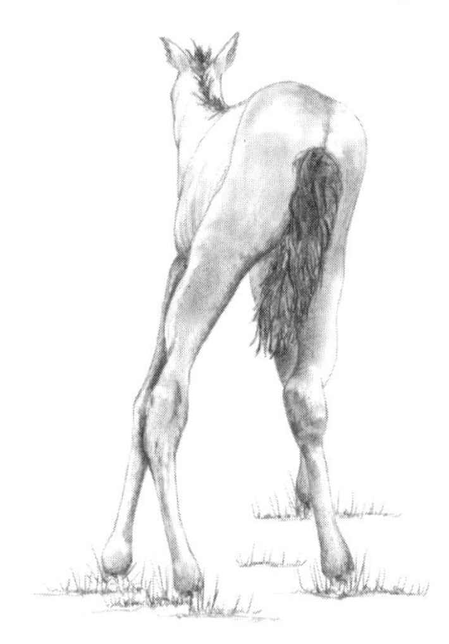

Windswept foal is a congenital condition that may resolve on its own. If it doesn't, correction is difficult.

what appears above is theory and conjecture and maybe I'm wrong, but until someone disproves what I have to say, I stand behind my theories and conjecture.

Hermaphrodites

MOST DAYS ABOUT 9 A.M. OR SO, I stop somewhere to buy a soft drink and a bag of peanuts. It's my "coffee break."

One spring morning many years ago, as I was waiting in line to pay fifty cents for a nickel bag of peanuts and seventy-five cents for a ten-cent soda, a client of mine who owned four mares came in. I wasn't scheduled to go to his farm that day, but when he saw me he asked if I could stop by.

"What's going on?" I asked.

"The gray mare foaled last night," he explained, "and the foal's got something wrong with him."

"Is he weak?"

"No, he's plenty strong. His . . . " — he seemed to be searching for the correct word, which he failed to find — " . . . 'thing' isn't right."

"What's wrong with it?" I had no trouble figuring out that he was referring to the foal's penis. For some reason it's a word that many people can't seem to say.

"It's not in the right place. Can you come and see him?"

His farm was less than a mile from the store, so I told him we would go right then. Once there, he showed me a vigorous, healthy-acting, normal-looking foal — normal-looking, that is, until you looked under its tail. There the normality ended.

There beneath the anus was what appeared to be a vulva, but from the lower end of this hung an eight- or nine-inch-long structure strongly resembling a penis.

"I'll be darned," I said. "A hermaphrodite!"

"No, it's not a filly," my client corrected. "It's a colt."

"I didn't say it was a filly," I rejoined.

"You called it a her," the client said.

"No. I said 'hermaphrodite.' That's an individual that has characteristics of both a male and a female."

I proceeded to explain the situation and told him that hermaphrodites were usually very studdish, and this one would probably be a serious problem for him in time unless something was done.

Incidence and Contributing Factors

Hermaphrodites are rare. Most people, even veterinarians, will never see one, but this was the third I had seen. I guess I just have a knack for being in the right place at the right time.

The first one I saw long before I was a veterinarian, actually before I had even returned to undergraduate school. I went to a California farm that had a mare for sale that I was interested in, and while there I saw them tease. The teaser was a hermaphrodite. And he was a handful.

The second one was a young horse an old farmer brought in to the equine clinic at veterinary school. Another student and I were working at the clinic that day, and our job was to take down the information on all horses being admitted, including the reason the animal was brought in.

"What's the complaint?" my classmate asked.

"I got nothin' to complain about," the old gentleman replied.

"That's great, sir," my classmate continued, "but why is the horse here?"

"His tool's in the wrong place. And he ain't got no balls. And he's meaner'n a snake."

He was right on all three counts.

Why hermaphrodites occur is unclear. The prevailing theory blames the phenomenon on errors in mitosis during early embryonic development. The result is either a true hermaphrodite, which is said not to occur in the horse, or a pseudohermaphrodite. A true hermaphrodite has both ovaries and testes or *ovotestes,* which are reproductive organs that produce both sperm and eggs.

A pseudohermaphrodite can be male, which looks like a female but has testes, or female, which looks like a male but has ovaries. Female pseudohermaphrodites reportedly are rare, but some researchers feel that exposure to androgenic substances (natural or synthetic steroids that act like sex hormones) during embryonic life can cause this phenomenon.

The male pseudohermaphrodite is by far the more common. External genital organs that resemble a female are present, but usually with a greatly enlarged clitoral structure that is mistaken for a penis. The urethral orifice may be located as in a normal female or in the penis-resembling clitoris.

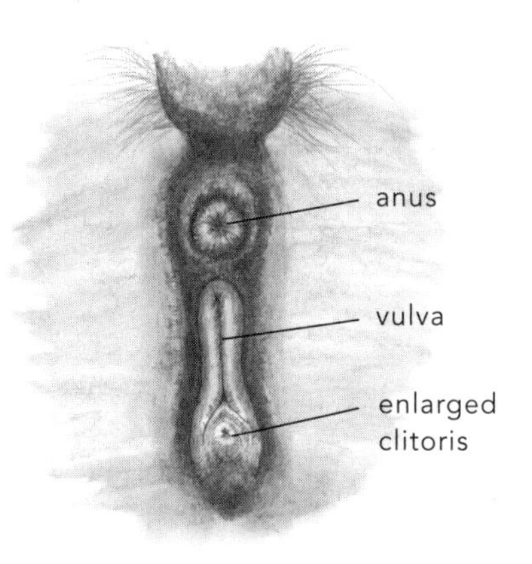

Hermaphrodites are rare. Most people, even veterinarians, will never see one.

These animals have testes retained in the body cavity or beneath the skin in the scrotal region and are extremely studdish, frequently dangerously so. The three that I have seen fall into this category.

Back to the foal with which we began this epistle.

The next morning I was scheduled to be at that farm. Tommy, my client, had taken a mare to be bred, so his wife was there to take notes on what we found on our examinations of the remaining mares.

"I don't understand about this new foal," she said. "Tommy tried to tell me what you said, but I don't really think he understood, either. He said you kept calling him 'her' but he's got a . . . a . . ."

This apparently was a difficult word for this family. "Penis?" I offered.

She blushed. "Well . . . yeah." She averted her eyes.

"That's not really a penis," I continued. "It's really a super-sized clitoris."

I decided I'd better lay off the anatomically correct words when she blushed again.

"So that's why you call him 'her'?" she asked.

"I don't call him — it — 'her.' The foal is a *her*maphrodite." I proceeded to give a brilliant explanation of Greek mythology and the origin of the word.

"Hermaphroditus," I told her, "was the son of Hermes, the messenger of the gods, and Aphrodite, the goddess of love." After her responses to the mention of genitals, I chose not to go into the fact that Aphrodite slept with most of the gods and that Hermes was her half brother.

"Hermaphroditus took a bath in a pool and was somehow welded with Salmacis, the nymph of the spring, who wrapped herself around him, into a body with both sexes. That event gave us our word for what you have here: a hermaphrodite." (Lest you think that I am a Greek mythology scholar, nothing could be further from the truth. I looked this up when I saw the one in veterinary school.)

She had appeared to be listening intently and, after all, the explanation had been crystal clear.

"So," she said, "you're saying this foal is both sexes?"

"Well, yes," I responded. "More or less."

"Then why do you call him 'her'?"

Treatment

In the case of a male pseudohermaphrodite, the testicles can be removed with the same basic surgery used in dealing with a ridgling, which improves the animal's disposition and is recommended. (See page 316 for more on this topic.) The elongated clitoral structure can be amputated, which will get it out of the way, although this is not really necessary. In many male pseudohermaphrodites, this does not dangle; it is merely an enlarged bulbous structure, and amputation is not needed.

Tommy chose to ignore the problem with his foal. They called the foal He-she, and He-she grew and thrived and attempted to strike, kick, or eat everything that came within twenty feet. By eight months old, He-she was unmanageable.

What eventually became of He-she I don't know, because at that point Tommy fired me because a mare that I had called "in foal" came up empty. None of us veterinarians would have any clients if that happened every time a mare lost her foal.

Wobbler Syndrome

A WOMAN CALLED AND INTRODUCED HERSELF, then said, "I'm not pleased with my present veterinarian and a friend recommended you. I have only two mares, but will you do my work?"

Around here, some of my colleagues will accept clients only if they have a certain number of mares, say five or ten. I've never understood that; a person with one mare may own two next year, maybe five in two or three years, and someday perhaps many. But even if the herd remains at one or two, they need veterinary attention just as the farms that have a hundred mares do. (This woman and her husband now have eight mares, and I imagine that today most of my colleagues would accept them as clients.) I told her I would, and she asked me to come that day to see a yearling that was "moving funny."

When I arrived, she brought out a beautiful, large chestnut Thoroughbred colt. It was February; most yearlings at that time of year are not much more than big weanlings, but this guy was already the size you'd expect to see in maybe May or June. I asked if she was sure that he was a yearling or did she perhaps mean to say two-year-old?

"No, he's a yearling," she replied. "He was born last March."

I didn't know his pedigree, but from his appearance he would bring top dollar at a sale no matter what pedigree he had.

"What's his problem?" I asked.

"He moves funny in his rear end," she said.

I was afraid I knew the answer then, but I told her to walk him away from me and turn him in a tight circle. It was difficult for him; his turn was erratic and uncoordinated.

"How long has this been going on?" I asked.

"We first noticed it about three weeks ago. He seems to be getting worse."

I had her turn him loose in a small paddock and we watched him trot off. When he tried to stop, his front end cooperated but his rear didn't. It went first to one side and then to the other. He was a wobbler.

What Is Wobbler Syndrome?

Wobbler syndrome is a manifestation of malformations of the cervical vertebrae that cause compression of the spinal cord. In reference books, it is also known as *cervical stenotic myelopathy,* but I don't know of anyone who calls it that in real life. It was first recognized in the United States in 1938 but has undoubtedly been around for a lot longer. It occurs in all breeds and all ages but is more common in young Thoroughbreds and Quarter Horses (and crosses of these breeds with other breeds) from six months to three years of age (usually less than two years, though). Colts seem to be more frequently affected than fillies.

Typically, an affected horse is a large, rapidly growing, otherwise healthy colt. There is a genetic tendency toward the condition. There was a stallion standing in the area where I worked when I first got out of school that sired perhaps 5 percent wobblers, an outrageously high percentage, so I learned about the problem early in my veterinary career.

Trauma can cause it, too, but that is far less common than the familial cases. Other suggested causes are mineral imbalance and overfeeding, but these have not been proved.

Clinical Signs

The clinical signs, primarily rear ataxia (stumbling), are the result of compression of the spinal cord. The nerves that go to the rear of the horse are on the outside of the cord; therefore they are damaged by compression, and proper nerve connection to the hind limbs is lost. Ataxia eventually progresses to the point where the horse goes down and is unable to rise again.

X-rays of the neck will usually show bony abnormalities in the cervical vertebral column. A definitive diagnosis may be made by demonstrating a reduction in the vertebral column dimensions by positive contrast myelography, but this requires general anesthesia at a university or large equine referral facility.

FETAL MALFORMATION

Do you know the original meaning of the word *monster*? It was a medical term denoting a congenital anomaly: a birth defect that distorts the newborn and is frequently not compatible with life. I once saw a monster.

Many years ago a client called and said a mare had foaled and that there was something wrong with the foal. I went immediately and he was right. There was something very wrong. For one thing, it was dead. For another, its face was pretty doggoned ugly. The upper jaw and nose were almost nonexistent and the lower jaw was also shortened but still longer than the upper. It stuck upward in front of what should have been the nose.

In veterinary school we learned that this fetal malformation occurs commonly in calves (although not so often that you have to lose sleep over it) but is rare in other species. Because the newborn's face looks something like that of a bulldog, that's the term given to it: bulldog calf. Except, in this case, it was a bulldog foal.

I have never read about this anomaly occurring in horses, so I don't know if this was a once-in-a-lifetime event, but I suspect it wasn't. To be sure that it's not something that every other vet sees daily, however, I checked a list of the common developmental anomalies occurring in horses. It wasn't on the list. When it does occur, the newborn, be it calf or whatever, doesn't survive for long, if at all.

My client was concerned that the mare might have another one, and I told him that it was unlikely. But we will never know if she would have; we only know that she didn't. She never got in foal again.

Treatment

Steroids and nonsteroidal anti-inflammatory drugs will reduce inflammation and give temporary relief, but the result is only temporary. Dimethyl sulfoxide (DMSO) given intravenously seems to help in the early stages, but it, too, provides only temporary benefits. In my experience, treatment has been unsuccessful. Euthanasia is the common course.

Surgery to stabilize the vertebral column by fusing some of the vertebrae is reported as being successful in selected cases, but the horse

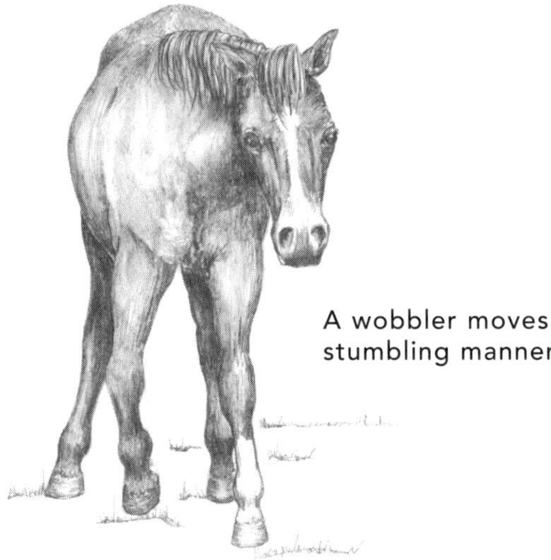

A wobbler moves in an uncoordinated, stumbling manner.

must have considerable value to justify this extreme. The cost of the surgery is great and the recuperative time is lengthy; in addition, surgery is not always successful.

Equine Degenerative Myeloencephalopathy

There is another condition that must be considered when signs of the wobbler syndrome are apparent. This is equine degenerative myeloencephalopathy. This condition was not described until the late 1970s, but, like wobblers, has most certainly been around for a lot longer than that. Many cases were probably misdiagnosed as wobblers. This is a degenerative disease of young horses of any breed that causes ataxia through its effect on the spinal cord and parts of the brain. There is a familial predisposition, but there is a higher incidence in horses deprived of pasture and raised on hay and/or pellets.

The typical age when symptoms appear is between four months and three years; the onset is insidious and progressive. The big difference between this and the wobbler syndrome is that this is treatable. Massive doses of vitamin E given early appear to reduce the signs. Also, the clinical signs plateau as maturity is reached at age three to five years.

As I suggested, wobbler syndrome and equine degenerative myeloencephalopathy were probably misdiagnosed one for the other for years, but that rarely happens today because of improved diagnostic techniques and increased experience.

I saw the colt we began this with just about the time that equine degenerative myeloencephalopathy was being discovered, and I didn't know anything about it. The colt continued to grow more ataxic in spite of being treated, and he fell often. The decision was made to put him down, and on postmortem examination the diagnosis of wobbler was verified.

Handling Foals

I WAS CLOBBERED BY A YEARLING a few years ago; he got me good. I was laid up for several weeks. I later learned that he had been allowed to run out since birth and had never been handled, except to manhandle a halter on him.

I am continually surprised — nay, amazed — by how some foals are handled. Or, rather, not handled — that is, ever.

Many horse owners, for various reasons, such as lack of personnel, lack of knowledge, lack of heart, lack of interest, lack of time, and laziness, either don't handle their foals or handle them improperly. As a veterinarian, I frequently receive the brunt of this mishandling, and I don't like it. And there is really no excuse for it.

Start Early, Handle Often

The first problem is the reluctance or refusal by some people to put halters on their foals. In my opinion, a foal should be haltered as soon as its head emerges from its dam. I would do it sooner except the placenta gets in the way.

Even though many people do halter their foals, they will not lead them. Sure, it's easier to let them follow Mom, but it is a whole lot easier to teach a 125-pound suckling to lead than it is a 400-pound weanling. Short-handed farms tell me one person can't lead both a mare and a foal at the same time. Hogwash. It takes a little effort, a little coordination, and perhaps a slight toll in bruised toes, but it can be done. And there is absolutely no excuse if two or more people are available.

Of course, there is more to foal handling than just leading. A foal must learn that people are friends and that he *will* be touched. And that touching will not hurt. On too many horse operations, big and small, the only time a foal is handled is when something mildly unpleasant must be done (trimming, worming, vaccinating), and before long the foal associates people with unpleasant things.

The reason usually offered for not giving a foal some attention is lack of time. Hogwash again. Most foals go out in the morning and come back in the evening, so they may be led at those times. When brought in at night, or whenever, the foal can be held an extra minute or two and petted and rubbed. He may not like it at first but eventually he will. Rub his face and head, gently handle his ears, rub his sides and

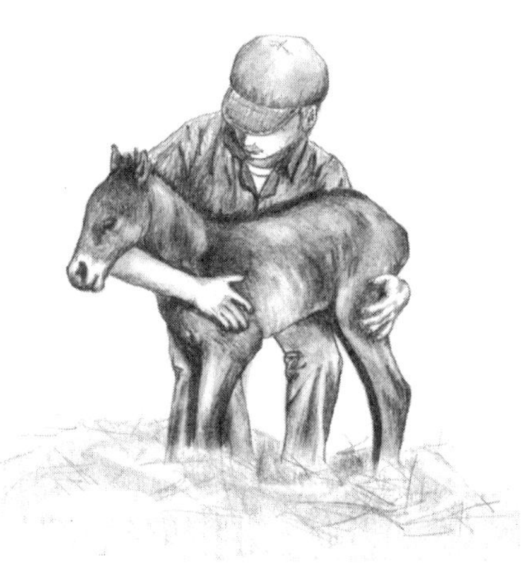

This is the proper way to hold and restrain a foal.

belly, run your hands down his legs. The whole procedure will only take a minute or two. In no time, most foals become agreeable and easy to handle. If there isn't time to spend two minutes a day per foal, the farm should not have horses.

The Problems

What follow are some examples of problems resulting from not handling foals; it's to the foal's benefit to be handled early and often.

A MAN DROVE UP TO THE HOUSE ONE DAY and asked if I was the veterinarian. I admitted it, and he told me that he had bred a pony and he kept the foal for his kids, but he thought the foal, now two, should be gelded because he was a "little wild."

We set a time for the following afternoon. I arrived on time and was met by the man and two boys at a small barn.

"Where's the pony?" I asked, glancing into the barn's only two stalls and finding them empty.

"He's out there," the guy said, pointing to a large field.

"I'll need him in here," I said. "Go get him."

"We can't catch him."

Naively, I thought maybe he had gotten worked up or this was not the time of day he was normally brought in, so I said, "Let's give him a few minutes to settle down, then we can try again."

"We can't never catch him," said the larger of the two boys.

Upon further questioning I learned that the pony had never been caught, indeed, had never even been in the barn. Weaning had consisted of selling his dam and shipping her away a year before.

I'm not sure how I was expected to geld him at sixty paces (if we could get even that close). For all I know, that pony, now pushing twenty, is still a stallion and still running free out there in the south forty.

Another time I was called upon to tend to a small cut on the shoulder of a six-month-old Clydesdale foal. If you have never seen a six-month-old Clydesdale foal, picture a 1958 Buick without power steering. And no brakes. This kid was as cute as she could be but completely unhandled, not even halter broke (or even haltered). She had just been running loose with her dam since birth.

Even though they ran her into a cattle barn, laying hands on her was not possible. I guess the laceration healed and she did not contract tetanus because I pass there frequently and she (now fully grown) and her mom are still there, running wild.

Another shoulder laceration occurred, this one on a Thoroughbred yearling colt, apparently the result of a nail backing out of the fence. This farm's horses — mares, foals, yearlings, everybody — were turned out by opening the stall doors and standing back. Strategic placement of gates and fences allowed the different classes of animals to be directed to the appropriate fields.

By "yearling," I mean barely. It was January. Another of the operation's more endearing management ploys was foot care: foals were first trimmed in the spring of their yearling year. Worming by the farm was done routinely, except in this guy's case; he was hard to catch in the stall so he was wormed maybe every third time.

When the lesion was discovered, they chased him into a stall and called me. It was a cut that needed to be sutured, but it wasn't. Even in a stall, it was three days before anyone could catch him, and by then it was too late to close it. It left an ugly L-shaped scar.

Other mishandled horses, such as the one we began this with, have been catchable, and I have the scars to prove it. I could continue to go on at length about lack of handling, but I won't. Suffice it to say, 90 percent or more of these problems could have been eliminated had someone been willing to take two minutes a day to handle these animals when they were babies.

Remember: even though the mare may be domesticated, her foal is born a wild animal. You like the little guy, sure, but he has no reason to like you. Minimal time and effort on your part or on the part of your employees can educate any foal and save a lot of wear and tear on you, your horses, and anyone who must deal with them. Like me.

Weaning

Weaning is one of my least favorite undertakings, whether it's being done by me or by one of my clients. Every year, a baby or two injures itself and every now and then a mare gets hurt, too.

There are a lot of theories on weaning, most of them centering on how and when to go about it. Each person is convinced that his method and timing is best and will readily condemn the procedures followed by others, but in truth there is no best way or time.

How to Wean

The "hows" range from "Nature's way," that is, leaving the foal on the mare indefinitely, to closing the foal alone in a darkened stall. Another method involves moving mare or foal to the other side of the farm, out of earshot of one another. You need a large farm for this. Then there are those who move one or the other to another farm until the weaning process is complete.

Possibly the least traumatic method is the one in which a mare is unobtrusively removed from a field of mares and foals. In theory, the foal to be weaned does not get upset because all the other foals around it, which still have their dams with them, are not upset. What works in theory, however, does not always work in practice, but generally this seems to be the most satisfactory way to wean.

When to Wean

The "whens" vary even more widely than the "hows." Again, there is "Nature's way," in which the mare and foal stay together until either the mare cannot tolerate a full-grown horse trying to nurse her, or the grown "foal" gets a sore neck from trying to bend it enough to get to the mare's bag.

For years, perhaps aeons, six months was the target age for weaning. I don't think anyone knows why, other than it is a nice, easy-to-remember number. Most programs, fortunately, now involve weaning at a younger age. September 1 (or some other date) is popular; every foal on the farm is weaned that day. This is one of the worst weaning "whens"; on September 1, a farm could have foals ranging from nine months of age down to younger than two months.

One of the issues to consider with six-month or September 1 weaning is the foal's nutritional needs. After four months of age, the mare's milk simply does not supply the dietary needs of the foal. By this age, the foal should be on a properly balanced grain and roughage (hay, pasture) ration.

Toward this end, my preference for a weaning "when" is at the age of fourteen to eighteen weeks. It is my opinion, although I have never seen or done any formal research to support this, that foals weaned at this age grow and develop better. (Bear in mind that this is an opinion.)

Weaning Woes

Back now to the first paragraph, wherein the possibility of injury to mare and foal was mentioned. Foals or mares closed in stalls often bounce off the walls, buckets, feed tubs, and anything else in there with them. Foals left in fields with other mares and foals often attempt to jump the fences between them and their dam, regardless of how many and how high they may be, and so will the mare. Now, jumping a fence or two is okay but all too frequently the horse jumps only *half* of the fence, which is not okay. (I once owned a mare that missed her calling. She was well bred and beautiful, but she could not outrun me or you and she passed this endearing trait on to her offspring. At weaning, however, she could clear, with room to spare, any and all fences between her and her foal.)

Other sources of potential injury to a weaned foal are the unweaned mares that may be in the field with it. A weaned foal may not accept the fact that its milk supply has ended, and it may try to nurse another mare. Occasionally a mare will allow a foal to do this, but more often than not she won't allow it and, if the foal is persistent, she will kick. I have seen one foal killed this way.

Many years ago, a client had a two-month-old foal in a field of about ten mares and foals that was weaned suddenly: his dam

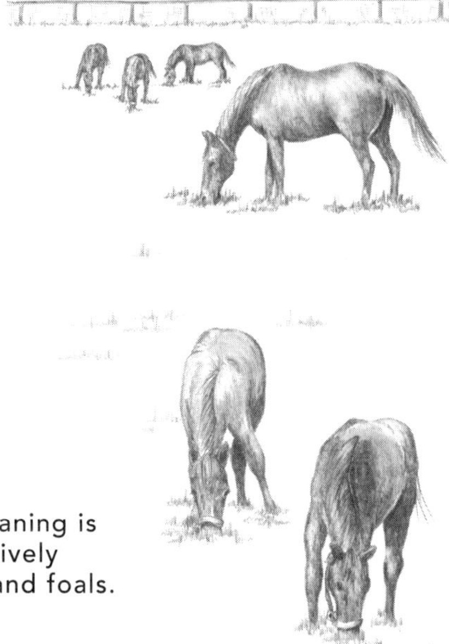

Possibly the best method of weaning is one in which a mare is unobtrusively removed from a field of mares and foals.

died. Not the best horseman in the world, the client reasoned that the colt was too old (and I know he was too cheap) to justify a nurse mare. Also, he did not want the work involved in giving the foal extra care, so he just left him to fend for himself with the other mares and foals.

The little guy wanted his milk. At first, the mares pushed him away and kicked at him, but after two days his hunger got the best of him. He stuck his head under a mare and she kicked. He pinned his ears, turned around, and kicked back. And kicked. And kicked. After about six or seven violent shots at the mare, he turned around and stuck his head back under her. She just stood there and let him nurse.

One day I weaned a foal. Even though the mare and foal were out of earshot, they both began to run the respective fences immediately, although neither tried to jump. This went on night and day, along with hollering and crying, for several days.

"This is the part of horse breeding I really hate," I said to my wife. "Weaning is almost cruel."

"The part I hate," she said, "is that they won't know each other if they ever meet again in the future. It's very sad."

I realize I anthropomorphize a lot, and I often criticize others for doing the same thing, but we really have no idea what goes on in a horse's head. My wife was right, though. I have seen many fillies enter the broodmare bands of which their dams were members, and there was not a flicker of recognition by mother or daughter.

But, as with all things, there are exceptions.

A client owned four mares and twelve acres, not nearly enough area to achieve the proper distance to ensure either out-of-sight or out-of-sound. He had a friend who had five mares and about fifteen acres, and the same problem existed there, so each year at weaning one would haul his foals to the other's farm and haul the friend's mares back to his. They would alternate mares and foals each year.

This client had a middle-aged mare (thirteen, I think) that had produced several foals, most of which were nondescript runners, if they ran at all. One, however, had run like the dickens, winning several stakes and several hundred thousand dollars. The year we are presently considering, this mare's foal was a full sister to this good horse and my client intended to race her and keep her as a broodmare.

Weaning was scheduled for August 15, when the foals ranged from three and a half to almost six months of age. At weaning, my client's four foals were vanned to his friend's farm and the friend's five mares were brought to my client's. Everything went well except for the mare and foal we are considering. At nearly six months, the filly was among the oldest. The mare hollered and screamed and ran for two weeks and reportedly her foal did the same at the friend's farm. Both were tranquilized a few times, but as soon as the tranquilizer wore off they were back at it.

After the first two weeks, the mare stopped running the fence and calling, switching instead to pacing and snorting. Her foal reportedly settled down a little, too. After thirty days, each man's horses were returned to their owner's farm; this particular mare and foal had apparently accepted the situation and were acting roughly as one would expect at a month post-weaning.

The mares and foals were placed at opposite ends of the twelve acres, just as had been done each year with no problems for as long as I knew. The filly, however, although tranquilized for the vanning, began running and hollering almost immediately. Within a few minutes, the mare began, too, and later that afternoon she jumped the fence. Or most of it; she banged a hind ankle and needed a few stitches, for which she cared little.

The running and hollering went on for a couple of weeks with no improvement, so my client hauled the filly back to his friend's place for another month. Both mare and weanling seemed to settle in after about a week, but when the filly was brought home again, they started in again. Once more the mare jumped most of the fence, but this time only removed a plank and a little hide. Back the filly went, this time not returning until January.

This time, neither mare nor foal, now a yearling, did much more than stand at the fence and look across the farm and whinny occasionally, although this went on periodically until September, when the filly left to be broken. Perhaps if the mare had had another foal that year, the problem would have ended (or never begun), but she was barren so we will never know.

The filly broke and trained uneventfully and went on to a modest two-year racing career, during which she won three or four races and almost enough money to pay her training bills. An injury early as a four-year-old caused her retirement, and she was brought home in February to become a broodmare.

She was placed in a paddock next to the one in which her dam and the other pregnant mares resided. She ran to the fence almost right away and called. The now seventeen-year-old mare picked up her head and ran over to her.

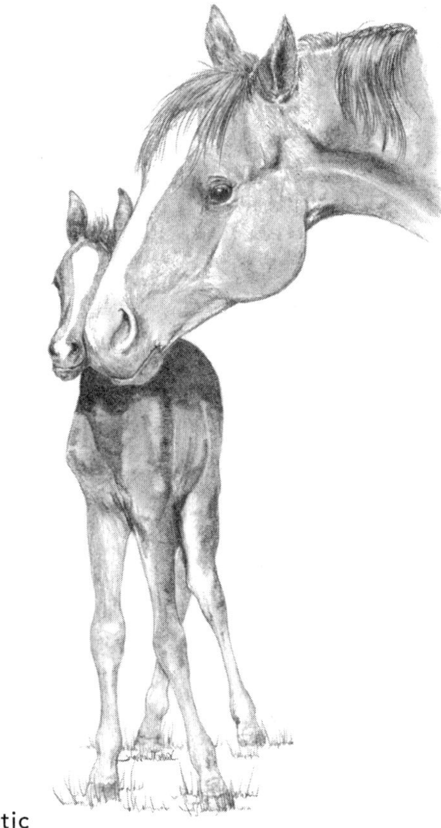

Weaning is traumatic to both mare and foal.

As I said, I tend to anthropomorphize, but I feel certain they knew each other. Eventually placed in a paddock together, the filly was subservient to the mare and still is, although I believe they are now eight and twenty-one, respectively. But they are very happy.

Whatever your weaning program, I don't think this will happen, but I really like it that at least one mother and daughter remembered each other.

It's too bad that the filly never knew her father.

Part IV

Care and Management

Horse handling and care advice, which is good to know even if you don't follow it

10

Farm and Stable Management

Safe Horse Handling

As I've said elsewhere in these pages, my wife used to be a manager of a horse farm but is now a physical therapist. In her former capacity, she had several employees get hurt on the job; in her present capacity she sees many, many horse farm employees who have been injured. Mostly it's backs and shoulders, but other parts suffer, too.

Horses are bigger and stronger than people, and in a one-on-one confrontation there's no contest: the horse wins. But there is never a need for a one-on-one; with a little care and some knowledge, anybody can get the upper hand.

Safe horse handling is a broad term that applies to horses, the people who handle them, and any other farm employees (mowers, stall muckers, and so on) who work with horses. It's a critically important but often overlooked subject that, if attended to, can result in considerable savings over a period of time. Properly executed, safe horse handling can result in decreases in veterinary bills (a sobering thought), insurance expenses, and lost staff hours. In the time I've been in practice in this area, there have been several deaths as a result of improper horse handling. (One was a veterinarian, and I find that real scary.)

In this section, we'll briefly review proper handling of the horses themselves; we won't be cover the subject in depth, but we will touch upon the most critical points. Some of what we'll review here is pretty basic, but I'm constantly amazed at how many veteran horse people either don't know or choose to ignore the horse-handling basics. By following these guidelines, handling horses will be made easier and safer.

Before we begin, familiarize yourself with these three truisms, each of which should be etched in stone:

- Accidents happen fast.
- Most accidents are avoidable.
- Most accidents occur when people are inattentive and in a hurry.

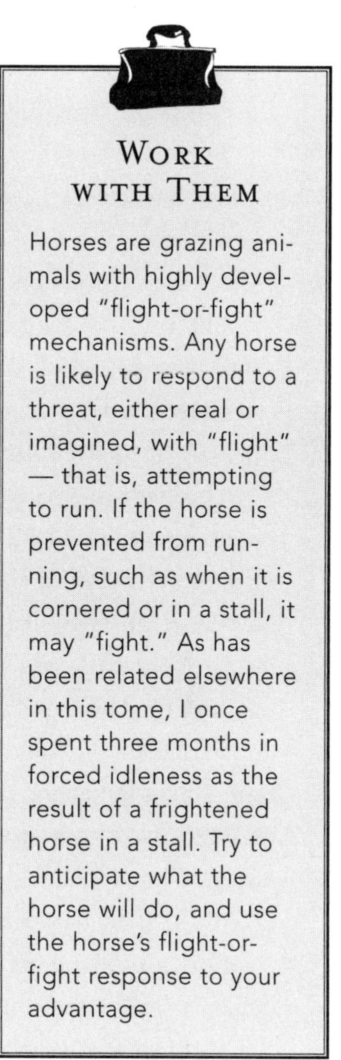

Work with Them

Horses are grazing animals with highly developed "flight-or-fight" mechanisms. Any horse is likely to respond to a threat, either real or imagined, with "flight" — that is, attempting to run. If the horse is prevented from running, such as when it is cornered or in a stall, it may "fight." As has been related elsewhere in this tome, I once spent three months in forced idleness as the result of a frightened horse in a stall. Try to anticipate what the horse will do, and use the horse's flight-or-fight response to your advantage.

Approaching a Horse

It's important to remember that a horse's vision differs from ours; a horse has a wider field of vision but sees with less acuity. While it's necessary for a horse to move its head to focus its vision, it is keenly aware of any movement within its field of vision.

Because of this heightened awareness, the moment just before you lay your hands on a horse's halter is a dangerous one. You have no control of the animal, but you are within range of its hooves and it can't see you clearly. The safest way to catch a horse is to approach from its left side, speaking softly and moving slowly. Reassure the horse and make it aware of your presence by first touching it gently yet firmly on the shoulder.

Next, slowly reach for the halter, holding the lead shank with the snap open in your other hand. It's best to attach the shank directly to the halter ring, but if you must hold on to the halter itself, loosely grasp the strap under the chin. Be prepared to let go if the horse jerks back or rears; the animal is stronger than you are, and there's great risk of injury to your shoulder, elbow, and back if you try to hold on or overpower it.

Catching an Unwilling Horse

These same techniques apply to catching a horse in the field, but if it plays hard to get, there are several strategies to use.

The simplest is to feign indifference or to simply squat down. Horses are curious and will often approach to see what's going on.

The use of a feed bucket will often attract a horse's attention and cause it to approach, but be careful. Other horses in the field will also recognize the bucket, and injury to the horses (or to you) can result if the boss of the field tries to hog the feed.

The last resort is cornering the horse. For this, involve as many people as possible and have each one carry a lead shank. Herd the horse into a corner slowly. Don't run or shout. The horse can outrun and outmaneuver an army if it gets excited (unless I've bet on it; then it can't outrun cold molasses). Tighten the line of people around it and speak soothingly. The nearest person should then approach the horse and attach the shank, then walk away without fuss or bother. This procedure may take several minutes or even the better part of an hour, and the temptation is great to jerk the shank and loudly discuss the horse's ancestry with it, but don't do it. It won't help matters, and it will just take longer the next time.

I once received a yearling filly to board, and nothing worked with her. As soon as she saw a person enter the paddock, she would take off for the farthest reaches and wouldn't stop running. Cornering her wasn't possible; no one could get close enough to her to close in on her. Finally, after two or three hours, she would get so tired of running that anyone could walk right up to her. After three sessions of this, she was confined to her stall until she became domesticated. She is an exception; you probably won't have one like her.

Turning Out a Horse

Okay, so now you have caught the horse. Next lesson: you eventually have to release it. When taking a horse out to a paddock, insist that it walk in a calm and collected manner. As you walk through the gate, keep the horse close to your right side, then proceed about fifteen or twenty feet into the field and turn it to face you. Step to its left side, hold the halter loosely by the chin strap with your left hand, and remove the shank with your right hand. Then stroke the horse's neck and step back. It's imperative that he not be allowed to bolt at the gate or in the paddock.

Before turning out several horses in a field, you should determine the pecking order for that field "herd." Always turn out the most submissive horse first and progress to the most dominant. If the "alpha" animal is turned out before the others, it may well try to kick at subordinate animals as they enter the field. Conversely, when bringing the horses in, attempt to bring the boss in first and work your way down the pecking order, bringing the most submissive horse in last.

Releasing a Horse into a Stall

When turning a horse loose in a stall, there are a few things to remember as well. First, be sure all door latches are retracted. I have sutured many lacerations resulting from latch bolts that have been run into, and a horse will remember things that cause pain. (In this instance the horse is less likely to associate pain with the door latch than with the stall door it had to walk through, which, for obvious reasons, is an association to be avoided.)

Head directly into the stall; don't angle in. The space appears larger to the horse head-on and there is less chance that it will run into the side of the doorway. Pass through with the horse at your side. Don't let it bolt, don't go in ahead of it because some horses will leap through doorways, and don't let it go in first because then you have absolutely no control over it and you're in a good position to be kicked. And absolutely, positively don't aim the horse at the doorway and turn it loose. That's a great way for a horse to get away.

Once in the stall, pull the door partially closed; some horses will attempt to leave, especially if excited. Release the horse as you would in a paddock.

There's much more to consider when leading and handling horses, but we'll leave that subject at this point and go on to restraint.

The Twitch

The main form of restraint is the twitch. The warning that follows shouldn't require discussion, but if I had a quarter for each time I've seen someone stand directly in front of a horse while twitching it, I wouldn't need the income I hope this book brings me. No, make that a dime.

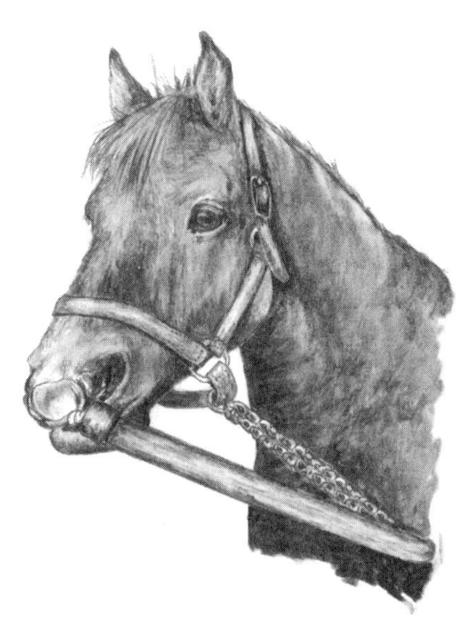

A twitch is very useful in controlling a horse.

Always stand on the left side of a horse, *never* in front of it, when applying a twitch.

Hold the twitch rope in your left hand with the loop between the thumb and index finger and between the ring and little fingers. Hold the twitch handle in your right hand or, preferably, have someone else, who should stand behind the horse's left shoulder, hold it. Reach to the horse's nose with your left hand, slip your thumb through the loop, and grasp the nose, slipping the loop over it. Quickly tighten the loop (or have the other person do it) while pulling back on it, staying close to the horse's left side (the other person is still just behind its left shoulder).

As the twitch is tightened, the horse may strike or rear, hence the need to be on its left side and not in front. If the twitch is pulled from your hands by a rearing horse, watch out for the swinging handle! It can break noses, knock out teeth, or just knock you silly. And speaking of twitch handles, always use a long-handled twitch. An ax handle or posthole digger handle makes a great handle for a twitch and will help keep you out of harm's way if you stand in the proper spot.

Help the Helpers

Last, deeply ingrained in the minds of many people is the idea that you're supposed to hold a horse from its left side, but when holding a horse for a veternarian or a farrier, *always* position yourself on the side of the animal on which the person is working. If the horse tries to kick or otherwise act up, pull its head *toward* you. This will take the horse's body (and hind legs) away from the person working on it, thereby decreasing the chance of injury. The veterinarian and farrier will thank you for your help.

Restraint

HORSES ARE BIG AND STRONG, a lot bigger and stronger than I am, and a lot bigger and stronger than their owners are. And, unfortunately, they don't always appreciate the things that we do to them.

Horses *must* be taught to behave and they *must* be disciplined when they don't. Too many horses, however, are *not* corrected and, worse, they're spoiled and allowed to get away with murder.

There was a trainer whose horses the exercise riders didn't want to ride. One day I was getting some medications from my car when an exercise boy came stomping out of a barn, muttering to himself.

"What's the problem, Red?" I asked.

"Man, Doc, it's that Tillman! If everybody's horses were like his, I'd find another way to make a living!"

"What's wrong with 'em?"

"They're crazy! They all act like they've never been touched before."

I had heard that before but it didn't affect me because I didn't do Tillman's veterinary work. But one day he came up to me. "Dr. Kelley, my regular vet hasn't come by today and I wanted my horses wormed and he knew it. Can you do it?"

I told him that I could and I'd see him in a few minutes. When I went to his barn, I had my worming equipment: wormer, bucket, pump, nasogastric tube, twitch.

He looked at the twitch. "Are you going to use that on my horses?" he asked.

"Yes. It's real hard to pass a tube unless they're twitched."

"Can we do it without the twitch?"

"Will they stand without it?"

"Oh, sure."

He put a shank on the first horse, then he petted him on the neck and whispered something I couldn't hear into the horse's ear. I reached up to put my right hand on top of the horse's nose and he hit the ceiling.

"Hold him!" I ordered.

"Okay, I got him." Then he *kissed* the horse!

After two more attempts to place my hand on the horse's nose and two more blowups, I finally got my hand there. Then I touched the tube to his nostril.

He absolutely exploded! All four feet left the ground and he came down right on top of my brand-new aluminum bucket, which flattened under the animal's weight.

That made me angry. As Tillman was kissing the horse again, I said, "If you'll let me twitch him, I'll try again. Otherwise, I'm through."

The horse was trying to get away from him, rearing and pawing. Tillman was whispering sweet nothings in his ear and letting the horse stomp on him.

"Just go," he told me. "I hope that bucket didn't hurt his feet."

I knew why his regular vet didn't show up that day, and I knew what Red was talking about. That horse was spoiled as badly as any I've ever seen.

Teaching Manners

No one likes to see ill-mannered, badly behaved children, and no one likes to see ill-mannered, badly behaved horses. A horse must be

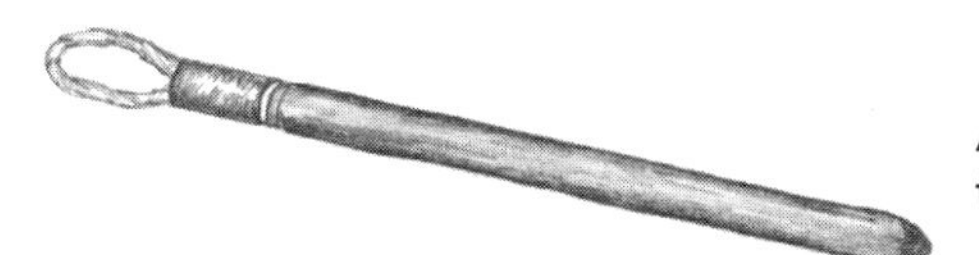

A typical twitch; long-handled twitches are best.

taught manners, just as children have to be taught manners. You don't have to be mean or heavy-handed; you just have to be firm and not let the horse get away with anything. Being firm in no way means you don't love your horse. No one loves horses more than my daughter does, and she allows no nonsense from them. And horses must be restrained when things they don't care for have to be done to them. Following are some common methods of restraint.

- **Twitch.** The twitch is the best tool for restraint. Its use is covered on page 284.
- **Tranquilizers and sedatives.** Other methods of restraint are pharmaceutical. There are tranquilizers and sedatives today that allow almost anything to be done to a horse. Unfortunately, too many people resort to these too quickly, and the vast majority of horses simply don't need them.
- **Chain over the nose.** A chain over the nose is effective, but don't maintain hard pressure on the chain. A series of short, quick, light jerks will do the job. For really difficult horses, placing the chain over the upper gums is extremely effective, but I don't like it. It hurts.
- **Lifting a leg.** This can help. A leg strap on the left foreleg is especially useful. Using a long belt, place it around the fetlock, run the end through the buckle, then lift the leg and wrap the belt around the upper arm and back around the fetlock and hold it. When you're through, just let go of the belt.

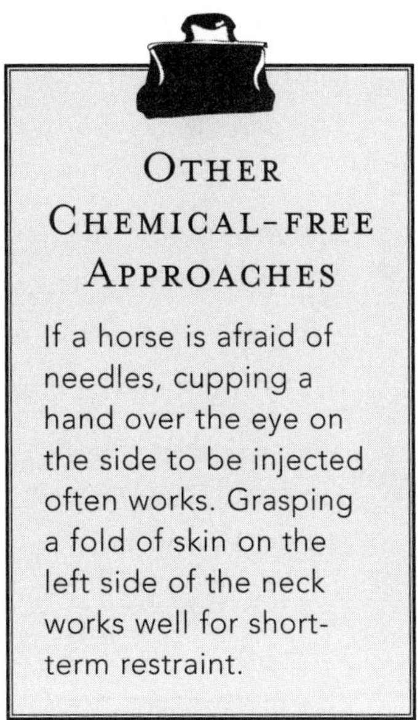

Other Chemical-free Approaches

If a horse is afraid of needles, cupping a hand over the eye on the side to be injected often works. Grasping a fold of skin on the left side of the neck works well for short-term restraint.

- **Ears as handles.** The ears are effective handles. Grasping them helps to control a horse, but, as with the chain over the gums, it hurts and it may make the horse leery of ear handling in the future. "Tailing" a horse really makes him stand still, but it takes a strong man to tail a full-grown horse. It does a great job with foals, however. Grasp the tail very close to the body and push it straight up over the back. It won't hurt but it sure makes a horse stand still.

- **Rope to tail.** A rope can be tied to the tail to restrain a kicker. Put the rope over a stall wall or rafter and pull. The weight is taken off the hind legs and the "kicker" is turned off.

But the twitch is still the best method of restraint for most relatively short procedures. To keep everyone safe, especially your veterinarian, teach your horse to tolerate the veterinary handling. Most veterinarians will be glad to offer some pointers.

Parasite Control

A CLIENT RECEIVED SEVERAL YEARLINGS to prepare for a sale. A few days after they arrived, one was found dead in its stall. The postmortem finding: a ruptured aortic aneurysm due to migrating strongyle larvae. The colt simply hadn't been wormed properly.

A new client had four mares. The first one foaled in mid-February. Around the first of April, I said, "It's time to worm your oldest foal."

"No," he replied. "I never worm foals before they're six months old."

I explained the damage that the parasites could do if he waited that long. He was unconvinced. I asked him to let me do a fecal exam to show him the parasite egg count in his foal. No. I told him I wouldn't charge to do the fecal exam. Well, okay.

The foal was seven weeks old by this time and the egg count was very high. He didn't believe me. "You're telling me that so you can charge for worming," he said.

I quit. I hope the next veterinarian convinced him, but obviously the one before me hadn't, so that client may have been a hopeless case.

I don't think we need to review the different kinds of internal parasites. Accept the fact that they are all bad and all do damage to your horse. And they can be killers, as evidenced in the first example.

Worming Schedules

A mare needs to be wormed the day after she foals. I don't worm a mare four to six weeks *before* she foals, because I feel that the medication is stressful, and a mare in late pregnancy doesn't need to be stressed. A foal, on the other hand, should first be wormed at four to six weeks of age (I always start at six weeks) and then every month until it is three years old. At that age, if it's being raced, shown, or otherwise used for some type of performance, a once-a-month schedule applies. If it's being used for breeding, pleasure, or simply pasture decoration, it goes on a sixty-day schedule.

For years it was accepted by many horse owners that a horse should be wormed every three months. That was wrong, but with some of the new deworming products, three-month intervals are okay. With the older products, sixty days was the proper interval. Read the label to see what the product manufacturer recommends.

Monitor Regularly

Even if parasites don't kill a horse as suddenly as they did in the case of the unfortunate yearling described above, they'll do it gradually. A heavy parasite load causes a horse to lose weight. Its coat is long and dull. The horse is depressed and more susceptible to disease.

And it's more expensive to keep because it requires more feed as you try to maintain its condition, which will be a losing battle unless the parasites are controlled.

It's a good idea to do periodic fecal egg counts to see how good a job your parasite-control program is doing. Depending on the number of horses per acre, choose a reasonable schedule. If you have only one horse per ten acres, you might want to do a fecal egg count every year and a half or two years. For five horses per acre, count those eggs at least once a year.

Proper parasite control will give you healthier, happier, better-performing, longer-living horses. Your veterinarian can help you to determine the best schedule and products for you and your horses.

Deworming the Farm

Over the years I have seen all levels of farm management. One "farm" consisted of about three acres and a dozen horses. Grass was scarce, and if a blade was brave enough to appear, all twelve horses leaped on it. The place was essentially fence-to-fence fecal matter, which also meant it was fence-to-fence parasites.

Parasite control in horses is important, as we've already discussed. Everyone who owns horses should know how to worm them, which includes familiarity with the deworming schedule, deworming products, and the importance of rotation. It's a favorite topic of veterinary advice columns in horse publications, and it's even written about frequently in professional veterinary journals.

Of course, advice can vary — different age to begin, different intervals, different rotation of products — but the key factors are a reasonable schedule and correct rotation. Keep in mind, though, that parasite control *in* horses is only half the battle. The horse's environment — that is, your farm — must also be the focus of parasite control.

Several steps can be taken to accomplish parasite control on the farm. Some are relatively simple and can be done in any horse operation, large or small, while others are more challenging and realistically cannot be done on many farms.

Fecal Check

I think the first, and certainly the easiest, step to take in ensuring you have a good parasite-control program is the routine examination of feces for parasite ova, also known as a *fecal check*.

The feces of every horse on the farm need not be examined, but a cross section should be. Let your veterinarian gather the samples. That way they will be fresh and of the necessary size. Over the years I have been handed many samples that were of no use. "Here, Doc, I picked this up last month and forgot to give it to you." "Here, Doc, I froze this, so it wouldn't go bad." Others have given me samples the size of a pinhead, while still others have provided piles the size of downtown Denver that I needed a forklift to pick up.

In small horse populations, check maybe one third of the animals; in larger populations, checking 10 to 20 percent of the animals is sufficient. It is important to test a reasonable sample from every sector of the farm; don't check samples from all four mares in Field A and none from the eight mares in Fields B and C and then assume you have correctly determined the parasite status.

The timing of the fecal samples is important. Taking them the day before or the day after worming tells you nothing. Ideally, the sample should be taken in spring and fall, fourteen to seventeen days after worming.

Your veterinarian will do the exam or take the samples to a lab and then report back to you. The results will be measured in ova per gram of feces. Zero parasite ova, the optimum goal, is impractical under most conditions, so the next best option is very few ova per gram. Your veterinarian will let you know if the counts are too high and will assist you in taking steps to correct the problem.

Management

Eight basic management techniques will help you to keep parasites to a minimum on your farm. We'll discuss them in order of increasing difficulty.

1. **Worm all horses kept together (same barn or paddock) at the same time.** This seems basic, yet many people will worm most of a barn and then decide to wait for assistance to worm that ornery mare and her nasty foal. Often the help doesn't show up until two or three days later.
2. **Maintain clean feed tubs and water buckets.** Wash and disinfect them once a week at least. If a horse should defecate in one, wash and disinfect it before using it again.

3. **Properly clean stalls *daily.*** Many small operations will try to economize by cleaning stalls every other day. Don't do it; it's a mistake.
4. **Harrow all paddocks and pastures each summer, when it's the hottest and driest.** This breaks up the feces and allows for desiccation of the parasite ova.
5. **Quarantine new horses, perform a fecal exam, and worm accordingly before turning in with resident horses.** A quarantine barn and paddock is nice, but just keeping the new horse in a stall until you've done what you need to is sufficient.
6. **Rotate pastures.** Obviously this cannot be done if land is limited, so it applies mainly to large operations. If it can be done, the longer a pasture stays idle, the better off it will be because the parasite ova will die out.
7. **Remove feces from fields.** Again, this is impractical or impossible in many situations, but if it can be done, compost the fecal matter or have it hauled off the farm.
8. **Dispose of manure properly.** Ideally, it should be hauled away or spread on idle fields. Alternatively, it may be composted for six months to a year and then spread on pastures. Spreading a wagonload of fresh manure on your pastures immediately after cleaning your stalls only serves to give your parasite ova a nice outing and further contaminates your fields.

Maintaining parasite-free horses and farms is probably impossible, but minimal infestations (contrary to common terminology, parasites *infest,* they do not *infect*) *can* be achieved. Good farm management will keep parasite problems to a minimum. Dutifully following these basic management steps will benefit your horse operation as well as your horses. You will have healthier, fitter horses that perform better whether they race, show, or are just ridden occasionally. Maintaining a parasite-free environment (or as close to that as practical) pays for itself in the long run.

Ticks

BEING A HORSE DOCTOR in the Thoroughbred capital of the world has its perks. Being invited to parties is considered by many to be a perk. My wife likes that one, but I don't like parties.

One perk I do like is being taken to foreign countries to look at or treat horses. Or just to consult. That's a great one.

My favorite location is Jamaica. I met a Jamaican horseman many years ago, and we became good friends. I've had the pleasure of visiting there at least a dozen times to help with and advise their horse-breeding operations.

On my first trip there, the manager of my host's farm asked, "Dr. Kelley, do you have a tick problem in Kentucky?"

Well, we do have ticks here, and sometimes they're a problem. I said as much.

"Look at this," he said, and pulled a mare's tail to one side.

Around the vulva and anus there must have been more than a hundred ticks. I had never seen anything like it. A groom began to remove them by hand.

"They'll be back just like that in two days," the manager said.

"Wow," was all I could say.

Ticks are external parasites of warm-blooded animals. They are disgusting little creatures that must have blood for survival. Heavy infestations can lead to anemia, but this is not the major problem ticks can cause.

Infestation and Disease Risks

Ticks are carriers for several diseases in both animals and humans, and this is the main reason that they must be controlled. And control is the only choice; while certain tick-borne diseases may be treated, there's no method for prevention of tick infestation.

There are many species of tick and most are not host specific. Mother Nature has made ticks a hardy life-form and has provided a wide variety, suited to a wide range of climatic conditions. There are

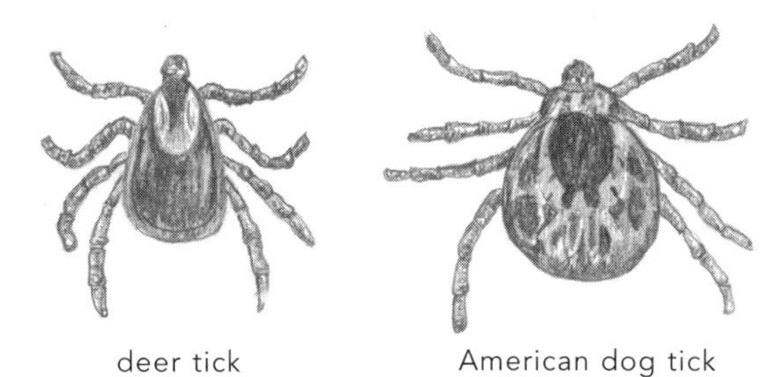

These are the two principal tick types in the United States, but there are many others.

winter ticks that range as far north as Canada, tropical ticks that live in Mexico and the Caribbean and as far north as Florida and Texas, and various other types that inhabit all areas in between, so wherever your horses are, ticks are waiting there for them.

The ear of a horse is a favorite site of attachment; indeed, one species is called the ear tick. Infestation here may be a main cause of tick-related suffering for horses. The ticks travel deep into the ear canal and create an irritation manifested by ear rubbing and head shaking. *Secondary bacterial otitis* (inflammation of the ear) frequently ensues. Diagnosis is made by finding the ticks in the ears through otoscopic examination under tranquilization or sedation. Treatment requires the introduction of a suitable pesticide into the ear canal, a procedure not particularly pleasurable to the horse. Be careful when doing this; a horse's swinging head weighs considerably more than your stationary one. If bacterial otitis exists, antibiotic or antibiotic/steroid ointments must also be used.

Tick paralysis, spread by a tick most commonly found in the western United States, is a problem in both horses and humans. The bite of a single infected tick can lead to paralysis, so this is a particularly threatening condition.

The two most common diseases horses can contract via ticks are Lyme disease and piroplasmosis. *Lyme disease* is caused by a bacterium carried by ticks of the genus *Ixodes,* while the causative agent of *piroplasmosis* is a protozoan carried by the tropical horse tick. Both conditions are treatable.

Lyme Disease

Lyme disease takes on added importance because it is increasingly becoming a serious problem in humans, especially in the Northeast and the West Coast of the United States. Signs of the disease in both humans and horses are nonspecific but include fever, muscle soreness, and stiffness of the joints. In people, it can easily be mistaken for a cold or flu in its early stages. In horses, diagnosis is made by clinical signs, history, and response to antibiotic therapy. The ticks responsible for Lyme disease are most commonly found in the tail and under the mane and, again, a topical pesticide is the treatment of choice to remove them.

Piroplasmosis

Piroplasmosis in the United States has occurred in Florida and probably in Texas (although it has been undiagnosed to date) but is most serious and widespread in the Caribbean. Horses exported from the United States to Caribbean nations must have a negative blood test for piroplasmosis. This must be for the purpose of protecting the native Caribbean infectious organisms from competition, because the first thing that happens to a horse when it steps off the plane on a Caribbean island is to be bitten by a tropical tick, thus contracting the disease.

Clinical signs vary in severity and include fever, depression, edema, weakness, and abortion in seriously affected pregnant mares. The causative organism destroys red blood cells, so anemia is evident in a blood count. There are drugs available now that can aid in the prevention of piroplasmosis, and treatment is also effective, but a persistent carrier state exists, so a "cured" horse may remain positive on a blood test.

Tick Control

Tick control is the key to minimizing tick-borne diseases. The tick population can be kept to a minimum by maintaining fields and paddocks in a closely mowed state, and horses should be kept out of wooded or overgrown areas.

Horses should be routinely checked for ticks. The primary sites of tick infestation are the ears, mane, tail, and under the tail around the anus and vulva. I have already said how many I've seen in that area on a single mare in Jamaica.

Manually removing the ticks is tedious and may well not be fully appreciated by the horse, especially in the anal-vulvar area, so the proper use of parasiticides or pesticides is the treatment of choice. A tick is an arachnid, not an insect; therefore, most insecticides are of no help. Pyrethrins and permethrins are effective, but it's essential to strictly follow the instructions on the label. Ivermectin will kill ticks, so the use of that product as a dewormer is helpful. The ivermectin enters the circulatory system, so when a tick bites it gets a mouthful of blood that proves lethal to it.

The life cycle of some ticks is two or three years, so if you choose to remove them manually (which you may well do in the case of only a few ticks), don't just flick them onto the ground or stall floor. Do something to kill them. The brick-and-hammer method is especially effective, but much easier and more convenient is the maintenance of a small bucket (or coffee can) of water, into which you can drop the removed ticks. They are notoriously poor swimmers.

Isolation Barn

A NEW CLIENT BOUGHT A BROODMARE at a breeding stock sale. He took her home and put her in his broodmare barn with fourteen other pregnant mares. The next morning she had aborted. Over the next ten days, thirteen of the other fourteen mares also aborted.

The cause was virus abortion (equine rhinopneumonitis) brought in by the sale mare.

Two yearling fillies shipped in from out of state, about a 600-mile trip. My client put them in a barn with eight other yearling fillies that were being prepared for sale. The next day one of the new arrivals was depressed and had a fever of 105 degrees. The day after that a thick nasal discharge appeared. The day after that, the other new arrival was depressed and febrile, too. Within a week the other eight were doing the same. Four of the ten had to be scratched from the sale.

It was strangles.

A client bought a weanling colt from a sale. He had three fillies and one colt, and he wanted another colt to keep the first company when he separated the sexes. Fearing the possibility of the new colt bringing something in to infect the resident weanlings, he stuck the new guy in his other barn, the one that housed his four broodmares. All four were in foal, and over the next two weeks all four aborted; three aborted in one night.

The cause was virus abortion, a respiratory disease typically seen in young horses.

All of the aborting mares in this case had received virus abortion vaccinations. Vaccination is essential, but I personally do not feel that *any* vaccination can withstand a really hot bug. These sure couldn't.

And the strangles vaccine makes some horses sick, so it's rarely given unless there is an outbreak in the area. Exposed horses should not be vaccinated. Also, be aware that it's one of the least effective vaccines we have.

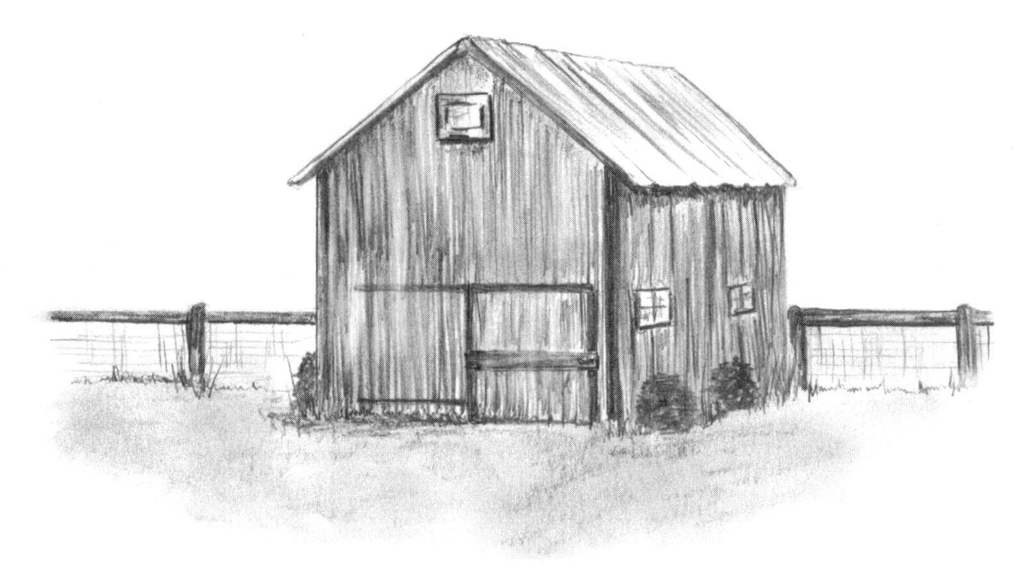

A small barn separate from other barns makes a good isolation facility.

Fortunately, all introductions of new horses do not end so tragically, but it can happen. And it doesn't have to happen. An isolation facility of some sort would have prevented all of those problems. A barn located away from the other barns and with its own paddock works well. But an isolation facility can be as simple as a shed in a distant paddock. Or, if it is an area of the country or a time of year when the weather is decent, isolation in a distant paddock will suffice.

In a perfect world (but, goodness knows, we do not live in a perfect world), new horses should be isolated for a month at least. Two weeks is the absolute minimum.

Containing Contamination

The benefits of isolation are lost if farm personnel spread contamination from the isolation facility to the other horses on the farm. Again, in a perfect world, one person or crew should care for the isolated animals and not have contact with others on the farm, but this is usually not possible or practical.

So take care of the non-isolated horses first, and then designate a person (or persons, if necessary) to tend to the isolates.

Before entering the isolation area, these people should don coveralls and disposable booties and gloves. When finished, the coveralls should be removed and left in the isolation barn until next time; booties and gloves should be removed and disposed of. The workers should wash and disinfect before returning to the rest of the farm.

Cleaning the Isolation Barn

When the time comes that the isolated animals can join the other horses, the isolation stalls should be cleaned thoroughly and left idle for at least two weeks. If disease was present, disinfecting is essential and the stalls involved need to be left empty for a minimum of eight to ten weeks.

Ideally, the muck from the isolation barn should be burned. If disease is present, muck *must* be burned. I once had a client with a nice isolation facility: a six-stall barn and two paddocks far removed from the rest of the farm. He had his crew place the muck from the isolation barn with the muck from the other barns and spread it on the horse fields — not good.

A further word of warning concerning strangles: the literature tells us that the causative organism *(Streptococcus equi)* can live in an environment for as long as two months after an outbreak. Hogwash. It can live for at least two years. There are at least two barns that housed severe outbreaks of strangles and were disinfected and left empty for two years. Shortly after healthy horses were introduced to the barns, strangles reappeared.

Another neat thing about strangles: moisture somehow protects the organism so after disinfecting, which is wet, there must be thorough drying. Burning the barn works well, but most people find that a little drastic. Good ventilation and time are the only reasonable alternatives.

I don't mean to imply that virus abortion and strangles are the only two threats from the introduction of outside horses to your farm. These two just happen to be the most dramatic. Flu is another disease easily introduced by stressed horses that have been shipped.

A Risky Proposition

The greatest risk for bad things is to place a horse from a sale with your resident horses. I firmly believe that every disease known to veterinary science plus several that are not known are passed around at sales. Many of the horses there have not been vaccinated — "I'm selling her; I'm not wasting money on vaccines" — and that fact, combined with the extremely high level of stress that the animals are under at sales (noise, strange people, in and out of stalls, and so forth), can spell disaster if precautions are not taken.

Shows, race meets, fairs, rodeos, trail rides, and any other place that horses gather are also marvelous sites for picking up undesirable bugs. You can't control what others do with their horses, but you can safeguard yours: a properly maintained vaccination program is absolutely essential (see page 2 for more on vaccinations).

Fruit Tree Toxicity

When I was in college, we had a small (stress "small") farm where we kept two broodmares and their foals. We didn't make much money with them because they weren't real high-quality mares, but they were the best we could afford, and they did manage to pay their way from the sales of their offspring.

In one paddock there was a pear tree. I went to the library and read up on pear trees to see whether there was any danger to the horses from it. There wasn't, and they *loved* it. That is, they loved the leaves. They ate the leaves as high as they could reach, then they reared up on their hind legs to reach higher. They preferred the leaves to their grain ration.

Since then, here in Kentucky, I have discovered that horses like apple leaves equally well. We have both apple and pear trees here, but they aren't in any of the paddocks, so for a treat every once in a while I'll lead a mare out and let her nibble on the leaves. They also love apples.

Beware, Peaches, Plums, and Cherries

But all fruit trees, although just as desirable to the horses, are not so harmless Apples, peaches, plums, and cherries belong to the same family, *Rosaceae*. The latter three, however, are members of the genus *Prunus*, and as such they produce hydrocyanic acid. If this is ingested by horses, the chief sign of a problem is sudden death, although there are other problems. Its effect is dose related.

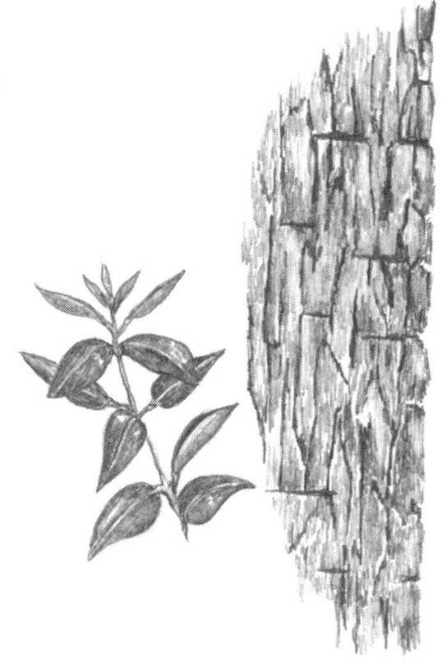

Wild cherry trees are most easily identified by their rough bark with distinctive horizontal slashes.

The hydrocyanic acid is formed as a decomposition product as the result of enzymatic action on the glycoside amygdalin found in the leaves, twigs, and bark of these trees. The chief source of the acid is wilted leaves due to frost, drought, or broken branches, but occasionally fresh leaves may be ingested and the acid will form in the stomach after the leaves are chewed. Usually death occurs less than an hour after ingestion of a sufficient amount; prior to death there is labored breathing, spasms, and coma. Ingestion of small amounts is suspected to cause abortions in cows.

In late spring and early summer 2001, there was a serious problem of fetal and foal losses here in Kentucky; abortions and foal deaths occurred on a widespread basis due to mare reproductive loss syndrome.

This was initially blamed on the ingestion of tent caterpillars that had eaten cherry leaves. Another possibility is that after the tent caterpillars, which were numerous that year, fed on the cherry leaves, they meandered into the horse fields. The horses then unwittingly ingested the caterpillar excrement. In either case, toxicity was secondary. The precise cause of the problem has yet to be determined, but apparently abortion in mares is also caused by the plants.

Treatment

If horses are known to have eaten leaves of these trees, treatment must be immediate and consists of intravenous sodium nitrite followed by sodium thiosulfate. An ounce of prevention is worth a pound of cure, however, and the best way to keep your horses from eating these potentially toxic trees is to deny them access to them.

The problem we had here in Kentucky didn't originate with trees in the horses' fields, but with trees outside the fence lines. The safest way to go is not to have any of these trees on your property.

Goats

WHEN I WAS A LITTLE BOY, my older brother always had at least one show horse, and we always had a couple of goats around the place. When I was about five, he had a five-year-old, five-gaited Saddlebred mare named Charming Joanne.

Joanne was beautiful and a marvelous show mare (she won just about every time out), but I didn't like her very much because she was a nut. She was kept in her stall most of the time because she was shown almost every weekend.

She didn't like being in a stall. She walked constantly and jumped up and down. One day at dinner my brother said to Mom, "Joanne needs company. I think I'll put one of the goats in with her."

He did, and within about two or three days Joanne stopped walking and jumping.

That's one thing that I don't like about how performance horses are kept. They spend most of their time in stalls. It may be as much as twenty-three hours a day for a healthy, sound horse. An injured or sick horse actually may be confined to its stall for weeks while it heals. They get lonely and bored, and they respond to that boredom in different ways. Some constantly walk circles in the stall; some kick the walls; some weave; some rear in an effort to see the horse in the next stall; some become mean; some become cribbers; some even bite themselves. It's something to do.

Companion Animals

One of the often-used methods to stop all of this (nothing is foolproof, however) is to do what my brother did: give the lonely horse a companion. Another horse would be ideal, of course, but that's impractical and, besides, two horses will hardly fit in a twelve-foot-square box stall. Therefore, other, smaller species are used. Over the years I've seen dozens of horses with such smaller companions. One horse had a rooster, another a hen. One had a duck, one had a sheep, and one had — believe it or not — a de-scented skunk. Another had a miniature donkey for a companion. A few had cats, but cats seem to be the least satisfactory because they roam too much.

I remember one that had a dog. One night I was called to the training barn to treat a case of colic and passed the stall of this horse and "his" dog companion. They were both lying down asleep; the little dog was curled up under the horse's throat, his head resting on the horse's.

The most common companion by far, though, is a goat. I'm not sure why this is; maybe it's because goats are cheap and easy to care for. I imagine over the years I've seen forty or fifty horses with goat companions. The horses come to depend on their goats, and vice versa.

Faithful Friends

A training center is just that, a place to train horses, and if a horse is to race it has to be vanned to the track where the race is being run. The race may be at a local track, where the horse has to van only twenty minutes or so, but some are vanned one hundred miles or more to race and then vanned back after the race. I have known a dozen horses that had to have their goats vanned with them.

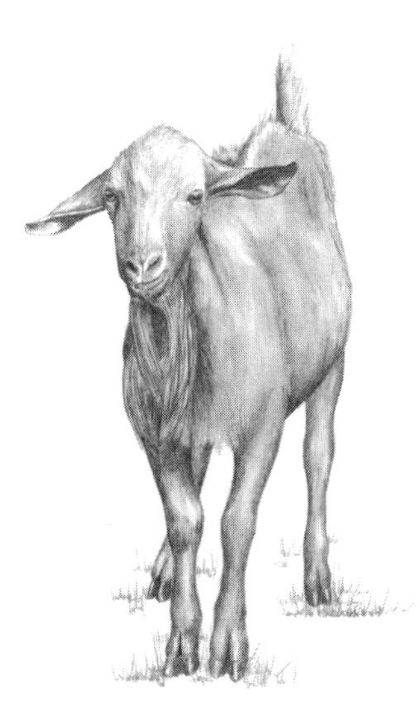

By far, the most common companion animal for horses is the goat.

And most of their goat companions don't like it when their horses leave. They cry and bleat and run in circles until their friends return. Once a goat that dearly loved her horse got out of the stall somehow after her horse had left for a race. She ran throughout the entire training center crying for him. No one could catch her until six hours later, when her horse returned. Then she ran right up to him and followed him back to their stall. On race days after that, she rode along with him.

There was one goat that was extremely protective of her horse. Her name was Molly; she wore a dog collar and had to be tied or held whenever her filly left the stall for any reason. Also, she had a reputation for attacking anyone who she thought was doing a disservice to her filly. This filly had been a terrible stall walker before Molly, but when the goat joined her she settled down nicely and became a very useful runner.

I was the trainer's veterinarian, and whenever I or the farrier needed to work on the filly, he would either tie up Molly or have one of his grooms hold her. Usually he snapped a rope, which was attached to one of the rings that supported the feed tub, to the goat's collar. She hopped about and bleated and even turned somersaults in an attempt to get free to "protect" her filly.

One day the filly came back from her morning workout with a slight limp. Her trainer asked me to look at her. With a groom holding Molly, he led the filly out and I saw she was slightly off in her right fore. I told him to put her back in the stall and I would examine her further there. The first thing he did when he reentered the stall was attach the rope to Molly's collar. "Okay, Doc, now you can come in."

I bent down to feel the filly's ankle and foot for heat. As soon as I touched her, Molly began jumping and bleating frantically and straining against the rope. I picked up the foot and the next thing I knew I felt excruciating pain and, just as in the comics, I saw stars — briefly. Then everything went black.

When I saw light again, I was sitting back against a bale of hay in the aisle outside the stall.

"Are you okay?" the trainer asked.

It took a second but I finally replied. "What the heck happened? Did she cow-kick me?" My head and neck hurt, especially the top of my head.

It seems that Molly's collar broke as she was flipping around, and she "protected" her filly. She butted me on the top of my head as I was bending over looking at the foot. The trainer said I "went down like a sack of potatoes and was out like a light"; not very original but his words, nonetheless.

Once Molly had been recollared (they had an extra one so this must have happened before) and I had taken a couple of aspirin, we determined that the filly had a very small but deep quarter crack that caused her to be stall-bound for several weeks. She was relatively content because she had Molly, and Molly loved it because her filly was not taken away for any reason.

Someday someone will come up with a method of showing or keeping horses in training without condemning them to solitary confinement. I don't think the goat industry will feel the pinch. In the meantime, consider your stalled horses with vices or nervous dispositions. Maybe a goat or another animal might help.

The Barn Cat

In this section, we digress from actual horse stuff to discuss a very important member of most horse farm operations: the barn cat. Too often people don't respect their barn cat or care for it in a manner befitting such an integral part of their operation. The fact that these felines spend their lives in a barn among other four-legged critters and are not welcome in a house (in most cases they wouldn't want to be invited in, anyway) doesn't change their wants and needs.

A New Cat

In introducing a new cat to a barn, care must be taken to keep it from running away. There's less danger of this with a small kitten, but a half-grown or adult cat is likely to be frightened by the strange, new surroundings and take off at the first opportunity.

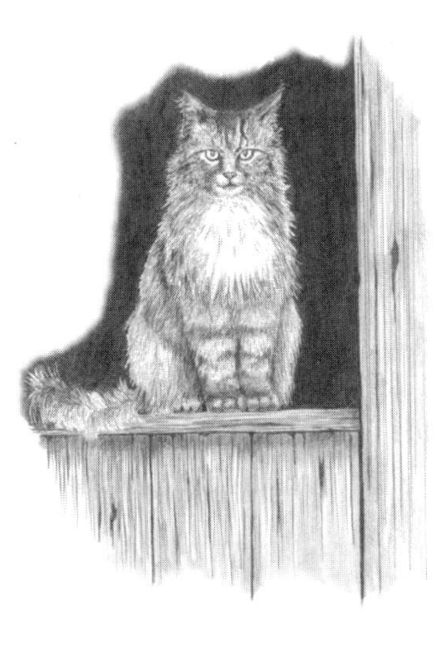

To let the cat familiarize itself with its new home, it should be restricted for a few days to the area that is to become its territory. This should be a feed room, warm-up room, or storage room, *not* an entire barn. Ample food and water must be supplied, as well as a litter box.

Be mindful of windows. They should be closed; a window screen is no match for a desperate cat, and a scared, confused cat in a new environment is indeed desperate. And as the door is opened, care must be taken that the newcomer doesn't shoot out. Whenever barn personnel are in the room, the cat should be handled and reassured.

After three or four days, most cats will have settled down to their new home; then they can be allowed to roam the entire barn, and the litter box can be eliminated. The feed and water must remain, however. More on this in a bit.

On-the-Job Training

The cat must be given free access to the area that it is to police. Feed and storage areas are the raisons d'être for a barn cat, but if it can't get to these areas its function is greatly reduced. A small hole, just large enough for the cat to get through, should be cut in the bottom of the door on the hinge side. The latch side of the door has too much give, especially if the door is hollow, and a determined dog can break through if it's given a toehold like that.

The area that the cat is expected to protect is where its food and water should be placed. Feeding a cat in the barn aisle or on a ledge in a stall is counterproductive for two reasons: (1) the cat has no reason to spend time where you want it to, and (2) leaving food in the open attracts unwanted visitors — dogs, raccoons, skunks, opossums, among others.

Food and Water

Many people don't feed their barn cats. This at best is counterproductive and at worst, cruel and inhumane. They reason that the cat will kill mice and rats if it's hungry, and they feel the price of cat food is too high. It's very true that a hungry cat will kill for its food, but a hungry cat doesn't want to waste its time chasing mice among feed bags, bins, shelves, and wall cracks; instead, it will go to the fields to hunt quarry that can't elude it as easily. The result: barn mice proliferate and the owner curses the cat that is only trying to survive.

A well-fed, contented cat that knows where its next meal is coming from may not eat mice, but by instinct will still hunt and kill them. It makes a game out of pursuing the rodents in the more sporting environment of the feed room. And its mere presence may be enough to deter many mice. The cost of cat food is nothing compared to the cost of grain lost to rats and mice. This is a fact that should be etched in stone somewhere, but nonetheless escapes the grasp of many.

A source of water in the cat's feed area is essential. Even the most well intentioned and caring of people are sometimes guilty of not recognizing this. Obviously, the cat needs water, and if a clean, fresh source isn't available it will search some out. Frequently, this is a bucket or tank and, if a foot slips, the usual outcome is a drowned cat.

General Care

Just as with any cat, a barn cat needs protection from disease through vaccination. In fact, a barn cat has greater need for a rabies vaccination because it's much more apt to come in contact with wild animals than is a house cat. Protecting your cat may save your horses. (For more information, see page 8 on rabies.)

A barn cat has even more need than a house cat to be spayed or neutered. It may be the only known resident feline on the farm, but it's safe to say that lurking in the tall grass or stand of trees on the back of the farm are several less fortunate members of the species, and nature will have its way. As a result, spaying or neutering is absolutely essential. An argument put to me by a client (one who doesn't feed his cat) was that his cat was a male and therefore he wouldn't have any unwanted kittens. He doesn't understand the fact that his tomcat could (and would) sire dozens of wild kittens.

A very sad sight, one that I have seen too many times, is a mother cat in the corner of a stall or feed room with a litter of kittens, all with matted eyes and purulent nasal discharge. They are, for the most part, doomed. Proper vaccination of the mother would have done the trick. And spaying of the mother would have prevented these unwanted kittens and unnecessary deaths.

A barn cat is important to any farming operation that requires grain storage and, properly cared for, will more than pay for its upkeep. Just use a little common sense and the rest will take care of itself.

11

General Horse Care

Water

Horses — all animals for that matter — should always have access to clean, fresh water. I have seen water tanks from which horses were supposed to drink that contained water so full of foreign matter (dirt, leaves, dead birds, algae, and so on) that it could have been more easily chewed than swallowed. There is absolutely no excuse for this, other than pure laziness, and that's a poor excuse indeed.

It's equally important to keep water and feed tubs free from bird droppings. Bird droppings represent a special hazard. Several horse deaths in England were attributed to drinking water that had been contaminated by bird droppings. That alone should motivate you to maintain cleaner water supplies.

- **Water tanks.** I'm not a fan of water tanks because they're a challenge to clean and keep free of contaminants. Their size alone is intimidating; it's much easier, quicker, and more satisfying to clean a smaller container. If you must use a tank, empty it at least once a week and thoroughly clean it. Twice a week is better.
- **Ponds.** Several farms have ponds as a water supply for the horses. A

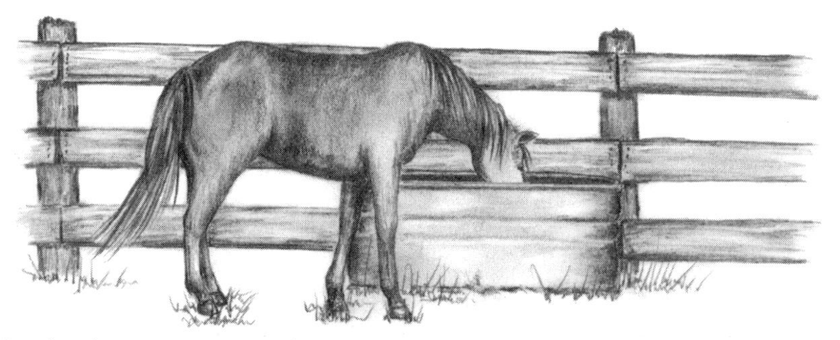

A fresh, clean water supply is essential.

pond is picturesque and a great place for ducks, but it's a lousy water source for horses. Even if the horses don't urinate and defecate directly into a pond, these materials are washed there by rain, along with lime, fertilizer, and any other pollutants that may be in the field.

- **Automatic waterers.** In the field, automatic waterers are the way to go. There are several on the market for field use, but I like the ones with the shiny little metal bowls because the bowls are easy to clean and you can tell when they're clean. It's a simple task to wipe them out every day.

These same waterers, or their first cousins, can also be used in stalls, but that's an expense that's probably unnecessary. Buckets do just fine, and they are easy to clean as well. A daily scrubbing with a brush and a weekly washing with soap and water will ensure that the horse drinking from it has a consistent supply of clean, fresh water. The same cleaning schedule should be maintained for feed tubs.

I don't know if anyone has ever researched water intake in horses offered clean water and horses offered different levels of contaminated water, but it doesn't take much thought to realize that the clean water would be preferred. And I suppose there is no way to know how many illnesses are attributable to water contamination, but I'll bet it's significant. A horse should drink at least a gallon of clean water daily.

There is no excuse for allowing your horses to drink dirty water. This is one aspect of horse health that can easily be controlled.

Managing Feed Intake

A CLIENT HAS A NICE FARM: a couple of hundred acres and about thirty quality mares. He makes a good living selling and racing their offspring, but he has a few with reproductive problems. They are difficult to get in foal.

In observing them, the problem is easy to spot, but somehow he doesn't see it. Even after having it pointed out to him, he refuses to acknowledge it, but here it is: two of the hard-to-conceive mares look as if they should have GOODYEAR painted on their sides and be floating over the Super Bowl. And two others look as if they could be skeletal specimens in an anatomy lab. The other two dozen or so look fine, plus or minus a pound or two.

He worries about the two skinny ones. He even acknowledges that they need to gain weight. One day he asked me about it.

"Feed them more," I advised him. It seemed to be a fairly simple solution.

"That can't be it," he said. "They get just as much as the others."

Surprisingly, he was not concerned about the two blimps, even though I told him they were way too fat to be efficient reproducers.

There is no man so blind as he who will not see. That's not original, but it sure is applicable. And this guy is not alone in his refusal to acknowledge weight problems.

There are two obvious issues with feed intake: too much and not enough. The former is pretty much a matter of management, and usually the latter is, too.

Preventing Obesity

The first thing to remember in feeding horses is this: horses have no self-regulatory mechanism to control their intake. In other words, they will eat themselves to death. Literally. In the wild this is not a problem; few mustangs encounter fifty-pound sacks of corn behind unsecured barn doors. The usual outcome is colic or founder or both, and either can be serious enough to cause the death of the animal.

Overeating at one sitting is readily controllable; simply make certain that your horses cannot get to your feed storage areas.

Although gaining access to feed in this manner is a very serious and tragic situation, it is not the main problem associated with overeating. The most common problem is strictly man-made: long-term overeating due to being fed too much and exercised too little. Or, sometimes, both. The result is obesity. Obesity is rarely the horse's fault; it's almost entirely the fault of the person responsible for its care.

If the feed is palatable, a horse will eat what it is given. To some horses, if it doesn't move (or moves slowly), it's palatable. Because the horse cleans up, that by no means indicates that it's still hungry. Each horse is an individual and must be fed as an individual. Just as there are varying requirements for food intake in a group of people, there are varying requirements in a group of horses.

Many times I have seen an otherwise knowledgeable horseman go through a barn and place the same amount of feed in each stall and then bring in a group of sixteen broodmares ranging in age from four to twenty years and in pregnancy status from empty to imminent. Fortunately, this feed regimen is probably appropriate for most of these mares, but in the group there will be a couple that are a few pounds underweight and two or three that are absolute butterballs. (The horseman in this section's opening paragraphs used this feeding method.)

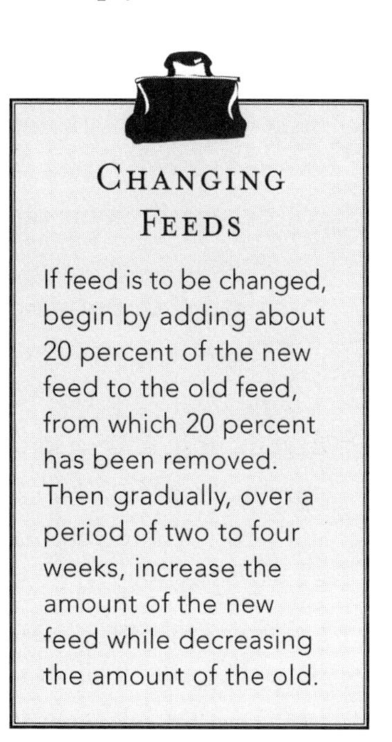

Changing Feeds

If feed is to be changed, begin by adding about 20 percent of the new feed to the old feed, from which 20 percent has been removed. Then gradually, over a period of two to four weeks, increase the amount of the new feed while decreasing the amount of the old.

Feeding outside using ground or fence feeders makes it impossible to regulate each horse's intake. Even if each horse is totally respectful (and if pigs fly) of its pasture mates' feeders, it cannot be known to which feeder a horse will go, and that makes it impossible to place varying amounts of feed in the different feeders. Often, you have the added issue of an aggressive, fast-eating horse hogging more than its share. (This is usually not the obese member of the group, however. This one works off excess intake by being bossy all the time.)

It is much easier to prevent obesity than it is to correct it; prevention requires knowing your horses, which, in turn, requires observing them. This is not difficult, yet too many people do not take the time to do it. Look at your horses. The 16.3-hand Belgian cross that looks as if he should be pulling a beer wagon probably needs more feed than the 14.3-half-Arab that looks too delicate ever to carry a full-sized person, but on many farms they are fed the same.

Once the weight is on, however, the problem becomes more difficult to manage. For proper health, you must get that extra weight off the fat animals, but this isn't as easy as it sounds. The temptation is there to starve it off, but you then run the risk of hyperlipemia, which is another subject and has its own section (see page 77). Suffice it to say, you don't want it.

To get the weight off, simply feed less of the grain ration and maintain a proper roughage level. Increased exercise is helpful, but in many cases (broodmares, for instance,) it's impractical. With stallions and riding horses, step up their exercise programs. The weight loss will not be noticed quickly, as anyone knows who ever tried to diet, but because your horse will rarely raid a refrigerator at midnight, the extra weight will eventually come off.

Correcting Underweight

There are also several reasons for a horse being underweight, among them improper feeding, parasitism, dental problems, endocrine dysfunction, and chronic disease. Your veterinarian can help in determining the cause. If it's too few groceries, the remedy is apparent: gradually increase the amount being fed and then maintain the horse at an appropriate ration.

Anorexia, or refusal to eat, has many causes and, knowing that a horse lives to eat, it should always be considered serious. To determine the cause in an otherwise normal-acting horse, evaluate the feed. It could be bad (moldy), or it could be from a new sack that was formulated slightly differently. Or poor eating could result from a switch in feeds, which should always be done gradually.

Other causes of anorexia include fever, pain, disease, colic, and disruption of routine (weaning, separation from a buddy, moving to a new farm, and so on). Address the cause and remove it if possible, and the horse will eat again. In extreme cases, nutritional supplementation may be necessary to get a horse over anorexia. This is best done under the care of a veterinarian in an equine hospital.

To sum up, all feeding problems must first be acknowledged before they can be corrected. Even though management is frequently at fault, your veterinarian can help you understand the problem and guide you in its correction.

Equine Supplements

Veterinary equine supplements can and should be an important part of a horse's regular care. These supplements range from the general to the very specific and are tailored to a horse's needs. One of the keys to learning what your horses require is to ask a veterinarian whether the horses need anything to help them in their appointed use. It is the veterinarian's job to inform you about and recommend supplements.

The dictionary defines *supplement* as follows:

- Something added to complete a thing
- Something added to supply a deficiency

At first glance, the definitions appear quite similar, but with further explanation the difference becomes apparent.

"Complete" Rations

Many horse feeds are promoted as "complete," and they are if the animals eating them have nothing else to do but exist or be taken for the occasional ride, but too many "complete" feeds fall short under the increased demands of training and reproduction. Most horses are asked to do more than lead a life of ease. From trail rides to shows to races, from breeding to pulling wagons and carts, most horses today are very active, justifying their existence for the pleasure and profit of their owners; the toll placed on them by these activities may well require more than a "complete" ration.

There are dozens of veterinary products available to assist you in bettering your horses' nutrition and, theoretically, performance, but these products compete with hundreds of over-the-counter products for sale in feed stores, catalogs, and tack shops. Ask your veterinarian what the most useful product for your horse might be.

As already mentioned, the veterinarian will consider the needs of your horses when making a recommendation. For horses under heavy stress, such as racing, there are supplements available that supply vitamins and minerals above those of the feed ration, and others that will replace electrolytes and amino acids depleted by heavy exercise. Other products provide an energy boost, and still others are metabolic enhancers, especially helpful to horses in heavy training.

For breeding stock, there are vitamin-mineral supplements, but additionally there are need-specific supplements that more directly address the requirements of the reproducing animal, such as vitamin E and selenium deficiencies — both frequently unrecognized problems.

So much for the first definition. The second definition — supplying a deficiency — is much more a function of veterinary medicine.

Addressing Deficiencies

Mineral deficiencies, especially in specific areas of the United States, are not uncommon. Diagnostic work has to be done to determine which mineral is low, and in most cases there is a veterinary product that may be used to correct the deficiency. The veterinarian can offer a real benefit in these cases by knowing which minerals are naturally deficient in his practice area (consult the soil science department of a local college or university or the Cooperative Extension office), thereby knowing what to test for and, consequently, what to recommend.

Also, certain hormonal imbalances can be aided by supplementation. Again, these require diagnostic procedures and later monitoring, but the horse and ultimately the owner will benefit.

There are a number of supplements designed for hoof and foot care, for problems ranging from dry hooves to laminitis. Several of these products function as preventatives as well as remedies.

There is supplementation available for debilitated horses and horses that are otherwise in poor condition. The various vitamin-mineral–amino acid preparations are useful here, and there are also products that supply full nutritional needs for aphagic animals (animals that do not eat) or those that are unable to eat due to injury. Included here are enzymes and microorganism supplements for gastrointestinal and digestion maintenance and products to ensure proper nutrition in foals, whether they be orphaned or weaned.

Finally, there are fat and lipid supplements to improve coat health. These are especially useful in show horses and horses destined for sales, two areas where appearance is of paramount importance.

Administering Supplements

Most supplements are dispensable products that can be mixed with the feed or put in the drinking water, but the latter requires more careful management. Obviously, if the supplement is intended for one horse, the water source for a group of eight cannot be treated. The horse must be separated and have an easily monitored water supply.

Supplements added to the feed are easier to monitor, but here again it cannot be effectively done if a group of horses is fed in the field. A problem encountered in both delivery forms, feed and water, is the picky horse that will not ingest anything different. The addition of corn oil or corn syrup usually gets such a horse to eat. Supplements also come in other forms, some of which require the veterinarian for administration. These are the drenches (products given by tube or oral syringe) and the injectables, although there are those who say that if it has to be injected it isn't a supplement. Some supplements are prepared in paste form and administered much as deworming products are.

Gelding

HORSES ARE BIG AND STRONG, bigger and stronger than people are. And they can be ornery, especially stallions. Although I have known a few stallions that were practically puppy dogs, I have known a whole lot more that were just plain mean.

When I was younger I firmly believed that no horse was too tough for me to handle. I was wrong, of course, but that didn't stop me from going one-on-one with some awfully tough critters. Age works wonders, and as I look back I find it amazing how foolish I was.

For this reason, I don't understand why anyone other than a breeder would want a stallion other than a teaser. Sure, if he has an outstanding pedigree and a great future as a sire, I can understand why he should be left alone, but most don't fit that description. So, for the sake of safety and ease of handling and managing, the vast majority of stallions should be gelded at an early age: sixteen to eighteen months is a good time.

A gelding is calmer and more tractable than a stallion, and you don't have to worry about a mare in the next stall being in season. True, the occasional gelding will act a little studdish, but this behavior is mild when compared to how he would act if he were still a stallion.

There are two acceptable methods of gelding: up and down.

The "Up" Method

The "up" method is a standing castration performed under tranquilization, using a local anesthetic. Most horses tolerate this well, and it eliminates any danger from a general anesthetic. This method requires a competent horse handler to hold the horse while the veterinarian is performing the procedure.

I was once asked to geld a two-year-old racehorse that was known to be a handful, but they neglected to tell me he cow-kicked. I tranquilized him and started to reach under him to wash his scrotum and — *WHAM!* — he cow-kicked me square in my left knee. Boy, it hurt, but I was young at the time, and I was not going to be dissuaded.

For reasons I don't understand, if a horse is pulled up by his tail, his kicking mechanism is turned off. We tied a rope to his tail and hoisted him by it over the wall of the stall. We couldn't actually lift him, but we could take the weight off his hind legs a little. He was fine, and we finished the operation. (A horse's tail can hold ten times the horse's weight. I don't know how that was figured out, but it's the truth.)

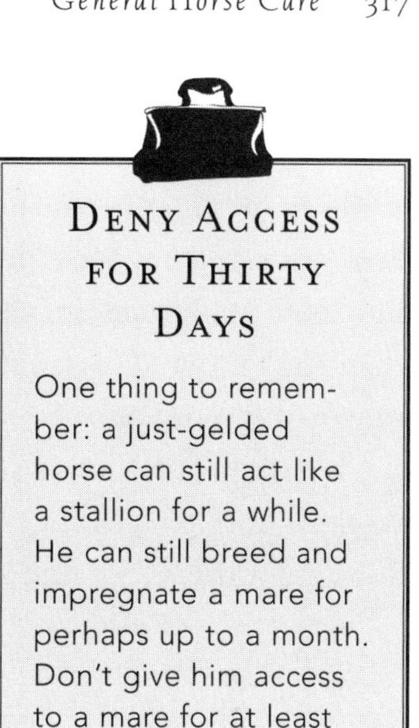

DENY ACCESS FOR THIRTY DAYS

One thing to remember: a just-gelded horse can still act like a stallion for a while. He can still breed and impregnate a mare for perhaps up to a month. Don't give him access to a mare for at least thirty days.

The "Down" Method

In this approach, the horse is laid down for gelding. There are drugs that can be used in the field that are short-acting and keep the horse down long enough to finish the job, but some veterinarians don't like them because they *are* short-acting and require a little more speed and efficiency during the procedure.

Then there are the general anesthetics that really should be used only in a clinic setting. The problem here is the same as any time a general anesthetic is used: there is always the risk, however slight, that an animal will not get up again.

Ridglings

While we're on the subject of stallions and geldings, let's consider ridglings (cryptorchids). A *cryptorchid* is a horse in which the testicles have not descended into the scrotum; if only one testicle has descended, he's called a *monorchid*. These guys *must* be gelded; they're often dangerous. The retained testicle(s) produces a high level of hormones because of the constant body heat, and the horse is usually downright mean. These operations must be done under general anesthesia because it's usually necessary to enter the abdominal cavity to get to the retained testicle(s).

Aftercare

Aftercare for a just-gelded horse is important. The horse must be made to move, or tremendous swelling will result and then there will be a real problem. Most gelded horses will move around if turned out, but some will just stand there. The reason is pretty simple: it hurts, so they don't move. This means the area will swell, so it will hurt more, so they will stand more.

It may be advisable to ride the horse a couple of times a day for a week or so after gelding, or he can be hand-walked twice a day. But absolutely, do *not* let him stand around.

Tying Up (Monday Morning Disease)

"Dr. Kelley, Hosey asked me to me to call you. He's got a horse that's bad tied up."

I've done veterinary work intermittently for Hosey (his name is actually José) for many years. He's a trainer with a few horses of moderate ability, which are pretty well on par with his training talents. I'm sure he avails himself of the services of other veterinarians as well as mine, but that's fine with me.

When I got to his barn at the track, I found Hosey forcing the poor filly to walk. A groom was leading her, and he was walking behind, hitting her with a broom so she would keep moving. Her legs trembled with each step and sweat was pouring off her. Her respiration was obviously greatly elevated. There were tears coming from her eyes. Maybe horses don't cry, but this one sure looked as if that was what she was doing.

I'm a tolerant and understanding person. Not necessarily tactful, but tolerant and understanding. I'm very proud, therefore, that I didn't say, "Hosey, how can you be so stupid?" But I did say something like, "Only a moron would walk a tied-up horse!" (Hosey's grasp of the English language isn't great. Maybe he didn't fully understand. I figured if he never called me again he did understand, but he has since called back.)

What Is "Tying Up"?

Tying up is what I have always called it, and I think most people call it that, but its official name is *exertional rhabdomyolysis*. It's also called *Monday morning disease* (because that's when it's often seen, after a horse has been given the weekend off), *paralytic hemoglobinuria, myositis,* and probably several other names. All breeds are known to tie up, and, although it affects both sexes, it's far more common in fillies.

Clinical Signs

The most commonly seen clinical signs are a function of muscle degeneration, which is what exertional rhabdomyolysis means. Typically, there is a stiff or rigid gait, most often involving the hind limbs and back. There is cramping that results in reluctance to move. An affected horse appears anxious, and the heart and respiratory rates and body temperature are all elevated. A tied-up horse should *not* be moved; it will cause further muscle damage.

The urine may be reddish or brownish due to the presence of myoglobin from muscle damage. Even if there isn't sufficient myoglobin present to discolor the urine, the urine of a tied-up horse will test positive for myoglobin. Other laboratory findings are elevated serum creatine kinase (the most specific indicator of muscle pathology), aspartate aminotransferase, and lactate dehydrogenase. These muscle enzymes, especially creatine kinase, are great indicators of the severity of the muscle damage.

Contributing Factors

There are several recognized causes of tying up.

- **Rest and feed.** A horse that is rested for a day or two and still fed a full ration is a prime candidate for tying up when exercised again, hence the moniker "Monday morning disease," as it's frequently seen after a weekend of rest.
- **Change in training.** A sudden increase in training or an inadequately trained horse asked to do more than it is prepared for will frequently tie up.

- **Endocrine problems.** Nervous fillies tie up more often than colts do. Also, horses with low thyroid seem to be more prone to tying up.
- **Genetics.** Some breeds and families seem to have a higher incidence of tying up.
- **Individual history.** Once a horse has tied up, it's probable that it will tie up again.

Even though we know what causes tying up, we don't know *why* it happens. Full feed while not being worked for a few days is the main factor in tying up, but why this is just isn't known.

It has been suggested that decreased blood supply to the locomotor muscles is a "why." It's possible that there are changes in fluid and electrolyte balance that result from exercise, training, diet, climate, or other factors, and these changes may cause fluctuations in local blood supply. It has also been shown that a horse subjected to the stress of heavy training or work has transient episodes of decreased thyroid function, and this also has been suggested as a "why" of tying up. These are only theories, however.

Treatment

If the horse is down, leave it there and don't force it to rise, which it may not be able to do anyway. Bed it, keep it warm, give it plenty of tender loving care, and begin the treatment regimen outlined below.

For treatment, high levels of nonsteroidal anti-inflammatory drugs should be administered, as well as xylazine, which will help to relieve the anxiety felt by the horse. Methocarbamol, a muscle relaxant, can be given every six to eight hours.

Vitamin E and selenium have been used as a treatment for tying up. There is no evidence that this does any good, but supplementation does seem to help as a preventive measure. It's not clear how. In horses prone to tying up, selenium fed at five times the recommended level seems to be beneficial, but to avoid the risk of selenium toxicity, don't do this unless the horse is a repeat offender.

In the case of hypothyroidism, giving the horse a thyroid supplement helps.

Prognosis and Prevention

The prognosis is good, providing proper time is allowed for the muscle damage to heal. This must be monitored by frequent measures of the muscle enzymes through blood samples, and exercise should *not* be resumed until the enzyme levels are back to normal.

Preventing a horse from tying up is difficult because so many factors may be involved. Proper dietary management is helpful; don't overfeed when a horse isn't going to be exercised.

WAY BACK WHEN I WAS A FLEDGLING veterinarian just out of school, I received a call to go to a place I had never been. The message was that they had a tied-up horse.

I arrived there and found no one at the barn, so I went to the house. There I found a very attractive middle-aged woman.

"Hi," I said. "I'm Dr. Kelley. I was told that you have a tied-up horse here."

"Oh, no," replied the pretty lady, straight-faced, "all of our horses are turned loose in the field. We don't tie any of them."

I eventually found her daughter in a riding ring with her tied-up horse. I asked her to explain things to her mother.

Arterial Hemorrhage

The main blood vessels, the arteries and the veins, are also the least prevalent; there are countless venules, arterioles, and capillaries that connect arteries and veins and distribute nutrients to the various and sundry parts of the body.

Arteries carry blood away from the heart, where it picks up, via the lungs, oxygen to deliver to the body's cells. Once the oxygen is depleted, the blood returns to the heart via the *veins,* where it once again picks up oxygen from the lungs.

The arteries, therefore, are closer to the heart's pumping action, and the blood therein is moving right along. The "oomph" has been lost by the time the blood gets to the veins and, as a result, it flows through the veins comparatively gently on its return trip to the heart.

When an artery is severed, blood shoots everywhere with force. Venous blood may gush if a large vein is cut, but it does not shoot out. Another difference: arterial blood is bright red because of the oxygen it is carrying. Some describe venous blood as "blue," but it is really only slightly purplish in the vein. Hemorrhage from a vein must be stopped, of course, but a little pressure and a few sutures will usually do it, unless it is a very large vein. The only problem I have ever had with a vein involved a cow, a creature of which I am not fond in the uncooked, mooing form.

IT WAS A WARM-WEATHER HOLIDAY a goodly number of years ago. I don't recall if it was Memorial Day, July 4, or Labor Day, but apparently all the non-horse vets had locked their doors and taken their telephones off the hook.

A man in a pickup pulled into our driveway at about 5 o'clock in the afternoon. I had just gotten home and had not even gone into the house yet.

He stuck his head out of the window. "You the vet?" he asked.

In retrospect I should have said no, but I admitted it.

"I got a cow that's hurt," he said. "Come look at her."

I explained that I was a horse doctor and he should try someone else.

"I've called every vet in the book. They either don't answer or won't come. She's bleedin' bad, Doc. She needs help."

No has never been my best word and a veterinarian *is* supposed to take care of animals (even cows), so I sighed and told him I'd follow.

He ran what was the last dairy in this area (it is now a housing development). The cow in question had suffered a large cut in a milk vein (the huge vein that runs forward from the udder on each side of the abdomen) when she ran into a manure spreader. Dark red blood was everywhere and it was still dripping slowly from the gash.

"When did this happen?" I asked as I waded through the clotted and unclotted blood that covered the milking room floor.

"When we brought her up to milk this morning."

"This has been going on for eight or ten hours?"

"More like twelve or so. We milk at 5 A.M."

The cow was agitated and I should have recognized what was going on, but I told the man I needed to tranquilize her. I went to my car, got the tranquilizer, and administered it to her. Then I went back to the car to get my suturing stuff.

When I got back to the cow she was dead. She had bled out. (One of the signs of bleeding to death is agitation shortly before the end.)

The owner soon thereafter told everyone that he had kept the cow alive all day and "the damn vet came and gave her one shot and she dropped dead." But this is about arteries and horses.

I had been out of school about six months when a client called shortly after midnight in early January. A mare was in labor and the foal was not coming.

How the guy even realized the mare was foaling I have never figured out. She was in a large field and there was no moon or stars. It was as dark a night as I have ever seen.

The man led me to her with the aid of a flashlight. When we approached she jumped up, but the fellow caught her. She wanted nothing to do with what I was trying to do with her, and the guy could not control her, even with a twitch.

I deemed that tranquilization was necessary, but the mare would not stand still so I could find a vein. Her owner, with flashlight in one hand and twitch in the other, was doing little good, so I told him to forget the flashlight and concentrate on the mare. I told him I could feel the vein well enough to inject her.

After several attempts at what was a very actively moving target, I felt warm, wet stuff on my hand. Assuming this was blood and that I was in the jugular vein, I injected the tranquilizer. The mare dropped like a sack of potatoes. You see, an artery is *not* a place in which to put something intended for a vein, and I apparently had gone through the vein and into the underlying artery. It can kill, but fortunately in this case it did not. It only knocked her out.

This made it pretty easy to straighten her foal's bent-back legs, and both mother and child were none the worse for the experience, although the owner was not happy when I (stupidly) told him why his mare had gone down as she did.

Okay, back to arteries. There is order in nature. Usually, for instance, in all mammals — horses, cows, dogs, cats, pangolins, and so on — veins, arteries, and nerves lie side by side. And in that sequence: vein, artery, nerve, front to back. Usually.

I was attempting to nerve a racehorse one day aeons ago. This is a pretty simple procedure: you make a small incision at the proper place and expose the vein, artery, and nerve. They can usually be differentiated. Usually. But when they cannot (rarely), you simply sever the one farthest back, which is the nerve. Usually.

However, this particular horse went vein, nerve, artery, which I learned when I cut what should have been the nerve. I got a face full of blood, as did the owner when I ducked. Proper repair was hastily performed, the nerve was severed, and the horse went on to win his next start a couple of months later.

A husband and wife, both music teachers at different schools, own a small farm where they keep a few horses. After school one day, they tried to load one of their critters onto their trailer, but the horse had other ideas. In fighting the procedure, he somehow became airborne and came down on top of the trailer's rear gate.

The metal did not give, but the flesh and underlying structures did. They called me immediately and said the blood was flowing freely. Fortunately, I lived a very few minutes from their place.

When I got there, blood was everywhere. It looked like a slaughterhouse. He had cut an artery in his shoulder, as well as a great deal of skin and muscle.

My first thought was *He's dead.* But he wasn't, and he didn't die. A great deal of pressure and a great deal of suturing worked wonders, and in a couple of weeks no one would ever know what had happened, except for a pencil-point scar that in no way indicated the mess that had been there.

The music teachers extolled my virtues as a great healer, which was fine with me, but in truth it was pure luck that first, their horse survived, and second, he healed.

There *is* one arterial problem that is more common than any of those I have just mentioned, but you will not see tons of blood associated with it. What you will see is a dead animal.

A client received five yearlings from an out-of-state farm for sales prep. He did this routinely for a number of farms, and it was his practice to give the new arrivals about a week to acclimate and then have me worm them.

But one of this group of five did not make it to his date with my nasogastric tube. He was found dead on the morning of the third day. The postmortem exam revealed a ruptured aortic aneurysm. The aorta is the body's number-one artery, running from the heart all the way to the tail. The other arteries branch off from it. An aneurysm is a weakening of the arterial wall caused by, in this case, migrating parasite larvae. Eventually this weakness will cause the wall to rupture. It may occur in weeks, or the horse may die of old age before it occurs, but it *will* happen if the animal lives long enough.

In this case, the victim was a thirteen-month-old colt in which someone had invested about $75,000 in a stud fee. To afford this, the owner had apparently saved money by neglecting the expense of proper parasite control (see page 288 on parasite control). The vast majority of aneurysms are caused by migrating parasite larvae.

The main point of this section is to inform you of the potential dangers of arterial injury or invasion. If you ever encounter arterial injury that you can see, apply forceful pressure, call for immediate help, and cross your fingers (figuratively, that is: it is difficult to cross your fingers and apply pressure at the same time). If it is one of those situations you cannot see, you won't know about it until it's too late, so don't worry about it. But most of these unseen cases can be avoided by proper parasite control.

Anhydrosis

"NO SWEAT" MEANS THE TASK IS SIMPLE, but if you have just run six furlongs in Florida in August, it means anhydrosis.

On perhaps my first trip to Jamaica, and at the request of my host, I went to the racetrack to look at his best horse's foot. I was shown to a stall that had been completely enclosed; there was an air conditioner installed in the window.

"Why?" I asked, motioning to the air conditioner.

"He's a non-sweater," the trainer explained.

We don't see many of these in Kentucky; at that point I had only seen one and he had just come up from Florida. Since then, I've seen maybe five more, most of them from Florida, too.

Incidence

Although the condition can occur in any horse, anywhere, at any time, it's most commonly seen in horses trained in hot, humid areas. It has been estimated that 20 to 33 percent of Thoroughbreds in training suffer from some degree of anhydrosis (failure to sweat) during the July to September period. But it isn't limited to racehorses. I bought a beautiful three-year-old filly, which was to be used as a show jumper, for the daughter of a friend who lives in Florida. The horse turned out great (state champion; I paid $3,000 for her and he later turned down $50,000), but she stopped sweating after two years there. She, too, had her stall air-conditioned.

Clinical Signs

Two theories have been postulated to explain anhydrosis. Both theories state, in complex terms, that the sweat glands don't work properly. It doesn't take an advanced degree to figure that out.

Sweating, of course, is necessary to cool the body, and the lack of it is the chief sign of anhydrosis. Total lack of sweating may not occur; rather, sweating may be patchy, occurring only between the legs and under the mane. Some horses are reported as unfit because their breathing is labored following exercise, but the real problem is that they aren't sweating. In other cases, the lack of sweating is ignored (or just not seen; pay attention to your horse) by the person responsible for the care of the animal. Also, after anhydrosis has existed for a while in a horse, the hair will be dull and dry. Long-term anhydrosis may lead to hair loss and severe scaliness of the skin. (Overworking a horse with anydrosis can elevate body temperature, so be careful. Bathe the horse with cool water to reduce the elevated temperature.)

Diagnosis and Treatment

Tests can be performed to confirm anhydrosis, but if a horse exhibits the signs previously described, further diagnostics are unnecessary. There is no definitive treatment, although electrolytes and reduction of feed concentrates have been suggested. Maintaining the horse in a cool environment is probably the best approach. Fans to promote air circulation are helpful, but an air-conditioned stall is the best solution. Many stalls (most, perhaps) aren't suitable for this, but a stall that can be enclosed should be.

Also, a fit horse is less apt to develop anhydrosis, and relocating anhydrotic horses to cooler, less humid areas often solves the problem.

Sudden Death

MANY YEARS AGO A WOMAN living in New Hampshire sent a twenty-year-old mare to board at a client's farm. The mare had not had a foal in four years, but in her younger days she had produced three or four stakes winners, so a foal out of her would be worth something.

The old mare arrived in October so she could be placed under lights and we could have plenty of time to work on her, which we did. To make a long story short, the mare conceived on an April cover. (See page 178 for more on the influence of lights on cycling.) Everyone concerned was ecstatic.

These were the days before paste wormers and before vaccines were readily available. Around the first of June, it was time to worm and vaccinate all the horses on this client's farm. There were about sixty head, so I usually allowed a few hours for this task. Worming was done on a sixty-day schedule for the adult horses, and at least some vaccinations were done on a quarterly schedule.

I arrived a little late that morning due to another client's emergency, but we got right to it. First, we went through the barns and wormed the horses. The old mare's stall was the second one we came to, so she was done early.

At the end of the line of four barns, we reversed and went back and vaccinated all the horses. This time the old mare's stall was the next to last we visited.

When that was finished, we still had to culture a couple of mares that refused to get in foal, but because of our late start it was nearly 1 P.M. and everyone was hungry. The farm manager told his crew to take a quick lunch and, after they had eaten, to turn out the horses. He asked me to come to his house and his wife would feed us. The old mare watched us walk down the lane.

Twenty minutes later everyone returned to the barn that housed the old girl. The manager told his crew to turn out all the horses except the two we were going to culture.

A minute later, a voice yelled out, "Come here! Quick!"

As it turned out, there was no need to hurry. The old mare was dead.

Another client was notified that a van would pick up a mare early in the afternoon to return her to her owner. This mare was particularly hard to catch and made a major mess when left in a stall, so rather than turn her out in the field she was normally in or leave her in her stall all morning, he placed her in a small catch pen he had behind one barn. It was a barn where little occurred, so after she was put in the pen my client and his employee left and spent the next few hours at his other barn. They both noted that she was "acting much quieter and calmer than normal" when they left her, but they thought little of it.

When the van arrived shortly after noon, they went to get her. She was dead.

A client with a slipshod operation called and said a yearling filly was in his yard, where she obviously didn't belong. Somehow she had crossed a cattle guard in the driveway, probably in an attempt to get some grazing; the horse field was eaten down to the dirt. (Cattle guards and horses don't mix, but somehow this man's horses never got caught in one.) She had been fine in the field that morning when he checked them three hours before, but now she was dead.

Causes

The reasons for the above deaths, as determined by postmortem exams, were anaphylactic shock, endotoxemia, and Japanese yew poisoning, respectively. These are only three of the many possible causes of sudden death in horses. The accompanying chart lists the most common causes, which fall into two categories: preventable and not preventable. It's pretty obvious which is which.

Although space doesn't permit a discussion of the mechanism or agent that causes death for each item in the chart, I will discuss the causes of death in the three cases previously mentioned. If it's any consolation (and it certainly isn't), most causes of sudden death do not require the horse to suffer. It's exactly what it sounds like: sudden.

I was present at one case of sudden death. The client's two-year-old colt was being worked on the track, seemingly fine, then he fell. It was a heart attack.

Anaphylaxis

Anaphylaxis is an acute immune reaction — an allergy, if you will. The horse is vaccinated; the first is the sensitizing dose, which alerts the body to the foreign substance. Later, but only rarely, thank goodness, the horse is vaccinated again. There is no way to know that any particular horse has been sensitized; it is a random condition that can occur at any time in any vaccinated horse. This is termed the *shocking dose.* All species can experience anaphylaxis. Epinephrine is an antidote, but it must be given quickly. The initial signs of anaphylaxis are difficult to determine; the first thing usually seen is that the horse goes down.

Causes of Sudden Death in Horses	
Natural causes	**Drug accidents**
Aneurysm (from parasitism)	Cyanide
Cardiac conductive malfunction	Ionophones
Cerebral vascular accident	Anaphylaxis
Hyperkalemic periodic paralysis	Anesthetics
	Iron injections
Physical causes	Intra-arterial injections
Cardiac arrest due to stress	Leukoencephalomalacia
Gunshot	Succinylcholine
Heatstroke	Urea
Hemorrhage	
Lightning/electrocution	**Wanton poisoning**
Strangulation/choking/suffocation	Arsenic
Trauma	
	Accidental poisoning
Infectious causes	Barbiturates
Anthrax	Insulin
Clostridial infections	Iron
Equine protozoal encephalitis	Plants (hemlock, [water and poison], Japanese yew, oleander)
Salmonellosis	Blue-green algae
	Magnesium
Feed	Nicotine
Blister beetle ingestion	Pesticides
Colic-shock	Potassium
	Strychnine

Endotoxemia

Endotoxemia is by definition the presence of endotoxin in the blood. Endotoxin is widespread in the environment, but it enters the horse's circulatory system only when the gut wall integrity is compromised by parasitism, ulcers, inflammation, or other causes. Signs range from mild fever to organ failure to death, depending on the dose of endotoxin. Broad-spectrum antibiotics can be used in treatment if the condition is suspected.

Japanese Yew

Japanese yews (*Taxus* spp.) are ornamentals planted around many houses. (I don't think they grow in the Deep South.) They are especially

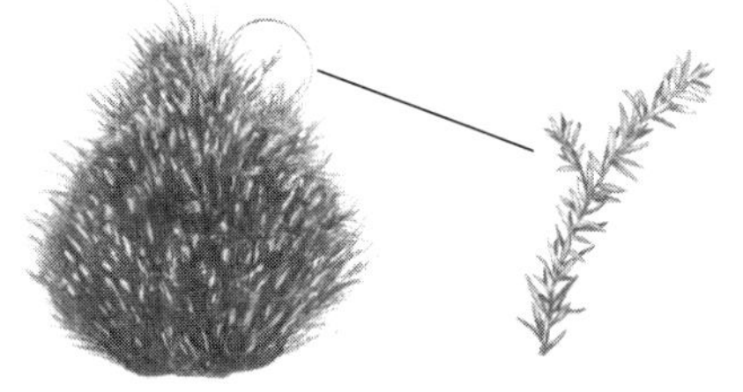

When ingested, Japanese yews can cause acute cardiac failure.

palatable, even more so when grazing is insufficient. The cause of death, which comes minutes after ingestion in most cases, is acute cardiac failure.

Proud Flesh (Exuberant Granulation Tissue)

A CLIENT WHO LIVES IN ANOTHER COUNTRY owns several mares, and he boarded them at three different farms in three different states. One of the farms was mine. One day he called and said, "Kelley, I want to keep all my mares in one place. Do you have room for all of them?"

Did I have room? I'd make room. This guy is a great person and he pays his bills, something that can't be said of everyone in the horse business.

Over the ensuing two weeks, vans full of horses from the other farms arrived at our farm. Upon arrival, I examined each mare for both my protection and that of the owner. One mare had a grapefruit-sized mass of proud flesh on her right hind cannon. It was as large and unsightly a mess as I had ever seen — a large, pink, rough nodule that bled freely when bumped. I called the farm from which she came and asked for a history of the lesion. "Oh, that just appeared there one day just before we shipped her to you," I was told. Baloney.

I've said this before: the horse is a good idea but the design leaves a lot to be desired. The obvious flaw is the great big body on those little skinny legs, but that's only the beginning. For instance, the layout of the intestinal tract is ridiculous. A gas bubble that would cause another species merely to burp sends a horse into paroxysms of agony. Things aren't even right in the beginning. The size of the offspring compared to the size of the mother is way out of line.

And a little nick on the ankle, if not tended to properly, will develop into an unattractive glob of proliferating tissue. The official name of the condition is *exuberant,* or excessive, *granulation tissue,* but I think only textbooks call it that. In the real world it's known as *proud flesh,* and it's a mess. How it came by the name "proud" is uncertain; you'd really have to dig into the *Oxford English Dictionary* to find a definition of the word that's even remotely applicable.

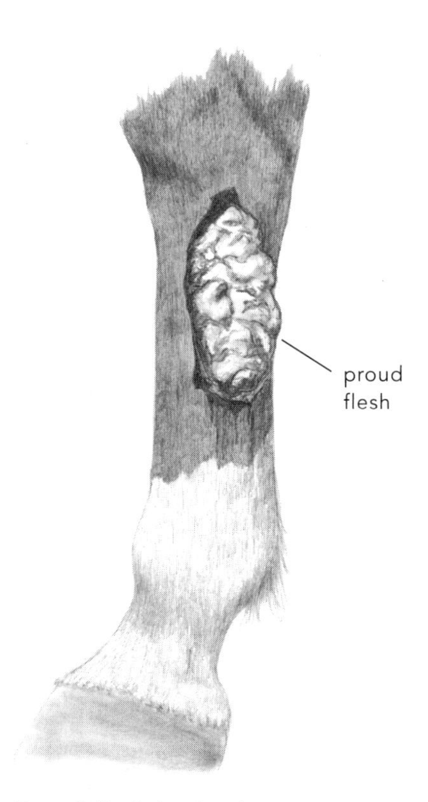

Proud flesh is simply a capillary bed out of control.

Contributing Factors

The exact cause of proud flesh isn't known but, although the books say it may occur anywhere on the animal, it's almost a certainty in unattended or improperly attended lesions of the legs below the knees and hocks. The fact that the areas in which it occurs most readily are those areas with the least fleshy tissue leads one to believe that this is significant, but I'm at a loss to explain why. One article stated that it is related to motion of the affected area. The lower limbs fit both scenarios: no underlying soft tissue to speak of and lots of motion.

Infection, contamination, and improper care are also contributing factors to proud flesh formation.

It's important to be sure of what you're dealing with because there are other conditions that may be confused with proud flesh. Some of these are sarcoids, squamous cell carcinoma, habronemiasis, and phycomycosis. Usually proud flesh is easily diagnosed by location and history, but occasionally a sample must be examined microscopically to be certain of a diagnosis.

Treatment and Prevention

The best treatment of anything is prevention. By this, I don't mean prevention of leg injuries; it's a good idea but not possible when dealing with horses. When leg injuries occur, prompt and effective treatment is essential. This means you must carefully look at all your horses, even those barren mares in the back field, every day. This should be done anyhow, but too many horses are only fed and never really looked over.

When any break in the skin is discovered, there are a few things that must be done. First, if the animal has not had a tetanus toxoid booster within the previous sixty to ninety days, one should be given. Don't administer tetanus antitoxin (TAT) unless the horse has never been vaccinated against tetanus before (see page 12 for more on tetanus).

Second, if the lesion can be sutured, have it sutured. Some obviously require sutures and some don't, but if there's a question, have your veterinarian decide. Successful suturing of lower extremity lesions must be done fairly soon after the injury occurs, so this qualifies as an emergency. Tell your veterinarian to come quickly. (An important note: Do *not* suture a puncture wound. To learn why, see page 8 on rabies.) If the lesion is not one that requires suturing or is too old to suture (an ankle cut that occurred at 8:00 P.M. is not a satisfactory suture candidate when found at 7:30 A.M. the next day, for example), there is still a need to give it proper attention. Cleanse it thoroughly and apply a topical antibacterial medication. Don't use any member of the furadantin family (the yellow stuff — nitrofurazone and its relatives): research has shown that those products retard the healing process and sustain some types of bacterial growth. If the lesion is below the knees or hocks where it can be bandaged, do so. Whether the lesion can be sutured or not, a systemic antibiotic should be administered.

In most cases, following this protocol will prevent proud flesh from forming. But sometimes it occurs regardless of what is done, or sometimes you acquire a horse on which proud flesh has already begun.

Fortunately, proud flesh is rather easy to treat, especially in the early stages of formation.

If the area of proud flesh is small, there are ointments available through your veterinarian that will take care of it very nicely. These are harsh, though, and they will damage any non–proud flesh areas if used incorrectly, so it's of paramount importance to follow the veterinarian's instructions very carefully.

A large area of proud flesh must be excised. There is no nerve involvement with proud flesh, since it's just a large capillary bed out of control, so your veterinarian can cut it right off with a scalpel blade and the horse won't bat an eye. It will bleed like a stuck pig, however, but this can be controlled with a little pressure.

Once the mass of proud flesh is removed, there will be quite a gap left in the skin where initially there was originally only a cut. This isn't suturable at this point and, if left, will either regrow the proud flesh or scar badly. A so-called pigskin graft may be used, and eventually the area will heal with minimal, if any, scarring. Again, your veterinarian can do this.

Proud flesh probably won't occur if you pay attention, but even in the best, most conscientiously run operation it may occasionally rear its ugly head. Proper care will reduce it to only a mild inconvenience.

In the mare we began with, proud flesh turned out to be more than a mild inconvenience, but she was an exception. The initial injury to her leg damaged the bone and under the proud flesh was a knot of exostosis (bone growth) that also had to be excised. With time (three months) and a pigskin graft, the leg healed but it never reached its original size again. Still, it was a definite improvement over how she shipped in, and there was no longer any proud flesh.

Warts

As far as being a health concern in horses, warts usually fall short. The real problem is in the eye of the beholder: they are ugly (the warts, not necessarily the beholder). Ugly, but uneventful.

I have known horses with warts practically all my life, and the warts never bothered me. They always went away eventually, and the horses were never any the worse for wear. The first case of warts I saw as a veterinarian, however, was quite traumatic.

A teenaged girl had her first horse, and she called one evening. "I came home from school and found *things* on Ballad's nose!" she exclaimed. "It's *awful!* Please come right away."

I was just sitting down to dinner and it had been a particularly bad day, but she sounded as if she was almost in tears. I had to go.

When I arrived at her place, she ran to the car. "Ballad's *ruined!* It's awful!"

I told her to calm down (I might just as well have told her to fly for all the good it did) and show me her horse.

Ballad had four warts on his muzzle below his right nostril. She hadn't seen him that morning or the previous evening because she had cheerleading practice and got home late, so I guess the warts could have been there for two days.

I took a pair of forceps and plucked them off. I told her that if that was the worst thing that ever happened to Ballad, he would live to be a hundred. She sniffled a "Thank you" as I left.

Clinical Signs

The official name of warts is *papillomatosis,* and the cause is the equine papillomavirus. The condition can occur in horses of any age but is most common in young animals, those younger than four years of age. The usual sites of occurrence are the lips, muzzle, and around the nostrils, and they may occur on the legs as a result of the horse rubbing its muzzle on them. Spread to other parts of the body and to other horses can occur via grooming, so routine cleansing of brushes and so forth is important.

Congenital warts (congenital cutaneous papillamotosis) occasionally occur and may be located in areas other than the typical ones. Although warts are usually an isolated problem occurring in one or a few horses, outbreaks do occur involving a whole farm.

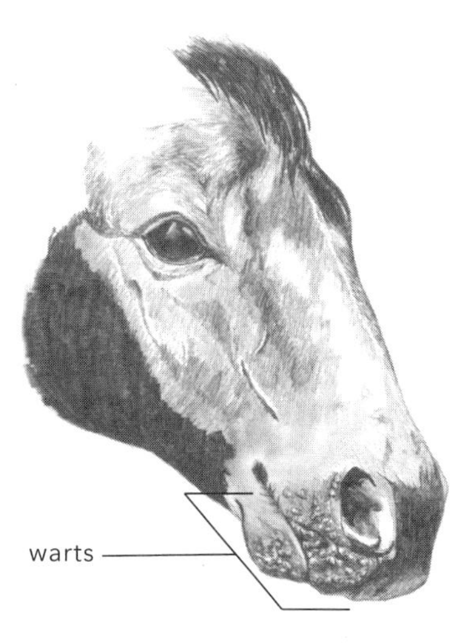

Warts are unsightly but un-eventful.

Incubation time is uncertain, but experimentally it is found to be six to eight weeks. The warts grow for another six to eight weeks and may eventually number more than one hundred. Most are small (a sixteenth of an inch or smaller), but some may reach a half-inch in diameter.

About the only thing that warts need to be differentiated from are verrucous-type sarcoids, which I have never seen so I can't discuss them intelligently. I have read that they occur more in saddle breeds than in racing breeds, which may help to account for the fact that I've been deprived of diagnosing them. The location of the growth is the key to identifying what the horse has, and the veterinarian can help to identify any questionable ones.

The two main problems I've seen with warts — and neither is damaging to a horse's health — are timing and bitting. By timing, I mean that they often seem to appear in late summer, around September. This way they can be present when you try to sell or show your otherwise perfect specimen. Buyers and judges, if not turned off, are definitely sidetracked.

Bitting problems involve the inability to properly seat a bit in the mouth of a horse with a heavy load of warts on its lips. This is a special inconvenience when trying to show or break a young horse.

Treatment

When a horse develops a heavy case of warts, the problem as perceived by many people is one of the horse's inability to eat or breathe because of interference by the warts. I really don't think that either of these actually happens, but if a client is honestly concerned, something needs to be done.

Warts are self-limiting (i.e., they leave of their own accord two or three weeks after maturing), but things can be done to hasten their departure. Cryosurgery and heating are both successful, as is the preparation of an autogenous vaccine, but these are a little on the heroic and expensive side. (An *autogenous vaccine* is made using some of the warts dissolved in an injectable solution.)

There are much easier and cheaper ways to handle warts. Some people advocate "smothering" them in petroleum jelly or some other thick goop. This may work; I don't know. In the case of only a few warts, as with Ballad, the easiest method of treatment is to simply pluck them off. An easy way to do this is to make a loop with some suture material, thread, or fishing line, then place the loop around a wart and yank it tight. Voilà! — no more wart.

In the case of many warts, removal of one at a time is still effective but time prohibitive. In these cases, the nature of the warts and the horse's body's response to the warts work in your favor. Take a hemostat or even a pair of pliers, choose two or three of the biggest warts, and crush them. Make them bleed. It won't hurt the horse unless you reach too low and pinch some skin. Within a few days to a week or so, the other warts will start dropping off.

I've been told the reason that this happens, but I won't swear to it. By making the area of the wart bleed, the virus causing the wart enters the horse's bloodstream, where evidently the body recognizes it as foreign and rejects it and all of its kind — the viruses within the remaining warts. In effect, it's an autogenous vaccine. I won't promise that this is exactly what happens within the horse, but the warts do leave and that's what counts.

Hematoma and Seroma

IN MY CAPACITY AS QUESTION-ANSWERER for the *Thoroughbred Times*, I get a wide variety of questions from readers. Some are easy to answer; I don't have to look anything up and can present a good, correct, and even scientific reply. I like those questions. Some are sort of easy, but I have to look the answers up in a book to be absolutely sure I'm answering correctly. I'm not as fond of them.

Some are real tough, and I must do a lot of digging to provide correct answers. I don't like those types of questions at all. And then some are *really* tough; I have no idea what the answers are and can't find anything about them in books. I have to consult other veterinarians, and sometimes I need to call experts. I hate those. Any veterinarian who says he knows it all isn't honest.

But some of the questions I receive are from people who just don't want to pay a veterinarian to look at a horse. For example: "I asked a friend and he had an idea but wasn't sure, so I asked a person I know who used to own a horse. He wasn't sure. What is it?" And then some obscure lameness or disease is poorly described. I, of course, have no idea either, so I tell them to call a veterinarian. That's not the answer the questioner is looking for, but that's life.

Occasionally, though, I'll answer one of these questions for two reasons: because I know the answer and I think it may hold interest for other readers. Such was the case when a reader asked about a filly with a fluid-filled lump on her back. It was obviously a hematoma or a seroma. These are more common than I ever thought before I became a veterinarian. I see six to eight cases per year.

Cause and Incidence

A *hematoma* is basically a big bruise. Due to trauma of some sort, a blood vessel (or vessels) has ruptured and blood has leaked out under the skin. A *seroma* is pretty much the same, but instead of blood it's serum that leaks from blood vessels and tissues. Both are surprisingly common; I see several each a year. I imagine the usual cause is a kick from a pasture mate, but I know of at least one that was the result of a tree limb falling on the horse (the owner saw it happen). Another cause is rolling on a stone or other object or, unfortunately, being hit by an ill-tempered handler.

Both can occur anywhere on the body, wherever the trauma occurs. If they occur on the side, gravity will usually pull the fluid down, but not always. Unlike edema, they are usually warm to the touch, and the fluid within can often be moved about, sort of like squeezing a filled hot-water bottle.

Treatment and Prognosis

The owner is always alarmed when one of these is found, but most times they will resolve themselves as the body reabsorbs the fluid. It's difficult to convince an owner of that in most cases, though; he wants *something* to be done. That something is usually lancing the hematoma or seroma and letting the fluid run out, which works pretty well, but if the leaking vessel hasn't yet healed, the fluid just keeps on coming.

This, obviously, presents a problem. I have had to pack some with sterile gauze to try to stop the leakage, and it has worked, but I shouldn't have opened them in the first place.

Hosing with cold water or placing cold packs on them will aid in stopping the leakage. This should be done early, but by the time they are noticed it's generally too late to do much good. Do it anyway. Once they stop enlarging (which is sometimes days later), lancing can be done, but I usually try to talk clients out of it for at least several days. Unfortunately, many folks take the lancing into their own hands and use a pocketknife or an ice pick to do the job. I can't express how unwise this is, but it happens.

The correct veterinary method is to clip the hair around the site to be lanced, scrub the area as if surgery is going to be performed, and use a sterile scalpel blade. The lancing should be done at the lowest point of

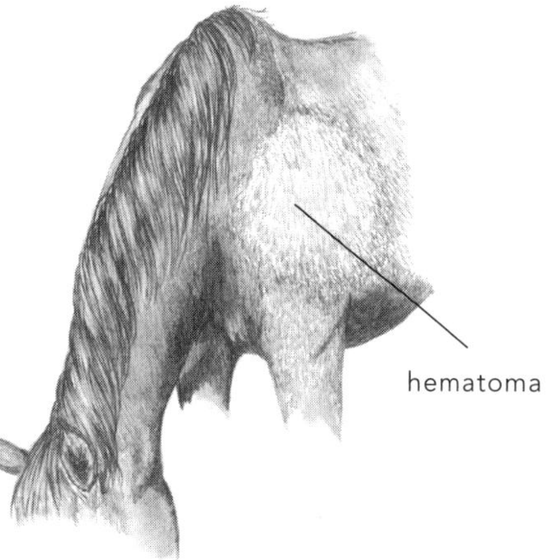

A hematoma, such as the one on this horse's shoulder, will be reabsorbed in time.

the swelling so gravity will assist in the drainage. The application of petroleum jelly on the area below the drainage site will help to prevent a mess on the horse. When a hematoma or seroma is lanced, by whatever method, a tetanus toxoid booster must be given. Some veterinarians routinely put a horse on antibiotics, but a properly performed lancing probably doesn't require it. A pocketknife lancing does.

The prognosis is always good to excellent. Every once in a while there will be a small knot remaining after it's healed. This is scar tissue and it doesn't bother the horse, so don't let it bother you.

Wind Problems

IT'S A GOOD THING THAT HIGH IQs aren't required for horse ownership. We horse doctors might not have many clients.

A trainer with four horses shipped in to the local training center. He was stabled next to one of my clients, and after a couple of days the new guy asked my client about a vet. "Doc Kelley will be by here this morning. I'll tell him to see you," my client told him.

When I came by that morning, I went to see the new fellow.

"Doc, I got a horse that runs out of gas after about a quarter-mile. He must have a wind problem," he said.

On questioning, I learned that this horse had no stamina at all. My mistake was in not asking how long he had been in training.

"It sure sounds like a wind problem," I said. "I'll scope him and see what his throat looks like."

I did and everything was perfectly normal.

"How long has this been going on?" I asked.

"Ever since I've had him," the trainer replied. "Almost a week now."

"Who had him before you?"

"Nobody. He was turned out on the farm since he was broken last year."

I thought he was kidding. No one works a horse just off the farm without first bringing him up to it gradually. It should be weeks before a workout. It had only been hours in this case. After further questioning, I found that he wasn't kidding. These four horses were the first he had ever trained.

I used to stay fit enough to go out and run a mile whenever I felt like it. All of a sudden, however, no matter how much I felt like it I couldn't run a mile. It was hard enough to walk a mile. Horses are that way, too. They have to get fit and be kept fit.

This trainer was, in effect, taking a couch potato and telling him to go out and run a half-mile. It just can't be done.

I told the guy to talk to my client who stabled next to him. Maybe he could give him some pointers. I don't know what happened; he shipped out at the end of the month and still owes me for scoping his horse. It's been more than fifteen years now, so I doubt that the money is coming.

The term *wind problem* covers a multitude of sins, from unfit horses to sick horses to those with conditions that can be repaired by surgery. We'll talk about the surgically correctable ones here. (Roaring, or *left laryngeal hemiplegia,* is discussed next; see page 342.)

• **Epiglottic entrapment.** This condition is fairly common in Thoroughbreds and Thoroughbred crosses. The epiglottis is caught in folds of mucous membranes that are attached to its lower surface. This results in an obstruction of the airflow. The main signs are respiratory noise on both inhalation and exhalation, reduced performance, and coughing, but in some horses there are no overt problems associated with the condition.

With those signs, other conditions must also be considered: soft palate displacement, roaring (left laryngeal hemiplegia), subepiglottic cysts, and several less common problems. Diagnosis, therefore, must be made by laryngoscopy.

As epiglottic entrapment may be an incidental finding on a routine examination, there is no treatment necessary if the horse's performance isn't affected. If performance is affected, the folds of mucous membranes must be separated, either by removal, laser therapy, or electrocautery.

• **Soft palate displacement.** In this condition, the soft palate is displaced from its normal position and blocks the opening of the larynx. The chief sign is a "gurgling" noise during rapid exercise and difficulty swallowing. Diagnosis is made by endoscopic examination, but in many cases the condition occurs only during rapid exercise.

A tongue tie often helps, and surgery often does no good. (A tongue tie is just that: the tongue is tied by a piece of gauze around the lower jaw to the floor of the mouth. It prevents it from raising and interfering with airflow and also prevents the rare instance of tongue swallowing.) Corrective surgery involves removal of certain muscles or removal of the rear portion of the soft palate. When all else fails, surgery is done.

• **Subepiglottic cysts.** These cysts cause respiratory noise and reduce performance. The difficulty in breathing increases as the level of exercise increases. Treatment consists of removal of the cysts.

All of these conditions are thought to be possibly congenital, and prognosis for return to intense training after surgery is fair at best. There is no reason that any affected horses can't be used for pleasure riding at gaits slower than a gallop, however.

Roaring

A YOUNG HUSBAND AND WIFE were big racing fans. They decided that they wanted to be more involved than just as two-dollar bettors, so they bought a two-year-old filly in training and found a trainer. As in everything, there are good trainers, there are bad trainers, and there are all manners of trainers in between. The trainer that they entrusted their horse to was in the lower half of the range, but he was honest (not a uniform characteristic among trainers) and he tried hard.

Someone recommended me to the couple. I wormed and vaccinated their filly and stopped by the trainer's barn every morning on my rounds. The filly seemed to be training well from what the trainer said, and she never seemed to have any problems.

One evening, though, the female half of the couple called. “Dr. Kelley, our trainer says our horse is a growler.”

I didn’t know what she meant. The only growlers I ever encountered were farm dogs that didn’t like me, which always hurt my feelings because I liked them.

I told her that I didn’t know what a growler was. She didn’t either, but she said that the exercise rider told the trainer that she growled when working out.

I thought I understood. “Did he by any chance say ‘roarer’?” I asked.

“Yes!” she answered. “I knew it was some kind of animal sound.”

I examined the filly’s throat with an endoscope, and the rider was right. Her left arytenoid cartilage (it’s always the left) wasn’t moving. I sent her to a fellow veterinarian who had done lots of these surgeries and he operated on her, tying the offending cartilage back out of the way and removing a portion of it. The surgery was a success, which is not always the case. She returned to training but because she was set back, she didn’t race until she was three. Eventually she won a couple of races.

What Is a Roarer?

A roarer is a horse whose left arytenoid cartilage is paralyzed and doesn’t open and close properly. As the air passes over the larynx, it makes a noise that is likened to a roar. Personally, although I had never thought about it before, I think *growl* may be a more apt description.

Incidence and Treatment

The fancy name for roaring is *laryngeal hemiplegia*, and it is estimated that up to 5 percent of Thoroughbreds are affected. Larger young colts are most commonly involved, and it seems to have a genetic basis, but the method of inheritance isn’t known. It occurs in other horses with Thoroughbred parentage. I’ve seen one Quarter Horse cross and two Thoroughbred-cross hunters that roared. All three had a Thoroughbred parent.

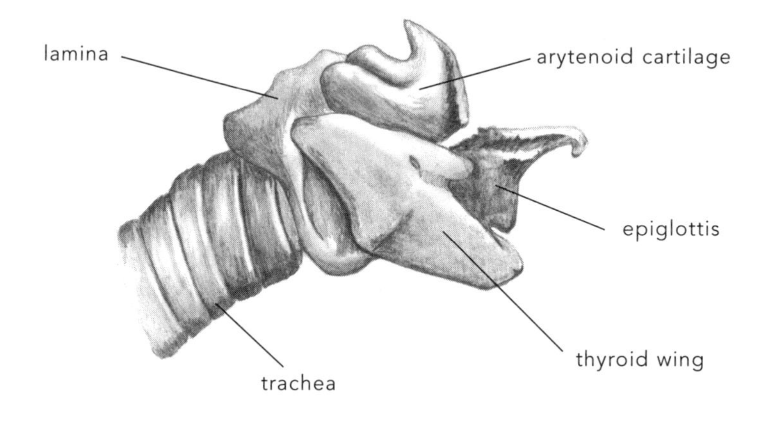

ANATOMY OF THE EQUINE THROAT

The malfunction of the larynx isn't cut and dried. A grading system has been proposed; see the box below.

Some say the condition can progress from one grade to the next, but others question this. I don't know. Grade IIs are not surgical candidates, some Grade IIIs need surgery, and Grade IVs must have surgery if they are ever going to perform satisfactorily. Grade IVs are the true roarers.

Each case must be evaluated thoroughly before surgery. As with any surgical procedure, repair isn't always successful, and I know of no way to predict the outcome beforehand. Grade IIs can be useful, if not great, horses; Grade IIIs are unlikely candidates to perform well. Normal breathing is not impaired.

Categories of Roaring

Grade	Status
Grade I	Normal
Grade II	Asynchronous, somewhat random movement of the left arytenoid cartilage; full movement of the cartilage can be induced
Grade III	Asynchronous movement of the left arytenoid cartilage; full movement cannot be induced
Grade IV	Asymmetry of the larynx; no movement of the left arytenoid cartilage

Tongue Lacerations

A CLIENT ONCE HAD A PARTICULARLY BAD-TEMPERED FOAL that was bent on self-destruction. I think anyone who has dealt with many foals has seen one like this guy, though it's difficult to imagine one as bad. He fought everything that anyone attempted to do with, on, or to him, and he was always banging himself up somehow.

The first time I saw him he was only six or eight hours old, and as I examined him he tried to bite both me and the person holding him. On being released, he spun around and tried to kick us. He came by his disposition naturally; his dam was a particularly ornery mare. Her sire was a horse that had been an excellent racehorse and very good sire but known far and wide for his meanness, and he passed that trait on to his offspring.

Over the next few months this colt only got worse. He would bite, strike, kick, rear — you name it. He wouldn't lead. He refused to be caught. A young woman was hired to work with the foals to gentle them, and she was very good at it, but she could do nothing with this one and eventually quit rather than have to deal with him. No one liked him and, indeed, most were afraid of him. In time he was nicknamed Misery.

This was back in the days when all worming was done by nasogastric tube, and I dreaded the third Tuesday of every month because that was the day that we wormed this farm's foals. We always got it done, but it took an army: a man on the twitch, a man on the ears, a man on the tail, and a man on his side pushing him against the stall wall. Tranquilization helped the first time but had no seeming effect on subsequent administrations.

Misery hurt himself several times, but we never learned how or where. He had nicks, bumps, and scratches on various parts of his anatomy at various times, and twice he came in with lacerations that should have been sutured but never were. One was about four inches long on his left shoulder; we treated it by spraying scarlet oil on it (a procedure he surprisingly didn't mind). The other was about two inches long, slightly above his left hock. No one had the heart to get close enough to his rear end to work on it, so we hosed it off (he *hated* that) and let it heal on its own.

Vaccinations were a barrel of laughs. This also required an army. I prayed that he would never get sick and require something like two- or three-times-a-day injections. He never did; I doubt any self-respecting bacterium or virus would have been brave enough to enter that nasty little body.

One day shortly after the breeding season ended, I was called by the farm. "Misery's bleeding from his mouth," the caller said.

My first thought was that he had been kicked in the mouth and lost some teeth, but with the assistance of the army of helpers we found that somehow he had cut his tongue nearly in two. About two inches from the tip of the tongue, there was a laceration about three fourths of the way through its width and completely through its thickness.

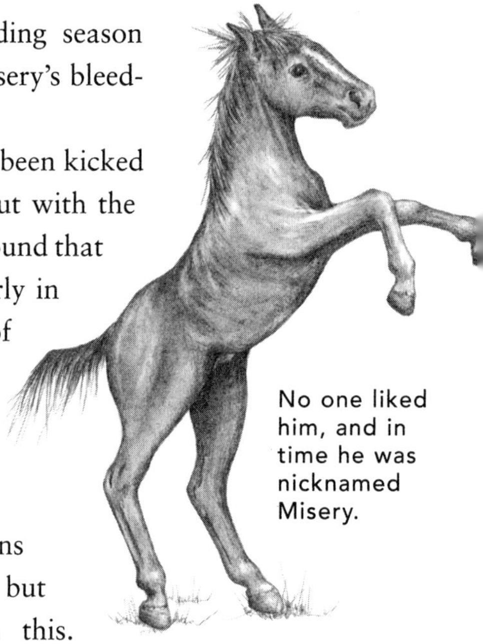

No one liked him, and in time he was nicknamed Misery.

I had seen a few tongue lacerations before that and I've seen some since, but none of them was anything like this. Scientific neglect and tender loving care took care of the others just fine. But this one needed sutures.

I had a young family at that time and I wanted to be around to watch them grow, so I suggested that we send him to a clinic where the suturing could be done "properly"; that is, with me far enough away to be safe.

The farm called the equine ambulance and asked for an extra man to help, but we still couldn't get him aboard. He bit one man, drawing blood, and kicked another in the knee and put him out of commission for several days. We were sure we would wear him down in time, but instead he wore us down.

The tongue continued to bleed (tongues have large blood supplies), although somewhat more slowly, so I steeled my courage and told the farm manager that we would lay him down there and put his tongue back together.

Have you ever bitten your tongue good and hard? Hurts like a son-of-a-gun, doesn't it? So we had a 400- or 500-pound colt that was meaner than any snake you could ever come across and who had just been wrestled for two hours in an attempt to get him into a conveyance that he chose not to enter. In addition, he was in serious pain from his cut tongue.

We gave him about thirty minutes to settle down a little (although he never really "settled down" in his life). Then, with considerable effort and the aid of the army, I got an injectable anesthetic in him, enough to hold a 500-pound horse down for about forty to sixty minutes. And down he went — for about three minutes.

I tried again, another 500-pound dose. This time all he did was get wobbly. He didn't go down.

I gave him another 300 pounds' worth. He just stood there glaring at us. I was afraid to give him any more for fear that it would kill him.

One groom suggested that we apply a tourniquet tightly around his neck and suspend him from a tree limb. We all agreed that would stop the bleeding, but the farm manager vetoed the idea.

Our only alternative, therefore, was to cross our fingers. He went off feed for a few days and periodically dripped a little blood, but within a week the lacerated tongue was healed, and outwardly one couldn't tell there had ever been an injury.

Incidence and Treatment

Tongue lacerations are not among the most common equine problems, but they occur often enough not to be considered rare or even unusual. It has been suggested that they occur more often than we know and we just never see them. The two most consistent signs indicating a possible tongue injury are blood or blood-tinged saliva coming from the mouth and reluctance or refusal to eat.

The major cause is trauma such as a kick, a foreign body (wire, nail, splinter), dental procedures, or too forceful a manipulation of the horse's tongue.

Treatment consists of ignoring it if it's a small laceration (the tongue heals marvelously well), suturing it if it's a larger one, or amputation if it's a severe cut involving only the tip. Foreign bodies should be located and removed, but I imagine this is pretty difficult. I've never had to do it. It's also a good idea to give antibiotics for several days.

Misery didn't receive antibiotics. No one wanted to inject him, so we tried putting some in his feed, but he wouldn't eat until his tongue was better and by then it wasn't necessary.

He continued to fight tooth-and-nail with everyone and everything. The decision was made to geld him, but no one knew how to get close enough to the necessary area to do it.

One day, when he was about eleven or twelve months old, he flipped over backward for no apparent reason (he never needed a reason for anything he did) and cracked his skull on a post. I wasn't there, but they told me he died instantly.

There's probably a moral here somewhere, but even if not, they almost certainly wouldn't have been able to train him. Or get him off the farm, for that matter.

Dental Care

"NEVER LOOK A GIFT HORSE IN THE MOUTH." But gift or not, checking the mouth must be done. Teeth are often the most neglected aspect of a horse's health care, even by knowledgeable, experienced horsemen.

The manager of a substantial farm that numbered about thirty mares with offspring of various ages complained to me that most of the mares were wasting feed. After each feeding, there was a large amount of grain on the floor beneath the feed tubs. Feed is expensive, and feed that never makes it into the horse is a terrible waste. Some horses are sloppy eaters by nature and some play with their feed and drop it, but 90 percent of a large group being playful and sloppy is unlikely. And a few of the mares were slightly underweight.

This was a fairly new client — I had been the veterinarian there for less than a year — and I was still not fully acquainted with the regular routine. They wormed on time and vaccinated as they should. And the horse's feet always seemed to be in good shape, so I figured the farrier made regular visits.

I asked the manager of the farm how often they floated the horses' teeth. He said it was an overrated procedure; they didn't bother with it.

The Mechanics of Chewing

Several dental problems may occur and we will cover most of them, but the primary issue is one that is a natural result of how a horse eats: the development of enamel points on the teeth. As I've said before, the design of the horse leaves much to be desired: a big body on little spindly legs, unreasonable intestinal arrangement, limited eyesight, among other things. Another design flaw is the teeth; they keep growing for the life of the horse. In domestic animals, this presents a problem.

A horse, of course, is an herbivore (although I have known a couple of stallions that could have been described as omnivores; they liked the occasional pound of flesh mixed in their diets) and, as such, must grind its feed for proper digestion. This is accomplished by a rotary chewing motion, and a horse's teeth are designed for grinding: the surfaces of the cheek teeth are flat, and the uppers slant down and out while the lowers slant up and in.

As the feed is ground, the outer edges of the upper teeth and the inner edges of the lower teeth have less contact with the opposing teeth and are not worn down by usage; as they keep growing, they form sharp edges (i.e., enamel points). After a while, the points of the upper teeth irritate the inside of the cheeks, and the points of the lower teeth do the same to the tongue. Eventually, it becomes painful to chew properly, so the horse does one of three things:

- **Stops eating or eats less.** This is pretty obvious because the feed tub is not emptied.
- **Stops chewing.** This is difficult to detect. All feed is ingested, but instead of being chewed properly (if at all), it is swallowed whole. Examination of the feces will reveal varying amounts of undigested, therefore unutilized, feed. Unground feed may lead to impaction and therefore colic.
- **Takes a mouthful of feed, chews a couple of times, says "ouch," and opens its mouth, at which point most of the feed falls out and onto the ground or stall floor.** If attention is paid, this is the most common and obvious sign of dental trouble. There is grain on the ground below and around the feed tub. Feed is wasted, and the horse suffers.

In time, all three will result in a horse in poor condition.

Floating

The problem the manager of the farm had could have been solved by floating the teeth to remove the enamel points. The general recommendation is to do this at six-month intervals, but that isn't necessary for all horses. In fact, some horses never seem to need it, so rather than routinely floating twice a year, a better plan is to have each horse's teeth checked every six months and float only those horses that need it. Proper attention to teeth floating will result in savings on your feed bill and horses that remain in good condition, which results in better performance and production.

Floating is a rather gentle name for rasping the points off the teeth. I don't know of any veterinarian who enjoys floating teeth. I know I don't. It is the closest thing to actual physical effort that our job requires, and if we had wanted to work up a sweat we would have chosen another line of work. Fortunately, in areas of large horse populations, there are "equine dentists" whose raison d'être is the teeth of the region's horses. Most of these dentists are honest, hardworking, capable, and possibly more knowledgeable than your veterinarian on the

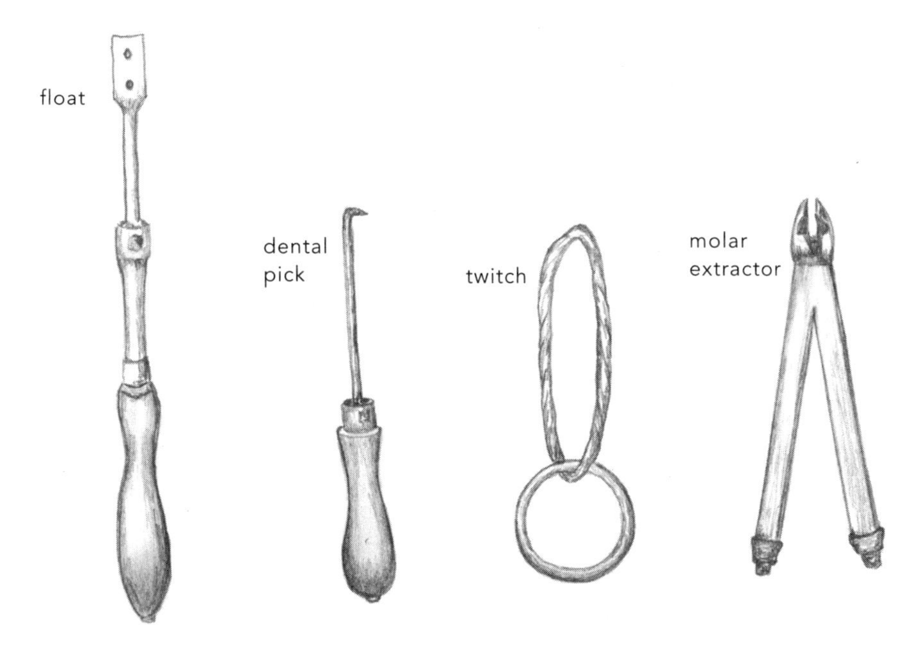

COMMON DENTAL TOOLS

subject of horse teeth. That said, this next statement will cause an angry response from some, if not all, of them.

Many dentists request that you allow them to do the floating alone; it's not necessary, or even desired, that anyone be present but the horses. I have found on two occasions that a dentist spent his time alone with the horses and billed my clients, but somehow neglected to do any floating. This is not a blanket indictment of these practitioners — far from it; it's merely a caveat, so pay attention.

I eventually convinced the farm manager to let me check his horses' teeth and float those that needed it. I ended up floating nearly thirty head, and I was worn out for a week, but the feed wasting stopped and most of those that were underweight gained condition over the ensuing weeks. Then I recommended an equine dentist whom I knew would do a good job for him. I wasn't about to float thirty head again.

Other Dental Problems

Most other dental conditions are associated with young horses.

- **Prognathism.** Prognathism, better known as parrot-mouth or overbite, is probably the most common congenital dental problem in horses and may be corrected in many cases if detected early. This necessitates, of course, looking at the teeth of a foal. If prognathism is present, the application of bite plates — horse "braces," in effect; they fit over the teeth and redirect them — may be started by six months of age.
- **Deciduous teeth and caps.** As the permanent teeth come in, the deciduous, or baby, teeth may not be shed, and they interfere with the horse's range of jaw motion. For this reason, it is sometimes necessary to remove them.

Also, caps may be retained, and these need to be removed. Exams should be performed during the time when permanent teeth normally erupt to determine if either of these conditions exists.

- **Wolf teeth.** Many horsemen advocate the routine removal of wolf teeth. Wolf teeth can interfere with a bit, but in many horses these teeth are not a problem. If desired, this should be done before the horse is broken or trained. In fact, it is best to do so at about one year of age (twelve to fifteen calendar months) for a couple of reasons: First, it's easier to do at this time because the periodontal membrane has not yet turned to stone; and second, healing can be completed and the rare infection controlled before a foreign object (a bit) needs to be forced in there.
- **Hooks.** Tooth problems later in a horse's life include the development of hooks, or curved edges, on the second premolar and/or third molar because of inadequate wear by the opposing teeth. This is primarily a problem in prognathic mouths. Without removal, these hooks can lead to even further bite abnormalities as the horse avoids chewing normally.
- **Canine teeth.** It is sometimes necessary to shorten canine teeth. With age, they may become abnormally long and interfere with bit placement. To correct this, they may be filed down.

- **Broken teeth/extra teeth.** Routine oral exams can reveal broken teeth; supernumerary, or extra, teeth (rare); gum problems; foreign bodies; tongue lacerations; and so on.
- **Abscesses.** Tooth abscesses can occur at any age. They may result from cavities or soft tissue infections. If the abscess is in an upper tooth, a classic sign is a unilateral nasal discharge that may be green or yellow or bloody and usually has a foul odor. Other conditions may also present with unilateral nasal discharges, but don't overlook the possibility of an abscessed tooth.

  If not tended to, an abscess can lead to infected sinuses or facial bones. The only course of action is removal of the abscessed tooth, because as long as it remains it will be a source of future infection. Antibiotics are indicated, too, but unless the affected tooth is removed, the infection will never be controlled.

Most dental and oral problems are readily corrected if detected early. This may be done by routine examinations beginning on day one and continuing on a twice-a-year basis. Unfortunately, the mouths of many horses are rarely looked into even if they are not gifts.

Behavioral Eating Problems

I HAVE BEEN ASKED TOO MANY TIMES TO COUNT why such-and-such a horse eats the way it does. Some bolt their feed, some fling it around, some take all day to eat their allotted ration, among other problems. I deal mostly with professional horse people, many of them second or third generation, and if *they* don't know the answers I don't know why they think I should. But they ask, so I try to answer. A lot of it is common sense, but the more I deal with people the less common sense I see.

As I said, many eating problems are not veterinary problems per se, but because I'm asked about them so often, I think they should be discussed, if only briefly.

Many horses, like many kids, have atrocious eating habits, and as in kids these habits can lead to health problems. As veterinarians, we have an appreciation for these health problems because they help us make our livings, but I personally feel that anyone who chooses to own horses has enough expenses without incurring others that may be avoided.

That said, there are several behavioral eating problems that can be eliminated or at least corrected somewhat, thereby preventing or reducing the frequency of problems such as colic and obesity, to name just two. The accompanying chart lists problems, their causes, and a prevention or treatment regimen.

Contributing Factors

Notice how many of the problems listed in the chart have "boredom" as a potential or contributing cause. There's a message here. Also, note the preponderance of "irregular feed schedule."

The life of a racehorse and most performance horses is incredibly boring. For a moment, let's imagine one of these horses as a professional baseball player. The first thing each morning, we take our ballplayer from his bedroom to the practice field and give him fifteen minutes of batting practice. Then we escort him back to his bedroom (which has not so much as a TV), where we lock him up, only bringing him meals at appointed times, plus or minus.

One morning we do not take him out for batting practice. Later that particular day, in the afternoon or evening, we take him not to the familiar practice field but to the playing field, where we tell him that it's now time to compete with and against other ballplayers brought in from their bedrooms. And after the competition, win or lose, we return him to his bedroom, where we again lock him up.

Now, suppose our ballplayer is used to getting his meals at 9 A.M., 1 P.M., and 7 P.M., but we have something to do one morning and his first meal isn't delivered until 10:30 A.M. Another day we run behind and his lunch doesn't come until 3 P.M. Then, still another day, we have somewhere to go in the evening, so we drop off his evening meal at 4:30 P.M. I can tell you one thing for certain: when his contract is up, he'll file for free agency.

I realize that I may be anthropomorphizing a little heavily here, but

Behavioral Eating Problems

Problem	Probable Cause(s)	Prevention/ Treatment
Gulping feed/rapid eating	Aggressive temperament Irregular feed schedule	Large stones in feed bucket to slow intake Feed hay before grain Feed on regular schedule
Eating slowly or picking at feed/poor appetite	Unpalatable feed Teeth problems Nervous disposition Respiratory problem	Check teeth (float) Change feed Treat respiratory problem
Scattering/dropping feed	Teeth problems Greed Boredom Feed change	Check teeth (float) Large stones in feed bucket Relieve boredom Change feed gradually Feed before other horses
Aggressive/impatient eating, kicking walls, pacing	Aggressive disposition Hunger Irregular feed schedule	Feed on regular schedule
Coprophagy	Boredom Unbalanced ration	Vitamin/mineral supplement Keep hay in front of horse
Wood chewing	Boredom Low-fiber diet Phosphate deficiency	Treat wood with "no chew" Increase hay intake Correct Ca:P ratio
Eating mane/tail/dirt/sand	Boredom Mineral deficiency	Cribbing strap (wide) Treat with "no chew" Avoid overgrazing
Cribbing/wind sucking	Boredom "Monkey-see, monkey-do"	Cribbing strap Treat with "no chew"
Weight gain/overeating	Too much feed in relation to exercise	Feed less Exercise more
Weight loss	Too little feed Parasites Teeth problems Disease	Feed more Worm Check teeth (float) Treat health problem

boredom and scheduling are important factors affecting equine behavior. The schedule is certainly an easy thing to control; if you routinely feed your horses at 8 A.M. and 4 P.M., be there (or have someone else be there) at 8 A.M. and 4 P.M.

The boredom is a bit more of a problem, but it, too, can be solved. If you can't turn the horse out, give him a window from which to see the world. Turn on a radio. Place a beach ball in the stall. Hang a couple of plastic milk jugs (empty) from the ceiling. Cut a hole in the wall of the stall so he can see the horse next door. Get a goat.

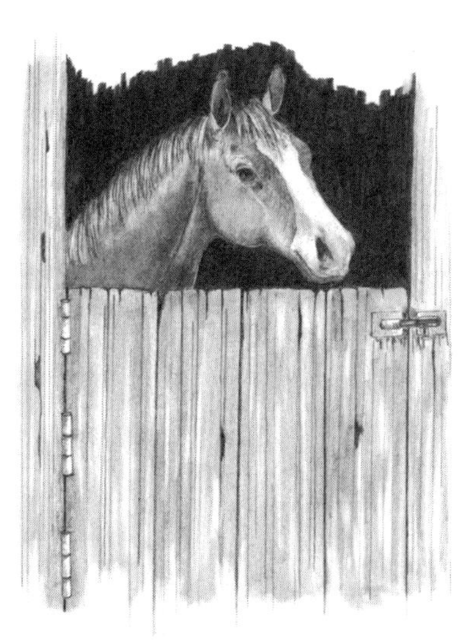

Give your horse a window from which to see the world.

Too many horse owners and managers accept these eating disorders as idiosyncrasies of certain horses, and it's true that some are ingrained habits that can't be changed. The owners fuss about them but rarely take action. But from the chart, you can see that the necessary actions don't require much effort at all, and the result will be a healthier and less aggravating horse.

Eyes and Eyelids

Eye problems are tough. Fortunately, there are veterinary ophthalmologists who can help horse doctors with the real challenges. This section is short because if your horse has an eye problem, you probably need a veterinarian. A horse's eyes should be looked at daily to determine whether there is cloudiness or excessive tearing, secretions, a closed eye, or anything else out of the ordinary.

Common Problems

• **Gunk.** In general, the most common problem with eyes is gunk or matter in the medial corner of the eye. This usually results from fly and dust irritation and is easy to treat (simply clean it out), but because it's sometimes difficult to tell whether the problem is caused by irritation or something else, if you are in doubt, call a veterinarian. A veterinarian should see any eye that appears to be abnormal.

- **Corneal lacerations and punctures.** The next most common eye injuries are corneal lacerations or punctures resulting from low tree limbs or woody weeds. The signs include blepharospasm, excessive tearing, and more gunk. These are very serious and, again, a veterinarian should be called immediately or sooner.
- **Laceration of the eyelid.** A fairly common problem is a laceration of the eyelid. It's surprising (to me, at least) how often this happens. I think the screens that are used as stall doors are one source of eyelid cuts; another one is the protrusions on clips and snaps with which buckets are hung. Clips and snaps should be hung with any protrusions safely concealed against the wall.

Because the lid is there to protect the delicate eye, an eyelid laceration must be sutured. If a cut is allowed to heal on its own, the area of the lesion will contract and the lid will no longer close properly. Any laceration around the eye is an emergency; get the veterinarian quickly, at least on the same day that it happens.

There are many other eye problems, and any abnormality should be shown to the veterinarian, but none is real common. They all need a vet's attention. For most eye problems, the veterinarian will dispense ointment or drops to be applied. The veterinarian may say to put it in twice a day or three times a day or every eight hours or even more often; follow the vet's instructions precisely. It's extremely important to medicate properly and at indicated intervals. Because

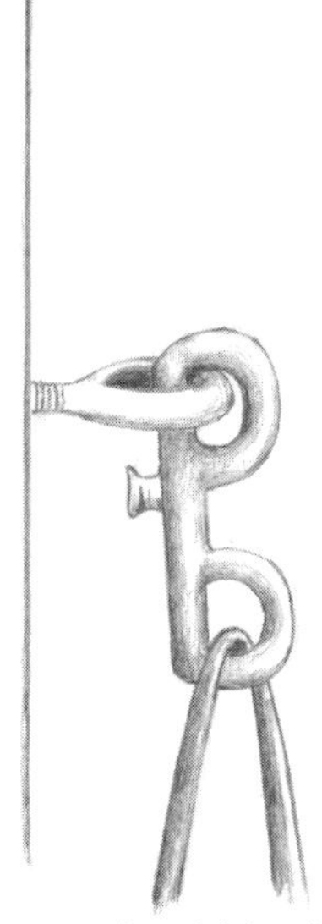

Snaps should be hung with the latch toward the wall.

tears wash away ointments and drops within seconds, I personally believe that you can't medicate an eye too often. Every ten minutes would be great but that doesn't fit the schedules of most people.

Applying Medication

Putting medication in a horse's eye isn't easy. Most horses don't like it and hold the eye tightly closed. A horse's eyelid is a lot stronger than it looks. Also, some horses will swing their heads, and there is nothing heavier than a horse's head when it smacks you in the face. Applying medication to a horse's eye is a two-person job and often requires a twitch. Be very careful with the medication applicator; the eye can accidentally be poked with it if the horse is uncooperative.

It isn't necessary to cover the entire surface of the eye with the medication or even the specific spot that needs it. Just get it in the eye and the natural tears will spread it over the entire surface.

To reiterate, if an eye appears abnormal (tightly closed, opaque, excessive discharge, blood, spot on the surface, etc.), consult a veterinarian immediately.

Stable Vices

A CLIENT WHO BOARDED MANY OUT-OF-STATE MARES every breeding season would send an information sheet to the owner of each mare that was coming to his farm for the first time. On this sheet he asked such routine things as age, pedigree, last breeding date, and so on. He also asked a few less common questions, such as: Does she tease? Does she trailer? Any vices?

He received mostly honest, forthright replies, except to that last question. Apparently, the owners of the mares thought he was asking whether *they* smoked or had an alcohol problem, because the answer was invariably "No." In several cases, it was amazing to see what some owners did not consider to be vices.

I don't know what percentage of horses has a vice. Maybe it's as high as 10 percent. Vices range from minor habits that only irritate the people who must deal with the horse to behaviors that are potentially life-threatening.

Vices are usually a result of inappropriate management. Horses are social, grazing animals, not intended to be isolated and pent up, and the stress thus caused is manifested in behavior that we find objectionable. Sometimes a companion animal relieves the stress (see page 301 on goats). There are several vices that are totally innocuous; others are stoppable or controllable, but most are not.

Minor Vices

The following vices fall into the innocuous category.

- **Defecating in feed tubs.** I once owned a mare that would situate herself so that she would defecate in her feed tub when she was kept in a stall. It didn't matter where the tub was located; she would back up to it and defecate in it all night. Of course, her stall was rather easy to clean, but the bucket was a mess. If you want to stop this behavior, simply remove the feed tub after the meal is completed.
- **Urinating in water buckets.** Other mares use their water buckets as toilets. Often this is accidental, but too many do it too often for it to be considered an accident all the time. It can be stopped by hanging the bucket higher, but if the stall contains a mare and foal, this is not a good solution, as the foal won't be able to reach the bucket. The only real solution in such a case might be to hang two water buckets far apart.
- **Spilling water.** Then there are the ones that bang their water buckets, spilling the contents. This can be prevented by immobilizing the buckets or installing automatic waterers; immobilization is considerably less expensive. One good sloshing of an immobilized bucket, however, will still waste a lot of water, create a mess in the stall, and cause the animal to go several hours without water, which is never a good idea.
- **Flinging feed.** Of more concern is the horse that flings its feed or bangs its feed tub. Feed is wasted and the animal doesn't get enough to eat. Immobilizing the tub helps, as does using one of the various

types of tub rings to make the feed more difficult to fling. Placing large rocks or bricks in the tub is also helpful.

• **Ingesting bedding.** Eating straw bedding can be stopped easily: bed with something else, if possible. I don't think eating the straw is particularly bad for the horse, unless the straw is dusty or the horse is in race training.

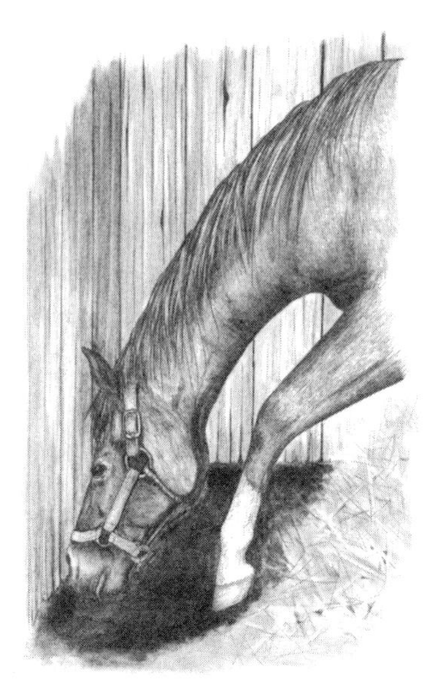

Digging is harmful mainly to the stall and your farrier bill. Some horses are so persistent they dig through asphalt.

• **Masturbating.** Masturbation is a vice of colts and stallions. It can be a problem if a stallion masturbates during the breeding season, but for the life of me I can't see what harm it does at other times. People want it stopped, however, and stallion cages, brushes, and rings are effective. A cage is placed so the penis cannot be made erect, and a brush is placed so the penis contacts it, causing slight pain. Rings, however, are very risky; there must be scrupulous attention to cleanliness and placement, and they should be checked at least every other day, if not daily. (See page 196, on penile trauma, for more information.)

• **Kicking.** Kicking the walls is a vice that can be expensive, due to the cost associated with repeated repair of stall walls, as well as dangerous, because a wall kicker will sometimes put a foot through a broken board, damaging its heels or coronet. I once tended a mare that fractured a coffin bone while kicking a wall made of cement blocks. It also seems to be contagious; one wall kicker in a barn will often be imitated by other horses living there. A suggested remedy is to tie heavy knotted ropes to the kicker's tail and turn him out; the theory goes, he will kick until, eventually, he tires himself out.

• **Tail rubbing.** Tail rubbing is generally considered to be a sign of some manner of parasite or skin problem — pinworms, ticks, a fungus, and so on — but I believe some horses do it because it feels good or otherwise fills some need. A tail board such as that used for Saddlebreds will stop it, but other than a rubbed tail, I don't know what harm it does unless the horse encounters a nail that has become exposed. To avoid accidental injury, all wooden structures should be checked periodically for exposed nail heads.

- **Digging.** Digging is damaging to the stall and to your farrier bill, and it's aggravating to the person who must attend to the holes thus created. I have seen a couple of horses that were so persistent that they dug through asphalt. Rubber mats will usually control the problem.

More-Serious Vices

Aside from the annoying behaviors just described, there are more-serious vices.

- **Weaving and stall walking.** Weaving and stall walking (swinging back and forth or pacing around a stall constantly) drive me crazy, but I also don't think a horse can remain in good physical condition if it

Common Vices and Their Treatments

Vice	Treatment
Defecating in bucket/tub	Remove bucket/tub; hang higher
Bucket banging	Secure bucket; tub rings or rocks
Eating straw	Bed with shavings
Masturbating	Stallion brush, cage, ring
Wall kicking	Knotted ropes in tail
Tail rubbing	Tail board; check for pinworms, ticks, etc.
Digging	Rubber mats
Weaving, stall walking	Allow visibility of other horses; jugs, tires, etc.
Eating manure or dirt	Evaluate feed ration
Self-mutilation	Bib, muzzle
Wood chewing	Treat lumber, muzzle
Cribbing	Cribbing strap, grazing muzzle

weaves or walks all the time it's in a stall. I knew one mare that was such an extreme stall walker that every night she ground her bedding into an unidentifiable pulp, even when she had a foal on her. The little guy was probably uncommonly fit just from trying to avoid being trod upon by Mom.

Suggested ways to stop weaving and walking include hanging things such as milk jugs in several places in the stall or placing tires or beach balls on the stall floor as a sort of entertainment center/obstacle course. Neither approach has ever worked for me. Giving a horse a pet or mascot (goat, sheep) occasionally helps, but some horses will abuse or even kill their companions, so it is neither a humane nor a lasting cure in such cases. Leaving a radio turned on while the horse is stalled is said to help and is also said to help control other vices, but I'm unconvinced. It could work for you, though.

What has worked in a couple of cases is allowing the horse to see the horse in the adjacent stall. If the walls are solid, cut a hole maybe six by twelve inches in the wall so the walker can see he is not alone in the world. I think weaving and walking are less of a problem in barns where the walls are only solid up to four feet and slatted above that level.

- **Eating manure and/or dirt.** Eating manure (coprophagy) and dirt is probably a sign of a dietary deficiency, and both can be harmful to the animals. (Eating manure is normal and accepted behavior in foals for the first few weeks of life, however.) Parasite ova ingestion and the accumulation of dirt in the gastrointestinal tract are the problems. A review of the feed ration is indicated; also make certain the horse has access to free-choice salt and trace mineral salt.
- **Self-mutilation.** Self-mutilation, where a horse will chew on itself (usually a leg), may be the most serious vice of them all. A bib or grazing muzzle will stop it.
- **Wood chewing.** Wood chewing is a real pain. It destroys the barn or fence, and ingested splinters can't be good for a digestive system, even one geared to roughage. There is the chance that a nail could be swallowed and that could be fatal, but this may be one of the easier vices

to control. Applying no-chew products to all chewable surfaces works well. Hardwood should be used in fence and barn construction; pine will be devoured in no time.

- **Cribbing.** Last but not least, the biggie: cribbing. A cribber grabs an inanimate, fixed object (such as a fence, feed tub, or stall door) with its upper teeth and sucks in air. The part most people find objectionable is the belching sound made when the air is swallowed. Cribbing straps and grazing muzzles are simple, moderately effective solutions. Cribbing is so widespread and universally detested that I devote an entire section to it (see below).

Fortunately, most vices are more offensive to us than they are harmful to the horses, and most of the time we can't alter the horses' inappropriate behavior. With that in mind, try the corrective measures outlined in the chart on page 361. Good luck.

Cribbing

First, some terminology. Cribbing is the act of a horse grasping a fixed object (fence plank or feed tub, for example) with its incisors, flexing its neck, and pulling back on the object, usually sucking in air (which is called *aerophagia*) as it does so. Some people refer to simple wood chewing as cribbing, but it isn't.

Predisposing Factors

The cause of cribbing varies with the horse. It's generally accepted that a foal of a cribbing mare learns the vice from its dam, and I firmly believe this. But there is possibly a genetic basis as well, because I have seen two orphaned foals from cribbing mares that never saw their dams crib and nevertheless became cribbers themselves. I have also seen foals of cribbing mares *not* become cribbers, so there is much to be learned here.

Another generally accepted root cause of cribbing is boredom, although I'm certain that the habit can be an accidental discovery, very

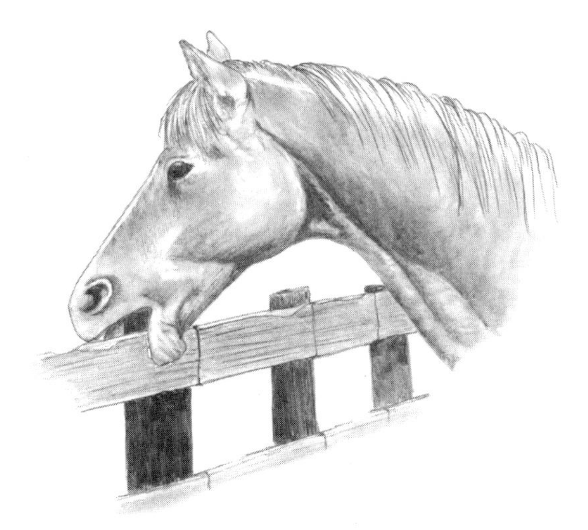

A cribber can destroy a fence.

likely a result of wood chewing. (I can't picture a bored horse saying to itself, "I think I'll bite this fixed object and suck air.")

Apparently gulping air is a pleasant sensation for the horse or the behavior wouldn't be continued. But it's not pleasant for the owner of the horse. The owner usually objects to the annoying sound of air being gulped, but more worrisome problems associated with cribbing are damage to fences and stalls, enlargement of the neck muscles, wear on the incisors, and weight loss as a result of reduced feed intake. A serious cribber prefers gulping in air to eating and often will not carry sufficient weight, but I've seen some pretty skinny cribbers that ate as much as their non-skinny stablemates. There is also the belief that cribbers have an increased incidence of colic, but there is no direct evidence that either weight loss or colic is related to cribbing. And it isn't necessarily the case that a wood chewer is likely to become a cribber.

Treatment

Cribbing in its early stages can be stopped by treating the surfaces the horse tends to grab with any of several no-chew substances. But once the habit is ingrained, it can become a real problem to overcome.

Cribbing straps are often helpful in stopping a cribber or lessening the severity of the behavior. These straps, made of leather or a leather-metal combination, are placed around the neck behind the jaw. There also is a new design in which part of the strap goes across the forehead. If secured too tightly they inhibit eating and drinking, and if secured too loosely they have no effect, so the correct adjustment is crucial to success. "On the tight side of snug" is probably the best way to describe how a cribbing strap should be adjusted. If you're not certain how far to tighten one, ask someone. Your veterinarian should be able to help. The straps function by preventing the arching of the neck necessary to suck in air satisfactorily.

If the standard narrow cribbing strap fails to work, there are two other designs, either of which may do the job. One has metal spikes on the lower portion. The spikes don't poke the horse unless the neck is arched in the air-gulping position.

The other is all leather but much wider — four inches — and has two buckles rather than one. I've seen confirmed cribbers that were unaffected by other straps quit when one of these was used. These versions aren't typically stock items at your local tack shop, though; they're usually made to order.

If cribbing straps are successful, they can't be left on and ignored. For one thing, they must be removed when the horse is exercised. Also, it's not uncommon for the straps, especially the ones with metal parts, to rub sores or for foreign material to work its way between the horse and the strap. For these reasons, it's a good idea to remove the strap at least once a week, preferably twice, to see if there's anything going on under it. A grazing muzzle will prevent cribbing, but it must be removed for the horse to eat grain, at which time it will crib.

There are those cribbers on which nothing works, however. Some are so bad that they no longer even require a stationary object to grasp. I once boarded a mare that I consider to be the all-time worst cribber. She would bite a plank and pull on it so hard that it would come off the posts. She would then carry it around in her teeth, sucking in air at her convenience. No kind of strap fazed her. She would remove, on the average, two planks a day and she rapidly plummeted to the bottom on my list of favorites.

Surgical Procedures

For horses such as this mare, or for any cribber for that matter, there are two surgical procedures that stop the horse from arching its neck and therefore prevent the action needed for cribbing to occur.

The neck muscles responsible for the actions required to crib are the sternocephalicus, omohyoid, and sternothyrohyoid. The paired sternocephalicus muscles flex the head and neck when working together, and they turn the head when acting alone. The sternocephalicus muscles receive motor impulses from the ventral branch of the spinal accessory nerve. The two omohyoid and sternothyrohyoid muscles are the swallowing muscles; they retract the hyoid bone, larynx, and base of the tongue. Of the two surgical procedures, a spinal accessory neurectomy is the simpler and quicker and is much less apt to cause neck disfiguration. This procedure involves removing a small segment (2–4 cm) of each spinal accessory nerve ventral branch.

A big advantage to this procedure over the other one is that it may be done under a local anesthetic. Incisions are required on both sides of the neck, but little time is lost from training because there are only skin and fascia sutures. Approximately 70 percent of horses in which this operation has been performed have shown complete (50 percent) or partial (20 percent) improvement in their cribbing.

The other surgery is much more invasive and often disfigures the neck. It's a triple myectomy. Sections of the six muscles previously described are removed and, if the neurectomy has not previously been done, the nerves are severed. This must be done under general anesthesia; three incisions are needed (one on each side and one on the ventral midline), and considerable time is lost during the healing process. The myectomies may be successful if the neurectomy wasn't, but the overall success rate is roughly the same as with the neurectomy.

The Last Resort

And if all else fails and the cribber is driving you crazy and pulling your farm apart, you can always sell the horse. But keep in mind that a cribber has to be so noted in sales catalogs.

Many years ago, a friend bought a nicely bred Thoroughbred mare — a steal at $37,000 — at a sale but learned when we went to the barn to check her that she was a cribber and it had not been announced. (It's a requirement at Thoroughbred auctions that it must be announced if a horse is a cribber.) He really wanted this mare, and he asked my opinion. Should he keep her or return her to be resold?

"Turn her back," I wisely advised. "They'll put her back through the ring at the end of the session and, when she's announced as a cribber, you can buy her again for a lot less."

He liked this idea, so he returned her. Later that day, after all the other horses had been sold, she was brought back in the ring and the announcement was made that she was a cribber.

Instead of the $37,000 that she had brought three hours earlier, she now sold for $53,000 and my friend was outbid. He rarely asks my advice anymore.

X-ray Safety

Many times I have had to take numerous X-rays of a broken bone to monitor its healing, and just about every time the owner or trainer has expressed concern over too many X-rays and the possibility of damage to the bone as a result. Rest assured, it won't happen. Radiation damage requires overwhelming doses of radiation that don't occur in routine, even repeated, radiographing. Bone damage results only when the supply of blood to the growth cartilage is impaired.

Every time this question is asked, though, I think of an event that occurred when I was a young veterinarian; I know better now.

I was doing the work for a trainer named Chester. He had very little veterinary work done and he rarely raced a horse; his income was derived from selling his horses in training. These were relatively cheap horses, and he relied on a quick turnover of lots of horses to stay afloat.

Shortly after I began doing his work, Chester told me he had a potential buyer for one of his horses, but the guy wanted X-rays of the horse's front legs. As I prepared to take them, Chester said, "Be sure you label the pictures with the horse's name: Blue Blue." And he watched carefully as I put the proper identification on the cassettes.

He brought out a nicely conformed, clean-legged bay and I X-rayed the legs, which were in fine shape. I let Chester have the films to show to his buyer, who was apparently satisfied, because he bought Blue Blue.

About two weeks later, Chester asked me to X-ray the front legs of Mountain Pass, again because a buyer had requested them. And again he stressed the need for proper identification on the films.

He brought out a nicely conformed, clean-legged bay and I X-rayed the legs, which were in fine shape. He showed the films to his buyer and Mountain Pass was sold.

In another week or two, Chester had a buyer for Flower Demon, pending the outcome of front leg X-rays. Once again, Chester insisted on proper identification and watched closely as I labeled the cassettes. And once again he brought out a nicely conformed, clean-legged bay. The horse looked familiar.

"Chester, didn't I X-ray this horse before?" I asked.

"Gosh, no, Doc," he answered in wide-eyed innocence. "You've never seen Flower Demon before."

Well, surprise, the X-rays were fine, and Flower Demon was sold.

Maybe a month later, he had a buyer for Greensong. I admit that occasionally I'm a little slow, but when he once again brought out a nicely conformed, clean-legged bay, I sensed something was amiss.

"Chester, you're having me X-ray the same horse each time," I said.

"Oh, c'mon, Doc . . ." he began, once again as naively as he could make himself sound.

"Doggone it, Chester, I'm not as dumb as I look. This is the same horse that I've radiographed three times before."

The innocence left his voice and face. "Look, you're getting paid. If I tell you this is Greensong, that's all you have to know."

I later learned that the nicely conformed, clean-legged bay was named Day Toy, a five-year-old gelding that couldn't outrun a tricycle with a bent axle. Day Toy earned his keep for Chester by being

X-rayed. Eventually I learned he had been known, at least on X-rays, by at least twenty different names over the previous two years.

Chester would show prospective buyers the correct horse, of course, whether it be Greensong or Blue Blue or whatever. The buyer would see the right horse move and work, but if and when X-rays were requested Chester would offer to supply them himself at no cost to the buyer. This is where Day Toy, whose legs didn't have a pimple on them, came in. No one can tell a horse's color and sex on radiographs; a person can only go by the name on the film.

Chester had been through several vets before me, but shortly after my refusal to do his work he found one he kept for years. I don't know if the guy was dishonest, stupid, or just didn't care.

Day Toy was X-rayed hundreds of times in his life and was none the worse for the experience. If X-rays didn't bother him, they won't bother any horse.

Care of Old Mares

When I was still in veterinary school, I took all our hard-earned savings and bought a Thoroughbred broodmare. My wife was less than thrilled (I was a student, so the hard-earned money was actually earned by her), but I explained that there are some things that a guy has to do. She still didn't understand.

The mare's name was Game Squaw, and she was twelve when we acquired her. She was thirty-two when her time ran out, but until she was thirty she was as spry as a youngster. All horses should have her disposition (she was a puppy dog), but all mares should not have her reproductive history — that's another story. Although what follows is written with broodmares in mind, much of it applies equally well to any old horse.

When we speak of "old" mares, we aren't necessarily referring to age in years. Just as some people are aware, active, and competitive at eighty while others are doddering, frail, and housebound at sixty, mares vary widely in their needs as they age. Basically, this is a play-it-by-ear situation: If an eighteen-year-old mare can't compete, treat her as "old"; if a twenty-four-year-old mare is holding her own, let her play on.

• **Competition with pasture mates.** Possibly the main problem encountered as a mare ages is her loss of ability to compete with her younger pasture mates. It isn't unusual for a group of broodmares to spend the vast majority of time outside, being fed in the field and having a shed for protection in inclement weather or for shade in the heat of summer.

An old mare that has lost her competitive edge may suffer seriously in a situation such as this. Other mares in the field, especially overly aggressive ones, may keep her from getting her feed or chase her from it after only a bite or two. If ground or fence feeders are used, it may be necessary to move the old mare's feeder a distance from those of the others. Preferable, of course, would be to take her to the barn and allow her to eat in peace. Note that access to hay is less of a problem if a sufficient amount is provided over a large enough area so that there's always an unguarded pile of hay for the old girl.

• **Dietary requirements.** Another problem with feeding in the field is not one necessarily limited to older mares. Just as all humans don't have the same dietary requirements, all mares do not have the same

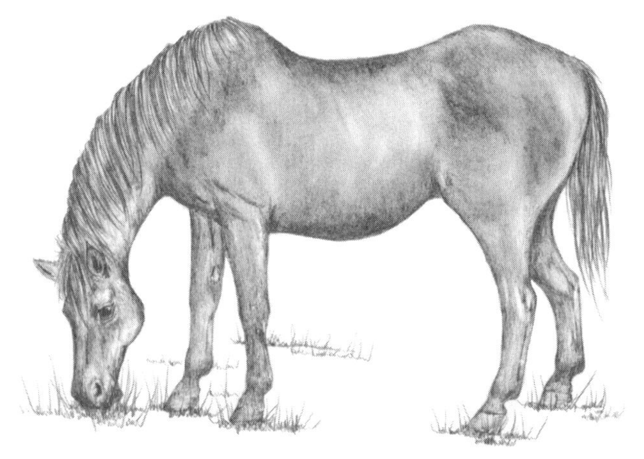

Possibly the main problem encountered as a mare ages is her loss of ability to compete with her younger pasture mates.

nutritional needs. Feeding in the field pretty much makes all their intakes the same, and this is especially unfair to an older individual that may need a greater amount just for maintenance. Even if the old mare is observed eating and not being chased by the younger ones, she may still lose condition simply because she needs more.

- **Shelter.** Shelter in this scenario may also be a problem for the old mare. Her younger companions will frequently bar her from the communal shed, thereby forcing her to stay unprotected in all types of weather. If no other solution is readily available, it will become necessary to keep the old girl in the barn during extremely hot, cold, or wet times. Ideally, a separate paddock will be provided as a sort of geriatric ward, where two or three old or aging mares can be kept together.
- **Water intake.** Water intake is always important in old mares. Adequate intake is especially a major concern in cold weather. I once read an article written by a man with a lot of initials after his name claiming that water intake in horses doesn't decrease in colder times. Hogwash. Horses do drink less when it's cold and this seems to be especially true of older ones. I'm not sure why this is, but this is a good reason either to ensure adequate access by having heated waterers or to bring the old mares inside at least once a day in winter.
- **Dental care.** Teeth care becomes a more serious issue as mares age. When young, floating may be necessary only every few years, but in aged animals it often becomes essential on an annual or semiannual basis. This is also play-by-ear; have the older mares' teeth checked twice a year and float as needed.
- **Disease resistance and skin care.** Depending on the condition of the individual, there may be less resistance to disease as a mare ages. Therefore, strict adherence to the vaccination and deworming schedules is essential. Also, for reasons that are not clear to me, mares seem to be more prone to skin disease as they age. General coat care — grooming, an occasional bath, etc. — will help greatly here.
- **Arthritis and hoof care.** The older a mare gets, the more apt she is to become arthritic, especially if she had a racing or other competitive career when she was young. There's not a lot that you can do about

this, other than give occasional anti-inflammatory drugs, but proper foot care can help reduce strain on joints. In many situations, the temptation is great to skip a trim during those times of the year when the hoof grows more slowly, but you can't do this with old mares. Trim regularly and faithfully.

• **Breeding.** A broodmare may remain productive even into her late twenties, and there is no reason to stop breeding just because she has gotten old if, of course, her health is good. A lot of top racehorses have come from old mares. The conformation of the mare's vulva may change drastically as she ages, however. A mare that never needed to be sutured may gradually develop the need as the years pass. One that needed the procedure when younger needs it more than ever as she gets older. (See page 174 on the Caslick procedure.)

• **Uterus.** Just as susceptibility to systemic disease seems to increase with age, so does the susceptibility of the uterus to insult increase. Bacteria accidentally introduced into a ten-year-old uterus and successfully defended against by the body's own responses may well set up housekeeping in a twenty-year-old uterus and prevent conception from occurring. Proper suturing can go far to ensure that this doesn't happen.

An old uterus just doesn't have the resiliency it once had. Where a ten-year-old uterus may be tight, firm, and back in conceiving condition on foal heat, a twenty-year-old uterus is usually still a floppy, flaccid bag at that point and not at all ready to accept a fertilized egg. Also, in this compromised uterus the normal contamination that occurs at breeding can easily lead to infection on a foal-heat cover, so it's a good idea just to pass and try on the twenty-eight-day (or whenever) heat.

• **Gestation period.** Length of pregnancy often increases in older mares. Some people deny this, but they have obviously never owned a mare over the age of eleven or twelve. It's not at all uncommon for a mare in her twenties to carry her foal a full year, occasionally even longer. This causes a number of problems. One is the frustration of looking for a foal at 340 days or so, only to have it continue to incubate another month. But it eventually arrives and all is well.

• **Other management issues.** The other problem, though, involves management decisions. Your twenty-two-year-old stakes producer foals on May 18 from a May 22 cover the previous year. We have just said that the chances for a successful cover on her foal heat are slim, so you must consider whether to breed her back in mid-June. You're then faced with the prospect of a June foal next year, or no foal. But she's twenty-two; will she even be around to produce a foal at twenty-four, which will be her foaling age if you skip this year? Personally, I'd breed her.

If an old mare becomes infertile, and this happens, she can still have a use. A quiet old mare that has seen it all makes a wonderful babysitter for a group of silly weanlings. This is a trying time for babies and a sensible old mare will have a marvelous calming effect on them. And the old mare will have learned long ago that being caught usually means dinner; the weanlings will come to the gate with her at these times, making it easier to catch and handle them.

Basically, then, an old mare may require a little more tender loving care than she once did, but there is no reason why she can't remain a productive member of your equine community.

At the age of thirty, old Game Squaw began slowing down. Getting around and competing got to be too much for her, so I kept her in a small catch pen adjoining a stall. She could go in the stall if she wanted, but she disliked being in the barn so she spent most of her time outside. From that vantage point she could see the other horses and that seemed to keep her happy.

At thirty-one, getting up and down became a real problem for her. At thirty-two, she had to be helped up, not an easy task because she was a large mare (probably 1,300 pounds). It got so I could just barely get her up, and she would then go back down in an hour or less. When winter was coming I decided that she couldn't make it through another cold spell. She needed to be put down.

I couldn't do it, though. I called a veterinarian friend and asked him to do it. I told him I wouldn't be there when he arrived. I called the guy who hauled dead horses to the lab and asked him to come out and get her.

I got the old girl up and told her good-bye and then I left. She wasn't there when I got back. I still shed a tear as I write about it.

Appendixes

Recommended Vaccination Schedule

Vaccination	Essential?
Viral encephalitis (eastern, western, Venezuelan)	Yes
Equine influenza	Yes
Rabies	Yes
Tetanus toxoid	Yes
Tetanus antitoxin	No; administered only when a broken skin lesion occurs and there is no history of previous tetanus toxoid vaccination or when tetanus toxoid status is unknown
Rhinopneumonitis	Yes
Potomac horse fever	Yes
Strangles	No
Botulism toxoid	No
Viral arteritis	No

*Foals receive a single dose at this time *only* if the dam was properly vaccinated. If not, vaccinate as if beginning at birth.

Beginning Dose	Booster Dose	Foals
Two doses, 3 weeks apart	Annually	90 days*
Two doses, 4 weeks apart	Annually	90 days*
One dose	Biannually or quarterly for horses racing or showing	
Two doses, 4 weeks apart	Annually	90 days
	When a horse receives broken skin lesion	
Two doses, 4 weeks apart	Annually Biannually or quarterly for horses racing or showing	90 days*
Two doses, 4 weeks apart in endemic areas	Biannually	90 days*
Different schedules for different products	Annually	Mares only
Mares at 8, 9, and 10 months of gestation	Annually in last month of pregnancy	Mares only
Mares at 90 days prior to breeding		

Equine Anatomy

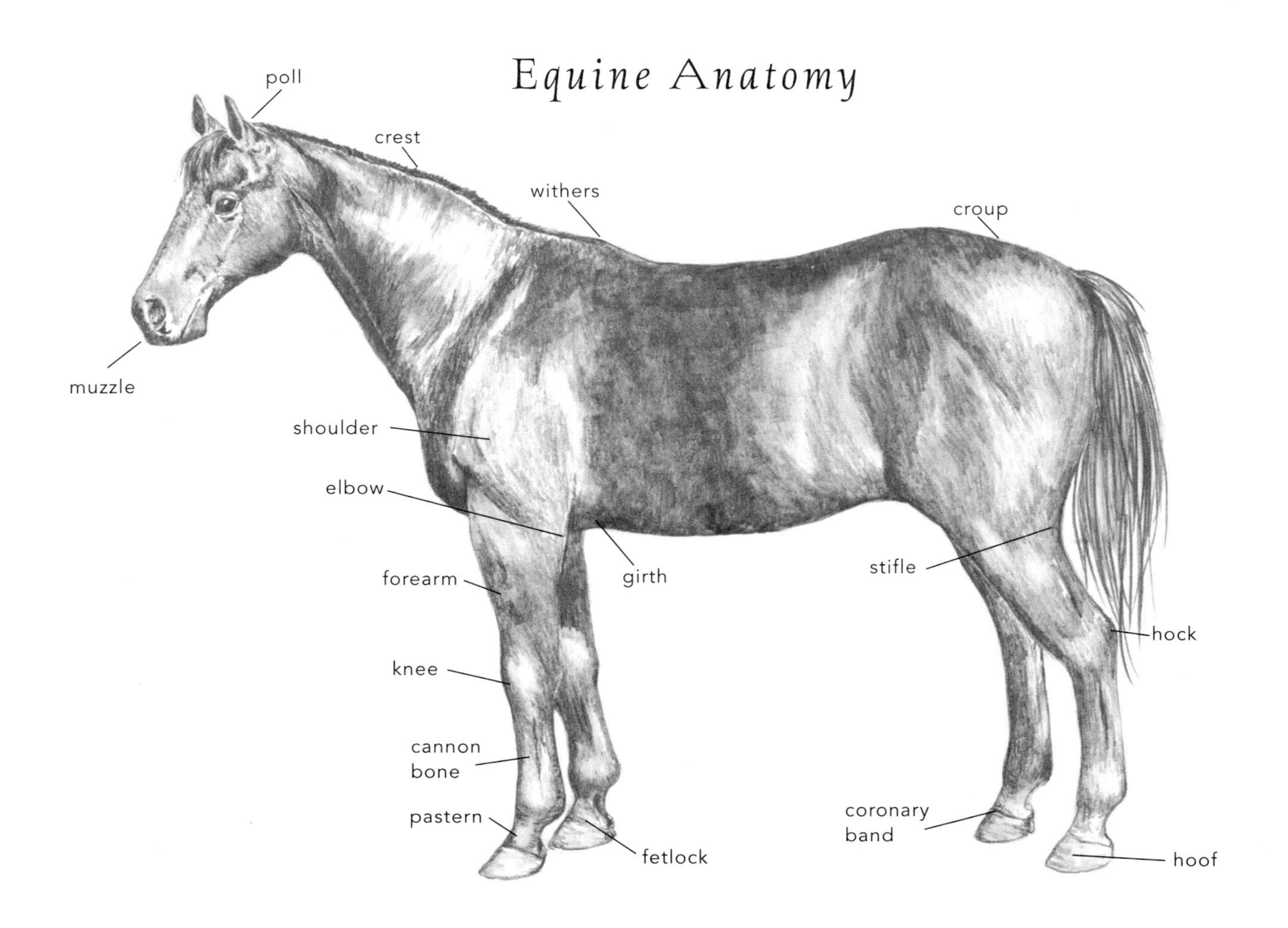

Skeletal Anatomy

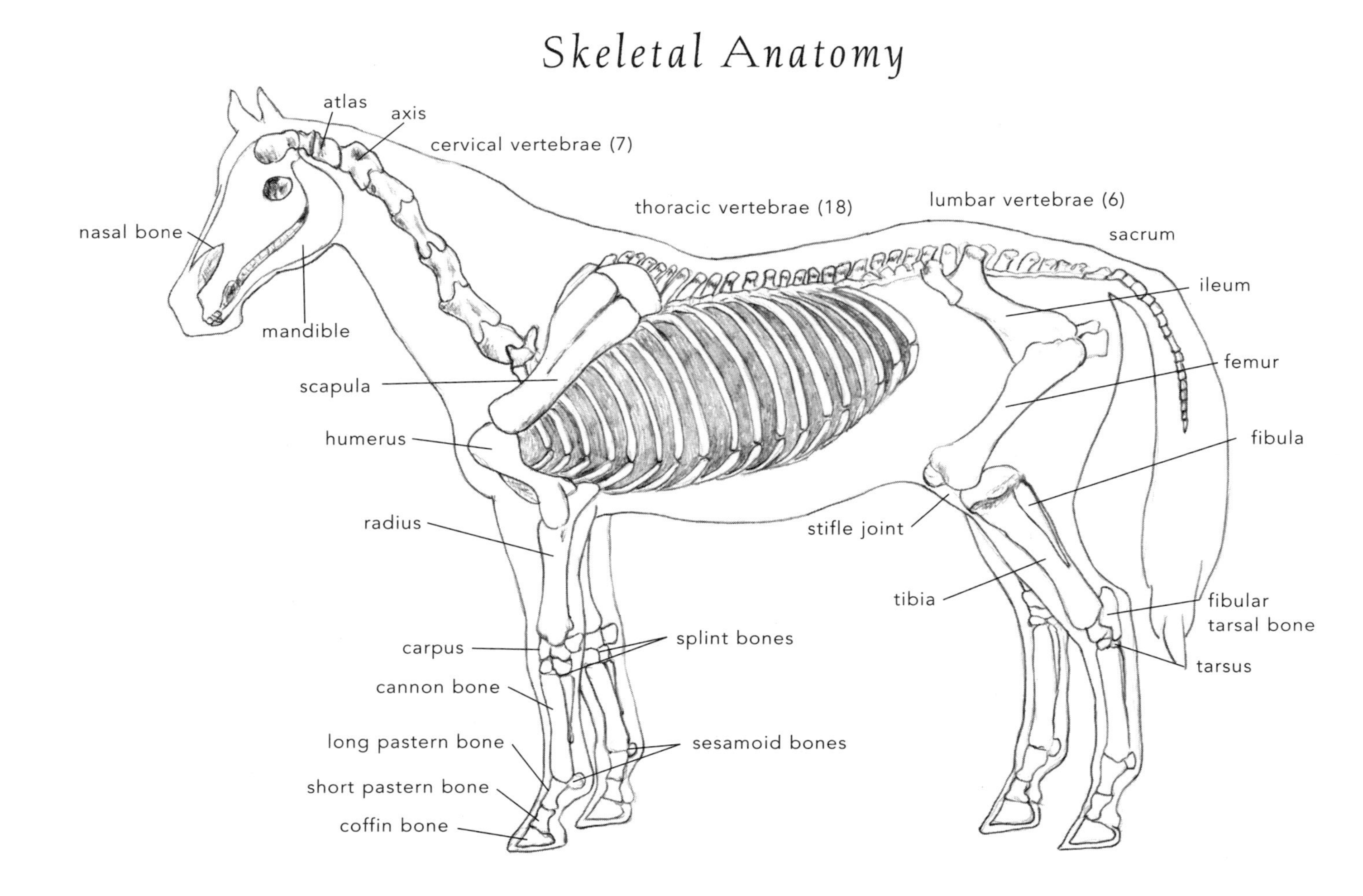

Glossary

abscess A circumscribed infection; a walled-off pocket of pus

acidosis A decrease in bicarbonate in the blood

actinomycete A microorganism

acute laminar degeneration Sudden disruption of the fingerlike projections that hold the coffin bone in place; occurs in laminitis

adipose tissue Fat

aerophagia Sucking in air during cribbing

aerosol Spread of disease through inhalation

afebrile Not having a fever

agalactia No milk production

albumin A simple protein found in blood

allantochorion The type of placentation in horses

alopecia Hair loss

amnion The thin white membrane surrounding the fetus

anabolic steroid A product that promotes muscle development

anaerobe Grows in the absence of oxygen

anaerobic In the absence of oxygen

anaphylaxis An acute immune reaction

anestrus The time of year when a mare does not cycle

aneurysm A weakening of the arterial wall

androgen A hormone that builds muscle

anhydrosis Failure to sweat

anorexia Refusal to eat; no appetite

anovulatory The stage of the ovaries when they do not produce eggs

anoxia Oxygen lack

anthelmintic A drug used to kill internal parasites

antibody A protein in the blood that reacts to an antigen

antibody titer The strength of the body's response to an antibody

antigen A foreign material (microorganism, toxoid, etc.) that stimulates an immune response in the body

antioxidant An agent that prevents oils and fats from becoming rancid

arthroscopy A type of surgery in which only a small incision is made; the operation is performed with the aid of a viewing apparatus called an *arthroscope*

articular Related to bone joints

aseptic peritonitis Peritonitis in which there is no living organism causing it

aspirate To suction off a liquid; the liquid suctioned off

ataxia Stumbling, unsteady gait

atrophy Wasting of tissues, organs, or the entire body

avulsion fracture A fracture in which a piece is pulled from the bone

azotemia Nitrogen in the blood

bacterial meningitis A bacterial infection of the meninges (a portion of the brain)

bacterial toxins Poisons produced by bacteria

barren Not pregnant after being bred

beta-hemolytic strep A type of bacterium

bicarbonate A compound in normal blood

bilateral Affecting both sides

bilirubin A red pigment found in bile

biopsy Microscopic examination of tissue taken from a living patient

blastocyst The fertilized ovum in the early stages of cell division

blepharospasm Spasmodic winking; involuntary closure of the eye

blind staggers *See* moldy corn poisoning

blood chemistry analysis A measure of elements other than blood cells found in blood

blood lipids Normal fat in the blood

bone spavin An arthritic condition of a horse's hocks

brachycephalic Having a disproportionately short head; "pug-nosed"
breakover The point of the toe of a horse where the hoof arc centers
broad-spectrum drug/antibiotic One that is effective against several microorganisms
"broken wind" Damage to the respiratory tract
bucked shins A condition of young horses exercised at high speeds; the cannon bones develop microfractures
"bute" Short for phenylbutazone, a nonsteroidal anti-inflammatory drug
cannon The "shin bone" of a horse
capillary refill time The amount of time it takes the capillaries to refill after pressure is placed on the mucous membranes; it is altered in certain conditions
cardiovascualr collapse Failure of the heart and blood vessels
carotid artery The main artery to the head region
carpal deviation Crooked knees
carpus The "knee" of a horse; analogous to the wrist of a human
cataract A loss of transparency of the lens of the eye
cauda equina neuritis An inflammation of the spinal nerves at the end of the spinal cord
cc Cubic centimeter; equal to one milliliter (mL)
cerebrospinal fluid The fluid surrounding the brain and spinal cord
cervical star The whitish area on the otherwise reddish brown placenta
cervix The tubelike structure between the vagina and the uterus
check ligament A ligament of a horse's leg
chorion The thick, heavy placental "bag"
clitoris A portion of the female reproductive tract; located at the lower end of the vulva in four-legged animals
Clostridium tetani The bacterium that causes tetanus
coffin bone The bone within a horse's hoof; pedal bone
coffin joint The joint between the coffin bone and the short pastern bone
Coggins test A blood test to determine whether a horse has or had equine infectious anemia
colic A set of signs that indicate pain or discomfort in a horse; usually abdominal in origin
colitis Inflammation of the large intestines
colostrum "First milk"; high in antibodies
complement fixation test A test that causes the substance (complement) in normal serum that is destructive to bacteria to set
conjunctiva Collective term for the tissue surrounding the eyeball
contracted tendon A tendon that is too tight or too short
coprophagy Eating manure or dirt
corpus hemorrhagicum The site on the ovary where a follicle has recently ovulated
corpus luteum Source of progesterone through the first 180 days of gestation
cow hocks Hocks that angle toward each other
cross match Comparing blood to see if it can be used for a transfusion
cryptorchid A male animal with both testicles retained within the body cavity
cunean tenectomy Severing the cunean tendon
cyst An abnormal sac containing gas or fluid
cystitis Infection of the urinary bladder
deciduous teeth The teeth in a young animal that are lost when permanent teeth come in
debride To excise devitalized tissue from a wound by scrubbing
deep digital flexor tendon A tendon of the lower leg of a horse
denuding Removing the covering of something
dermatitis Infection or inflammation of the skin
dermatophilosis *See* rain scald

dermatophytosis *See* ringworm
desmitis Inflammation of a ligament
desmotomy The cutting of a ligament
developmental orthopedic disease (DOD) Bone disease resulting when the process of converting cartilage to bone in growing horses is interfered with or altered
devitalized Dead
diaphragm The muscular structure that separates the thoracic and abdominal cavities
diarrhea Loose bowel movements
diestrus The length of time between a mare's heat cycles
differential diagnosis A list of possible diseases causing the signs that are seen in a sick animal
disseminated Widely scattered
distal Farthest from the body
DMSO Dimethyl sulfoxide; a topical drug to reduce swelling due to trauma
dysphagia Difficulty eating or chewing
dysplasia Abnormal tissue development
dystocia Difficult delivery
ectoparasite A parasite that feeds on the outer body of a host; e.g., a mosquito
edema An accumulation of clear, watery fluid
electrolyte Any of a number of compounds in the blood
ELISA Enzyme-linked immunosorbent assay; a method of testing for certain diseases
embryo The unborn young before it can be recognized as a specific species
empyema Pus in a body cavity
encephalatides Plural form of *encephalitis*
encephalitis Inflammation of the brain
encephalopathy Brain damage
endemic area An area in which a disease is common
endoscope Fiberoptic device used to see interior parts of a body
endotoxemia Endotoxins in the blood
enteritis Inflammation of the intestines
entropion Inverted eyelid
enzyme A naturally occurring protein that brings about chemical changes in the body
epidemiologist A scientist who studies epidemics
epipharyngeal orifice An opening from the throat to a guttural pouch
epithelial Pertaining to the epithelium, the covering of the free surfaces of the body
equine degenerative myeloencephalopathy A degenerative disease affecting the spinal cord and brain of young horses
equine herpesvirus An infectious agent of horses
equine infectious anemia An incurable anemic disease of horses; "swamp fever"
equine influenza Debilitating viral respiratory disease
equine pastern dermititis An infection of the skin of the pastern
equine recurrent uveitis An infection of the horse's eye that comes and goes, eventually ending in blindness; "moon blindness"
equine viral arteritis (EVA) A viral equine disease of the arteries
erythrocytes Red blood cells
Escherichia coli *E. coli;* a common bacterium found in the environment capable of causing infection
estrogen A female hormone
ethmoid hematoma A collection of blood in or around the ethmoid bone
Eustachian tube A tube leading from the inner ear to the pharynx
euthanasia Humane destruction
exertional rhabdomyelitis A muscular disorder of horses, also known as *tying up*
external nares Nostrils
exudate Fluid that comes from a lesion
febrile Having a fever
fecal check or exam A method to determine the amount of internal parasites
feces Manure
fetus The unborn young; in the horse, after about forty days of gestation

"finished up the track" Lay term for losing a race badly
FDA Food and Drug Administration; the federal agency that regulates and approves drugs
fetotomy Dismembering and removing a fetus to save the mare
flatulence Excessive gas production by the intestines
flexor cortical lesion A lesion of a flexor tendon
foal heat The mare's first heat period after foaling; usually at eight to twelve days
founder *See* laminitis
fungicide An agent that kills fungi
genus The classification of biological entities between family and species
globulin A protein in the blood, milk, and muscle
gluteal muscles Muscles of the buttocks
goiter A condition in which the thyroid gland swells; may be caused by too much iodine or not enough iodine
goniometer A device for measuring angles
granulate Forming into grains; "scabbing"
granulomatous enteritis An enteritis marked by granulation
grapes A lumpy infection of the pastern; severe equine pastern dermitis
gravel Hoof abscess that ruptures at the coronary band
gray matter The grayish tissue of the brain and spinal cord that contains nerve cells and some nerve fibers
grease Heavy fluid discharge from a wound, seen in greasy heels
gutteral pouch An enlargement in the throat region of equids; paired
habronemiasis A skin disease caused by *Habronema* spp.
heat cycle The length of time between heat periods; estrous cycle
hematuria Blood in the urine
hemoglobinuria Hemoglobin in the urine
hemolytic anemia An anemia caused by the destruction of red blood cells
heparin A blood-thinning drug
hepatic Pertaining to the liver
hepatitis Inflammation or disease of the liver
herpesvirus A family of viruses
histological exam Microsopic examination of slides prepared from tissue samples
histology The study of the body tissues on a cellular level
hoof angle The angle at which the hoof is trimmed
hoof tester A tool used to check for sensitivity in a horse's foot
hormone A chemical produced in one organ and carried by the blood to another organ to affect its function
hydrocephalus A condition in which there is an excess of fluid in the brain
hydrops An excessive accumulation of clear, watery fluid in any section of the body
hyoid bone A **U**-shaped bone between the jaw and the larynx
hyperlipemia Excessive fat in the blood
hyperplasia An increase in the number of cells
hypogalactia Reduced milk production
hypoglycemia Low blood sugar
hypothermic Having a lower than normal body temperature
hypothyroidism Reduced production of hormones by the thyroid gland
icterus *See* jaundice
idiopathic Denotes a disease of unknown cause
immune-mediated A disease that is combated with assistance from the immune system
impar ligament One of three ligaments that support the navicular bone; it runs from the coffin bone to the deep digital flexor tendon behind the navicular bone
in utero Gestation in the uterus
ingestion The introduction of food and drink into the stomach

inguinal hernia Intestine in the inguinal ring
inguinal ring The hole in the body cavity through which the testicles descend into the scrotum
integumentary Relating to the body covering
internal os of the cervix The opening of the cervix at the uterine end
intestinal inoculant A bacterial preparation used to resupply the normal bacteria of the intestines
intussusception Telescoping of the intestine into itself
involute Return to normal size
iodinated casein A drug used for thyroid supplementation
jaundice A yellowing of the skin and tissues
joint flush Rinsing out an infected joint with an antibiotic
kelp Seaweed; high in iodine
keratinization Development of a horny (hard) layer
knuckling Contraction of the posterior tendons resulting in walking on the front of the hooves
lacrimation Tear production; crying
lactic acid The muscular waste products produced during exercise
laminitis Inflammation and release of the hoof wall laminae in horses
larynx The upper part of the respira-tory tract between the pharynx and the trachea; the "voice box"
lay-up A horse that is temporarily taken out of training, often due to injury
lead The foot that hits the ground first in a three- or four-beat gait
leptospirosis A bacterial infection
leukopenia A decrease in the number of white blood cells (leukocytes) in the blood
lipemia Fat in the blood
lipid Fat
lymph node A structure where lymph (a clearish fluid from the tissues) is transported to the lymph vessels on its way to the venous system
lymphoid hyperplasia Abnormal growth of lymph tissue
marginal osteophytes Spurs on the edge of a bone
mastitis Infection of the mammary glands
meconium The hard feces in a foal's rectum at birth
melanoma Skin tumor containing melanin (a black pigment)
meniscus Cartilage that separates bones in joints
metabolism The result of ingestion; the utilization of nutrients
metacarpal bones The bones below the knee of a horse
metastasize Spread of cancerous cells from one area of the body to another
metatarsal bones The bones below the hock of a horse
microcotyledons The small, fingerlike projections that connect the placenta to the uterus
mitosis Cell division
moldy corn poisoning A disease of the liver and brain caused by ingestion of certain fungi growing on corn
Monday morning disease Lay term for tying up
monorchid One testicle retained within the body cavity
moon blindness Lay term for equine recurrent uveitis
morbidity The percentage of a population that is sick
mortality The percentage of a population that dies
mucoprotective mechanism A mechanism by which the mucous membranes are protected
mucous membranes The lining of the mouth, vagina, etc.
multifocal Occurring in many areas
myalgia Muscular pain
mycosis Any disease caused by fungi
mycotoxic encephalomalacia *See* moldy corn poisoning
myectomy The cutting of a muscle
myocardium The muscular substance of the heart

myoglobinuria Myoglobin in the urine
myopathy Damage to muscles
navicular bone A wedge-shaped bone within a horse's foot
navicular bursa A sac associated with the navicular bone
necropsy Postmortem exam
necrosis The pathologic death of tissue
neonatal isoerythrolysis Anemia (jaundice) in foals resulting from colostrum with incompatible antigens
neonatal maladjustment syndrome (NMS) Central nervous system disorder in foals
neoplasia A cancerous tumor
nerve axon The conducting portion of a nerve
neurectomy The cutting of a nerve
neurological Pertaining to the nervous system
neuron A nerve cell and its processes
neutrophil A type of white blood cell usually elevated in acute infections
nonspecific Unidentified
nonsteroidal Not containing or related to steroids
nonsteroidal anti-inflammatory drugs A class of drugs; phenylbutazone and flunixin meglumine are examples
normal horse temperature 100°F to 101°F
nuclear scintigraphy Diagnostic test based on the detection of a radiolabeled phosphate compound in bone and soft tissue
nurse mare A mare used to suckle an orphaned foal
open wound A lesion that has not been sutured
oral mucosa The lining of the mouth
os An anatomical opening
osselets Arthritis of the fetlock joint
osteoarthritis Cartilage covering the jointed surfaces of bones breaks down and underlying bone becomes thickened and distorted
osteochondrosis Results from a defect in the process of ossification of articular (joint) cartilage into bone
oxytocin The hormone responsible for milk production and release
paired serum sample Two blood samples taken at specific intervals to determine the presence of a disease
palpable Able to be felt by the hands
palpation The act of feeling something with the hands; in mares, it usually refers to the ovaries
papillomatosis Warts caused by the equine papillomavirus
parturition Birth
passive transfer The immunity acquired from the dam in the colostrum
patent ductus arteriosus A fetal blood vessel that connects the left pulmonary artery to the aorta; it should close at birth and is termed "patent" if it does not; the foal's blood is not properly oxygenated if it doesn't close
pathogen An organism with the capabilities of infecting
pathologist A person who studies diseases
PCV Packed cell volume; the percentage of cells in the blood
Penrose drain A section of material for fluid to leak out of the lesion and prevent it from closing
periodic ophthalmia Another name for equine recurrent uveitis
periosteal elevation (PE) In cases of bone abnormalities, the sheath covering a bone is cut to allow the bone to grow
periosteum The covering of a bone
peripheral nerve A nerve of the outer area of the body
peritonitis Inflammation of the lining of the abdominal cavity
pervious urachus Failure of the urachus to close, allowing urine to leak from the umbilical stump
petechial hemorrhage Minute hemorrhagic spots, usually seen on the mucous membranes of a horse in certain disease conditions
pharyngeal tonsil The tonsil in the region of the pharynx

pharynx The portion above the esophagus and below the mouth and nasal cavities

phenylbutozone "Bute"; nonsteroidal anti-inflammatory drug

photophobia Abnormal sensitivity to light

phycomycosis A fungal condition

physeal dysplasia Abnormal tissue formation in bones

physis The area near the end of a long bone where growth takes place

piroplasmosis Disease caused by a protozoan carried by the tropical horse tick

plasma transfer The immunity given by a transfusion of plasma

positive contrast myelography X-rays taken after an injection of a contrast medium

Potomac horse fever A disease usually found in areas near large waterways

prepuce The free fold of skin that covers the penis

primary disease A disease that occurs as the result of the invading micro-organism and not one that occurs after the body has been weakened by another organism

progesterone The hormone responsible for the maintenance of pregnancy

prognathism Upper jaw longer than the lower jaw; "buck teeth," or parrot mouth

prognosis The outlook for recovery from a disease or injury; a prognosis ranges from "excellent" to "poor"

prolactin A hormone that starts milk production

prolapse The falling or turning out of an organ

prolapsed uterus Inversion of the uterus

proteinuria Protein in the urine

prothrombin A clotting factor in the blood

proud flesh Excessive, or exuberant, granulation tissue on a wound

pruritus Itching

pulmonary abscess An abscess in the lungs

"put down" To put to sleep, euthanize

radiograph Technical term for an X-ray

radius One of the bones from the shoulder to the knee of a horse

rain scald A skin condition of horses

regimen A regulation of the diet, medication, exercise, etc.

renal filtration The act of the kidneys purifying the blood

reportable disease A disease that, because of its ability to spread, must be reported to public health officials

reservoir An area or host in which a disease survives without causing signs of illness

reticuloendothelial system A group of cells found in various organs responsible for destruction of foreign cells

retrograde axonal migration Moving along nerve axons

retropatellar fat pad A pad of fat behind the patella

retropharyngeal lymph node A lymph node located behind the pharynx

rhinopneumonitis A disease that affects both the nasal passages and the lungs

rhinovirus (EHV-1) A virus that affects the nasal passages

ridgling Lay term for a male horse with an undescended testicle (monorchid) or testicles (crypt-orchid)

rain scald A skin condition of horses

roaring A sound made by horses with laryngeal hemiplegia

rotavirus A virus that causes often fatal diarrhea in foals

ruminant An animal with a rumen; cow, sheep, etc.

salmonellosis A disease caused by *Salmonella*

sarcoids A bumpy skin disease of horses

sclera The white of the eye

scoliosis Crooked spine

scoping Using a fiberoptic endoscope for viewing internal structures

scours Lay term for diarrhea

scrotum The sac that contains the testicles

scurfing The production of a roughened surface
seborrhea Overaction of the sebaceous glands
sebum The secretion of the sebaceous glands
secondary bacterial infection An infection that occurs after the body has been weakened by a previous infection
seedy toe A lay term for the separation that occurs in the toe region of a foundered horse
selenium A trace mineral necessary in muscle function and reproduction
sepsis The presence of pathogens in the bloodstream
septicemia Pathogens circulating in the blood
septic shock Shock caused by pathogens in the bloodstream
serovar A subgroup in biological classification
serum The liquid portion of blood
serum hepatitis A disease of the liver
serum lipids Normal fat in the serum
serum neutralization test A diagnostic laboratory test
shear heel A greatly worn heel bulb caused by overuse of the opposite heel bulb
sickle hocks Hocks that cause the feet to be well forward
sinus A hollow in a tissue or organ
sinus cyst An abnormal sac within a sinus
sinusitis Inflammation or infection of a sinus
slipped Lay term for aborted
smooth muscle Muscles of the intestinal tract
spasmodic Marked by involuntary muscle contractions
splint The third or fifth metacarpal or metatarsal bone of a horse; an enlargement on one of those bones
stallion ring A ring that is put on a stallion's penis to prevent him from getting an erection
steatitis Inflammation of adipose tissue (fat)
stenotic myelopathy Cervical vertebral malformation commonly known as *wobbler syndrome*
stomatitis Inflammation of the tongue
"stop" a mare To impregnate a mare
strangles A contagious upper respiratory disease
Streptococcus equi Bacterium that causes strangles
streptomycin An antibiotic
striated muscle Muscle other than cardiac and smooth
strongyloides A type of internal parasite
strongylosis Infestation of stronglyes
Strongylus A genus of internal parasites; strongyles
subacute Between acute and chronic, referring to a disease
subacute hepatic necrosis Death of liver tissue that occurs quickly
subcutaneous Beneath the skin
subgroup A biological classification
submandibular lymph node A lymph node located below the jaw
sulci/sulcus The grooves on either side of the frog in a horse's foot
supernumerary digit Extra finger or toe
suture To sew together
synovial effusion Leaking of joint fluid into surrounding tissue
synovial fossa A hollow in a joint capsule
systemic Relating to the entire animal
tarsal bones The bones of the tarsus (hock)
tarsus The hock of a horse; analogous to the ankle of a human
teaser A stallion used to determine if a mare is in season
tenotomy Surgical division of a tendon
tetanospasmin Toxin released by the bacterium responsible for tetanus infection
tetanus antitoxin An antibody formed in response to the tetanus organism
tetanus toxoid A product capable of stimulating antibody production against tetanus

thermography The measurement of the heat of a part of the body

third eyelid In horses, an "eyelid" in the medial corner of each eye; nictitating membrane

thoracic abscess An abscess within the thoracic cavity

throatlatch The area of a horse where the head meets the neck

thrush An infection of the frog in a horse's foot

thymus A lymphoid organ located in the neck region of young animals, it disappears in maturity

thyroid A gland located in the neck regulating growth

titer The level of a reaction

total protein The amount of albumin and globulin in the blood

transplacental Crossing the placenta

Trichomona An organism that causes infection

trimester One third of pregnancy

tying up A disease of horses in which it is difficult to move the locomotor muscles

tympany Low-pitched, resonant sound characteristic of excessive intestinal gas production

ulcer A lesion on the surface of the skin or mucous membrane

ultrasound A technique using sound waves to visualize portions of the body

umbilical tape A type of wide suture material

underrun heels A condition that results from not trimming often enough; the toes grow long and the heels become crushed by the improper foot angle

urachus Umbilical cord structure that transports fetal urine

urticaria An eruption of itching wheals

verminous (parasitic) encephalitis A brain disease caused by parasites

vesicle A small, circumscribed elevation of the skin containing fluid

vestigial A small remnant

Viborg's triangle An area on each side of the throat of a horse bounded by the ramus of the mandible, the lingual facial vein, and the tendon of the insertion of the sternocephalicus muscle; just remember it's in the throatlatch region

vibrissae The sensitive hairs on a horse's muzzle

villi Small projections

viral encephalitis A virus infection of the brain

vitamin E A vitamin important in muscle function and reproduction

vitrectomy A procedure in which the vitreous humor is removed from the eye

volvulus Rotation or twisting of the small intestine

vulva The lips of the opening to the vagina

wax Dried droplets of milk on a mare's teats near foaling

white line The line in a horse's foot between the hoof wall and the sole

white muscle disease A disease caused by selenium deficiency in the young; the muscles lack color

windsucker A mare that pulls air into her vagina due to poor vulvar tone

Index

Note: Numbers in *italics* indicate illustrations; numbers in **boldface** indicate charts.